E.V.

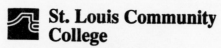

St. Louis Community College

Forest Park
Florissant Valley
Meramec

Instructional Resources
St. Louis, Missouri

COOK'S HEALTHY HANDBOOK

COOK'S HEALTHY HANDBOOK

Good Nutrition and Safety in Your Kitchen

❖ ❖ ❖

Karen Eich Drummond, R.D.
Joseph F. Vastano, R.D.
Josephine C. Vastano

John Wiley & Sons, Inc.
New York • Chichester • Brisbane • Toronto • Singapore

Library of Congress Cataloging-in-Publication Data

Drummond, Karen Eich.
    Cook's healthy handbook : good nutrition and safety in your kitchen / Karen
  Eich Drummond, Joseph F. Vastano, Josephine C. Vastano.
        p.   cm.
    ISBN 0-471-55608-4
    1. Cookery—Handbooks, manuals, etc.   2. Diet—Handbooks, manuals,
  etc.   I. Vastano, Joseph F.   II. Vastano, Josephine C.   III. Title.
  TX714.D78   1992
  641.5—dc20   92-21833
                                                                    CIP

Printed in the United States of America

10 9 8 7 6 5 4 3 2 1

❖ ❖ ❖

ACKNOWLEDGMENTS

Grateful acknowledgment is made for permission to use the following copyrighted recipes which are reprinted or adapted from the sources below.

"Baked Apples," "Bulgur with Parmesan," "Old-Fashioned Apple Pie," "Strawberry Sauce,"—*Controlling Your Fat Tooth* by Joseph C. Piscatella, New York: Workman Publishing, 1991.

"Basil-Baked Cod Fillets," "Italian Style Microwaved Halibut Steaks," and "Shark Kabobs" from the National Fisheries Institute.

"Braised Veal Steak with Vegetables"—National Live Stock & Meat Board.

"Chicken Stock" by Denise Webb, *New York Times*.

"Graham Cracker Crust" and "Peanut Butter Apple Muffins"—*The Joy of Snacks* by Nancy Cooper, Minnetonka: International Diabetes Center, 1987.

"Oat Bran Muffins" and "Lentil Burritos"—*Taste the Good Life* by Health Strategies, Wichita: Health Strategies, 1989.

"Orange Chiffon Cake"—*Eating Well* Magazine.

"Quick Meat Sauce for Pasta"—*Low Fat & Loving It* by Ruth Spear, New York: Warner Books, 1991.

"Quinoa Mexican Style" and "Carrot Cake" by Marian Burros, *New York Times*.

"Ready-Bake Bran Muffins"—*The Family Health Cookbook* by Alice White and the Society for Nutrition Education, New York: David McKay Company, 1980.

"Red Vegetable Stock" and "White Vegetable Stock"—*The Art of Nutritional Cooking* by Michael Baskette and Eleanor Mainella, New York: Van Nostrand Reinhold, 1992.

"White Sauce"—*The American Heart Association Low-Salt Cookbook* by R. Starke and M. Winston (Eds.), New York: Random House, 1990.

"Zucchini, Tomato, and Wheat Berry Slaw"—*The Grains Cookbook* by Bert Greene, New York: Workman Publishing, 1988.

Grateful acknowledgment is also made to the following groups for sharing a wealth of information that served as part of the resource base for this book as well as selected recipes.

American Dairy Association
American Dietetic Association
American Egg Board
American Lamb Council
American Mushroom Institute
California Iceberg Lettuce Commission
California Table Grape Commission
Idaho Bean Commission
Idaho Potato Commission
National Cancer Institute
National Coffee Association
National Fisheries Institute

Acknowledgments

National Live Stock and Meat Board
National Pasta Association
National Pork Producers Council
National Turkey Federation
National Yogurt Association
Produce Marketing Association, Inc.
Rice Council of America

Tea Council of the USA
United Fresh Fruit and Vegetable Association
USA Dry Pea & Lentil Industry
U.S. Department of Agriculture
U.S. Department of Commerce—National Fish
    and Seafood Promotional Council
Wheat Foods Council

Many illustrations of cooking equipment and foods are taken from the following books published by John Wiley and Sons Inc.

Professional Cooking (second edition) by Wayne Gisslen

Food Preparation for the Professional (second edition) by David A. Mizer, Mary Porter, and Beth Sonnier.

❖ ❖ ❖

CONTENTS

Contents

Contents

Contents

Contents

❖ ❖ ❖

PREFACE

In the 1990s, a discussion of foods and cooking would be incomplete without sensible and practical tips on selecting, preparing, and serving nutritious foods. That's what sets *Cook's Healthy Handbook* apart from other books—it explores the field of food and cooking from a new and timely viewpoint, that of health and nutrition. The traditional aspects of food and cooking are discussed and intertwined with pertinent nutritional information and over a thousand tips for selecting and preparing light and tasty foods. In addition to being an invaluable kitchen reference, *Cook's Healthy Handbook* is also a cookbook and contains over 100 easily prepared recipes for delicious, healthy foods that you and your family will enjoy. Each recipe lists the per-serving amounts of calories, carbohydrate, fiber, fat, cholesterol, and sodium.

To get the most out of *Cook's Healthy Handbook*, here are some of its major features to guide you.

- In Chapter 1, Nutrition in a Nutshell, specific eating practices are listed that can help you lower your risk of cancer, heart attack, stroke, and adult diabetes.
- Chapter 2 gives many tips on eating the high-carbohydrate way, and Chapter 3 explains 101 ways to eat less fat and cholesterol.
- Chapter 4 contains tips for planning nutritious menus that save time and money as well as guidelines to develop your own nutrition scorecard (including your daily needs for calories, fat, saturated fat, cholesterol, and sodium). You can use your personalized nutrition score-

card to compare your nutritional needs to the amounts provided by foods at the supermarket or recipes giving such information. Guidelines for reading the new food and nutrition labels are also discussed.
- Chapter 5 explains basic cooking how-tos, and Chapter 6 gives the latest information on timely food safety topics such as seafood safety, egg and poultry safety, and the possibility of lead contaminating your ceramic dishes.
- Chapter 7 has pointers for selecting appropriate cookware for your kitchen and describes kitchen equipment made with good nutrition in mind.
- The remaining 11 chapters explore different groups of food using, in most cases, the following format.
  - Purchasing information
  - Nutrition profile
  - Storing pointers
  - Tips for cooking in a light and healthy manner

These chapters use many quick-reference charts to help you choose, for example, a lean cut of beef, or decide how long to microwave fresh broccoli.

We hope this book will help you make better-informed food selections and use various cooking and baking techniques to prepare tasty and healthy meals.

Karen Eich Drummond,
Yardley, Pennsylvania
Joseph F. and Josephine Vastano,
Lanoka Harbor, New Jersey

COOK'S
HEALTHY
HANDBOOK

❖ ❖ ❖

CHAPTER ONE

NUTRITION IN A NUTSHELL

Nutrition is the science of food and the substances found in food, and how they relate to health and disease. Almost daily, we are bombarded with news reports that something in the food we eat (such as fat) is adversely affecting our health and that what we eat may indeed cause and complicate certain diseases. Heart disease and cancer, as well as stroke and diabetes, remain leading causes of death and disability in the United States. According to the *Surgeon General's Report on Nutrition and Health* (1988), two-thirds of Americans die of diseases linked to diet. The accompanying chart lists a variety of dietary changes you can make to lower your risk of cancer, heart attack, stroke, and adult diabetes.

Nutrition also examines the processes by which you choose different kinds and amounts of foods and the balance of foods and nutrients in your diet. A **balanced diet** is one with a variety of foods that does not emphasize certain foods at the expense of others. **Moderation** (eliminating excessive amounts of calories, fat, sugar, etc.) and **adequacy** (providing enough calories and nutrients) are also important and are a key to choosing a healthy diet.

Nutrients are substances in food that provide energy and promote the growth and maintenance of your body. Nutrients also regulate body processes, such as your heart beating and food being digested, and support the optimum health of your body. There are about 50 nutrients that can be arranged into six groups as follows.

1. Carbohydrate
2. Fat
3. Protein

❖ *Preventing Disease: A Menu of Health Saving Tactics* ❖

	No Tobacco	Low-Fat Diet	High-Fiber Diet	Avoid Alcohol	Avoid Salted, Pickled Foods	Diet High in Vegetables and Fruits	Exercise, Weight Control
Cancer							
Lung	✔✔✔	✔				✔	
Breast		✔✔✔	✔			✔✔	✔
Colon		✔✔✔	✔✔✔			✔✔✔	✔
Liver				✔✔✔	✔	✔✔	
Heart attack	✔✔✔	✔✔✔				✔✔	✔✔
Stroke	✔				✔✔✔	✔✔	✔✔
Adult diabetes		✔✔✔	✔			✔✔	✔✔

✔✔✔ *Highly effective*   ✔✔ *Moderately effective*   ✔ *Somewhat effective*
Source: American Medical Foundation

4. Vitamins
5. Minerals
6. Water

The functions of each group of nutrients are shown in Table 1. Most foods are a mixture of carbohydrate, fat, and protein.

It's been said many times: "You are what you eat." This is certainly true. The nutrients you eat are found in your body. Water is the most plentiful nutrient in the body and accounts for about 55 percent of your weight. Protein and fat each account for about 20 percent of your weight, while carbohydrate is only 0.5 percent of your weight. The remainder of your weight includes minerals, such as calcium in bones, and traces of vitamins.

Certain nutrients provide energy. The energy in food or the energy needs of the body are measured in units called **calories**. Of the nutrients, only carbohydrate, fat, and protein provide energy, as follows:

Carbohydrate:	4 calories per gram
Fat:	9 calories per gram
Protein:	4 calories per gram

❖ Table 1   Functions of Nutrients ❖

Nutrients	Functions
Carbohydrate	Provide energy, promote growth
Lipid (fats and oils)	and maintenance, regulate body
Protein	processes
Vitamins	Regulate body processes
Minerals	Promote growth and maintenance,
Water	regulate body processes

A gram is a unit of weight; there are 28 grams in 1 ounce. As you can see, fat has over double the number of calories of the other nutrients (that's why fat is fattening!). Vitamins, minerals, and water do not have any calories. Alcohol, although not a nutrient because it does not promote the growth and maintenance of the body, provides 7 calories per gram. Table 2 lists the daily calorie requirements for men and women.

THE ENERGY NUTRIENTS: CARBOHYDRATE, FAT, AND PROTEIN

Carbohydrate

Sugar, starch, and fiber are the main forms of carbohydrate in the foods we eat. Sugar occurs

❖ Table 2   Calories Needed Daily ❖

To determine how many calories you need daily, multiply your weight by the number below that matches your activity level.

Activity Level	Calories Needed/Pound/Day
Sedentary, inactive	11
(Example: has no aerobic activity)	
Moderately active	13
(Example: performs aerobic exercise 2 to 3 times each week)	
Active	15
(Example: performs aerobic exercise 4 to 5 times each week)	
Very active	18
(Example: performs aerobic exercise daily)	

EXAMPLE: 120-pound person who is moderately active

120 pounds × 13 calories needed/lb./day = 1560 calories needed daily

NOTE: If you are overweight, do not use your current weight. Instead, use the suggested weight for your height using the chart to the right. The higher weights in the ranges generally apply to men who tend to have more muscle and bone. The lower weights more often apply to women, who have less muscle and bone. Height does not include shoes and weight does not include any clothing.

❖ *Suggested Weights for Adults* ❖

Height	Weight in Pounds	
	19 to 34 Years	35 Years and Over
5'0"	97–128	108–138
5'1"	101–132	111–143
5'2"	104–137	115–148
5'3"	107–141	119–152
5'4"	111–146	122–157
5'5"	114–150	126–162
5'6"	118–155	130–167
5'7"	121–160	134–172
5'8"	125–164	138–178
5'9"	129–169	142–183
5'10"	132–174	146–188
5'11"	136–179	151–194
6'0"	140–184	155–199
6'1"	144–189	159–205
6'2"	148–195	164–210
6'3"	152–200	168–216
6'4"	156–205	173–222
6'5"	160–211	177–228
6'6"	164–216	182–234

naturally in fruits and milk and in a refined form, commonly known as table sugar, in soft drinks, cakes and other bakery products, candies, syrup, jams and jellies, and other sweetened foods. Refined sugar is unusual in that it is pure carbohydrate and contains no vitamins, minerals, protein, or fat. Although refined sugar seems to be responsible for only one health problem (causing cavities in your teeth), foods high in refined sugars, such as many cakes, contribute calories without providing much in the way of other nutrients. In addition, these foods are often high in fat and contribute excessive calories to the diet.

Grains, such as wheat, corn, rice, rye, barley, and oats, are rich sources of **starch**. Grains are used to make breads, breakfast cereals, and pastas. Besides grains, starches are also found in potatoes, vegetables, and dried beans and peas. Starchy foods, once avoided by dieters as fattening, are actually good choices for those who want to lose weight. Many people think that starchy foods such as bread and potatoes are high in fat and calories. They aren't—until the bread is thickly buttered and the potatoes generously

topped with sour cream. By eating more starchy foods, dieters (and anyone else for that matter) wind up consuming less fat and therefore fewer calories.

Like starch, **fiber** is found abundantly in plants, especially in the outer layers of cereal grains and the fibrous, chewy parts of fruits, legumes (dried beans and peas), vegetables, nuts, and seeds. Fiber is not found in animal products such as meat, poultry, fish, dairy products, and eggs. What's different about fiber is that it can't be broken down or digested in your digestive tract, like sugars and starches, so it passes through the stomach and intestines unchanged and is excreted. Fiber has received much good press because it has many desirable effects: it may lower your blood cholesterol level; eating high-fiber foods provides an increased sense of fullness; and fiber helps prevent constipation (to name a few desirable effects).

Carbohydrates are discussed in more detail, including tips to increase your intake of starch and fiber (and decrease your intake of sugar), in the next chapter.

Fat

The fat in your diet is both visible and invisible. When discussing fats, most people think about only the visible fats—butter, margarine, cooking and salad oils. But much of the fat in your diet comes from less visible sources—the fatty streaks in meat, the fat under the skin of poultry, the fat in milk and cheese, the fat in many baked products, fried foods, nuts, and the fat contained in many processed foods such as candy, chips, canned soups, and convenience frozen dinners. According to the U.S. Department of Agriculture (USDA), the top five sources of fat are:

1. Cheeseburgers, hamburgers, and meat loaf
2. Hot dogs, ham, and other processed meats
3. Whole milk dairy products such as cheese
4. Commercially baked goods, such as cakes, cookies, and doughnuts
5. Roast beef and beef steaks, french fries, and fried chicken

Unprocessed cereal grains, fruits and vegetables (except avocados and olives), flour, pasta, breads, and most cereals have little or no fat.

Although, for example, when wheat flour and apples are used to make apple pie, much fat is added (it's in the pie crust).

There are three different types of fats:

1. Saturated fats—These are found primarily in animal foods such as meats and whole-fat milk and cheeses.
2. Monounsaturated fats—These are found in plant oils such as olive oil, peanut oil, and canola oil.
3. Polyunsaturated fats—These are found primarily in plant foods such as soybean and corn oils.

Cholesterol is a fatlike substance that the human body needs, but too much of it is not desirable (as is the case with fat). Unlike fat, cholesterol is found only in food from animal sources. No plant foods, such as grains, fruits, or vegetables, contain any cholesterol.

Most health authorities recommend an American diet with less fat, saturated fat, and cholesterol. Populations like ours with diets high in fat have more obesity and certain types of cancer. The higher levels of saturated fat and cholesterol in our diets are also linked to an increased risk for heart disease.

A diet low in fat makes it easier for you to include the variety of foods you need for nutrients without exceeding your calorie needs because fat contains over twice the calories of an equal amount of carbohydrates or protein. For most people, a goal of consuming 30 percent or less of total calories from fat is reasonable (most Americans get about 37% of their calories from fat).

A diet low in fat, especially saturated fat, can help you maintain a desirable level of blood cholesterol. (Saturated fat raises your blood cholesterol more than anything else in your diet, even more than dietary cholesterol.) For adults, a desirable level of blood cholesterol is below 200 milligrams/deciliter. As blood cholesterol increases above this level, so does the risk of heart disease. Risk can also be increased by high blood pressure, cigarette smoking, diabetes, a family history of premature heart disease, obesity, and being a male.

Chapter 3 offers tips for reducing your intake of fat, saturated fat, and cholesterol.

Protein

Protein is present in almost all foods of animal and plant origin. Animal sources of protein in the American diet include meat, poultry, seafood, eggs, milk, cheese, and other dairy products (except butter—it's almost all fat!). Protein appears in plant foods in smaller quantities than in animal foods because plants have less protein in their tissues (and much less fat as well). Plant sources of protein include legumes, cereal grains and products made with them such as bread and ready-to-eat cereals, vegetables, nuts, and seeds. The legumes (beans, peas, and lentils) contain larger amounts and better quality protein than other plant sources. Fruits contain very little protein.

According to surveys conducted by the USDA, 14 percent to 18 percent of calories in the American diet come from protein. The recommended level is closer to 10–12 percent of calories. Eating too much protein has no benefits, and as a matter of fact, it can be harmful. Eating too much protein may:

- increase the loss of calcium in the urine
- increase the amount of fat in the diet when the protein comes from animal sources (this may increase blood cholesterol levels and contribute to heart disease)
- increase the chances of obesity
- create a deficiency of vitamin B6, which is needed to metabolize protein

To eat less protein, you should eat smaller servings of meat, poultry, fish, and eggs, and also eat meatless meals (such as pasta and marinara sauce).

THE REGULATOR NUTRIENTS: VITAMINS, MINERALS, AND WATER

Vitamins

Vitamins are organic nutrients found in foods that are essential for growth and good health. Although your body only needs small quantities of vitamins, the roles they play are enormously important. For instance, vitamin B12 and folacin are needed to make red blood cells that transport oxygen throughout the body, and vitamins A and D are needed for proper bone formation.

In the early 1900s, scientists thought they had found the compounds needed to prevent two diseases caused by vitamin deficiencies: scurvy and pellagra. These compounds originally were believed to belong to a class of chemical compounds called amines and were named from the Latin *vita*, or life, plus amine—vitamine. Later, the "e" was dropped when it was found that not all of the substances were amines. At first, no one knew what they were chemically, and they were identified by letters. Later, what was thought to be one vitamin turned out to be many, and numbers were added; the vitamin B complex is the best example (for example, vitamin B1 and vitamin B6).

Then some were found unnecessary for human needs and were removed from the list, which accounts for some of the gaps in the numbers. For example, vitamin B8, adenylic acid, was later found not to be a vitamin. Others, originally designated differently, were found to be the same. For example, vitamins H, M, S, W, and X were all

shown to be biotin. As the number of vitamins being discovered increased, scientists began naming them by their structure or function.

Today we know of 13 different vitamins, listed below. To look at a display of vitamins at the store, you would probably swear there were more. And there probably are many bottles labeled "vitamins" that indeed are not vitamins, or maybe we don't know they are vitamins yet. The vitamin supplement business is very big, and you have probably wondered if you should be taking a supplement. If you really feel you need additional vitamins, your best bet is to buy a multivitamin (and mineral) supplement that supplies 100 percent of the RDA for 10 or so essential nutrients. It can't hurt and may act as a safety net for individuals who eat haphazardly. But no such supplement can adequately take the place of food and serve as a permanent substitute for improving a poorly constructed diet, and too much supplementation can very often be dangerous to your health. Table 3 summarizes the functions and sources of vitamins.

Minerals

If you were to weigh all the minerals in your body, they would only amount to four or five pounds. You need only small amounts of different minerals in your diet, and these are given in the accompanying list, but they perform most important jobs in your body. For instance, calcium is necessary for healthy bones, and iron is essential for healthy red blood cells that transport oxygen within the body. Without enough calcium, you may experience osteoporosis or adult bone loss. Without enough iron, you may experience fatigue, a symptom of iron-deficiency anemia.

Minerals have some distinctive properties not shared by other nutrients. For example, whereas over 90 percent of the carbohydrate, fat, and protein in the diet is absorbed into the body, the percentage of minerals that are absorbed varies tremendously. As examples, only 5–10 percent of the iron in your diet is normally absorbed, about 30 percent of calcium is absorbed, and almost all the sodium you eat is absorbed. Unlike vitamins, minerals are not destroyed in food storage or prep-

❖ Vitamins and Minerals ❖

Vitamins	Minerals
Vitamin A	Calcium
Vitamin D	Chloride
Vitamin E	Magnesium
Vitamin K	Phosphorus
Vitamin C	Potassium
Thiamin	Sodium
Riboflavin	Sulfur
Niacin	Chromium
Vitamin B-6	Cobalt
Folate	Copper
Vitamin B-12	Fluoride
Pantothenic acid	Iodine
Biotin	Iron
	Manganese
	Molybdenum
	Selenium
	Zinc

❖ *Table 3 Vitamins* ❖

Vitamin	Functions	Sources
Vitamin A	Formation and maintenance of healthy skin and hair; proper bone growth and tooth development; proper functioning of immune system; maintain protective linings of lungs, intestines, urinary tract, and other organs; normal reproduction; possibly protects against cancer; proper sight	Dark green vegetables, deep orange fruits and vegetables, liver, egg yolk, milk, cream, cheese, fortified cereals
Vitamin D	Proper bone growth and teeth; helps absorb calcium and phosphorus from food into the body	Milk, liver, cod liver oil, sunshine
Vitamin E	Prevents oxidation (destruction) of fat, vitamin A, blood cells, and other important substances; important for the health of the cell and the proper functioning of the immune system	Vegetable oils, wheat germ, whole-grain cereals, legumes, nuts, seeds, green leafy vegetables
Vitamin K	Blood clotting	Green leafy vegetables, liver, tomatoes, egg yolk, vegetable oils
Vitamin C	Formation of collagen (a cement that holds together our cells and tissues); helps absorb iron into the body; prevents oxidation; helps wounds heal; may prevent cancer; strengthens resistance to infection	Citrus fruits, tomatoes, white potatoes, broccoli, other green and yellow vegetables, fortified juices and cereals
Thiamin (B-1)	Releases energy from the food we eat; normal functioning of the nervous system, digestion, and appetite	Pork, liver, dry beans and peas, peanuts, peanut butter, whole grains, enriched breads and cereals
Riboflavin (B-2)	Releases energy from the food we eat; healthy skin; normal functioning of the eyes	Milk, yogurt, cheese, organ meats, meat, poultry, dark green leafy vegetables, whole-grain and enriched breads and cereals
Niacin (B-3)	Releases energy from the food we eat; maintenance of healthy skin; normal functioning of the nervous system and digestive tract	Meat, poultry, fish, organ meats, milk, eggs, whole-grain and enriched breads and cereals
Vitamin (B-6)	Makes and breaks down proteins in the body; makes red blood cells to transport oxygen around the body	Organ meats, meat, poultry, fish, whole-grain breads and cereals, legumes
Folacin	Makes new cells during growth and pregnancy	Green leafy vegetables, organ meats, legumes, meat, poultry, seafood, whole-grain breads and cereals
Vitamin (B-12)	Makes new cells; growth of healthy red blood cells; normal functioning of the nervous system	Animal foods only
Pantothenic acid and biotin	Releases energy from nutrients	Widespread in foods

aration, except that they are water-soluble so there is some loss in cooking liquids. Like vitamins, minerals can be toxic when consumed in excessive amounts. Table 4 summarizes the functions and sources of minerals.

Water
Deny someone food and he or she can still live on for days, even weeks. But death comes quickly, in a matter of a few days, if you deprive a person of water. Nothing survives without water, and virtu-

❖ *Table 4 Minerals* ❖

Mineral	Functions	Sources
Calcium	Builds and rebuilds bones and teeth; helps blood to clot, muscles to contract, and nerves to transmit impulses; maintains normal blood pressure; aids in absorbing vitamin B-12	Milk and milk products, canned salmon and sardines (with bones), some greens (collards, kale, mustard greens, turnip greens), legumes
Phosphorus	Builds and rebuilds bones and teeth	Widely distributed in foods
Sodium	Water balance and acid-base balance in body; muscle contraction; nerve impulse transmission	Salt, many processed foods, MSG
Potassium	Water balance and acid-base balance in body; makes protein; helps release energy from nutrients; muscle contraction; nerve impulse transmission	Fruits and vegetables, milk, grains, meat, poultry, fish, legumes
Chloride	Water balance and acid-base balance in body; protein digestion; helps calcium and iron get absorbed	Salt
Magnesium	Builds bones and teeth; helps contract muscles and transmit nerve impulses; makes protein; maintains normal body temperature	Raw leafy green vegetables, nuts, dried beans, seeds, whole-grains, seafood
Sulfur	In hair, skin, and nails; part of thiamin and biotin	Protein foods
Fluoride	Solid tooth formation	Drinking water
Iodine	Maintain normal metabolic rate; normal growth and development	Iodized salt
Iron	Transport of oxygen to the cells; making use of oxygen when it arrives	Liver, meats, egg yolk, seafood, green leafy vegetables, legumes, dried fruits, whole-grain and enriched breads and cereals
Selenium	Prevents oxidation; essential for normal heart functioning	Seafood, meat, liver
Zinc	Formation of protein; wound healing; blood formation; general growth and maintenance of all tissues; taste perception; appetite; night vision	Meat, shellfish, eggs, milk, whole-grains, some legumes
Chromium	Helps insulin do its job	Liver, meat, dark meat of poultry, whole-grains
Cobalt	Part of vitamin B-12; red blood cell formation	Animal foods
Copper	Formation of hemoglobin that transports oxygen around the body; helps keep bones, blood vessels, and nerves healthy; part of many important enzymes that speed up reactions in the body	Organ meats, meats, shellfish, whole-grains, nuts, legumes
Manganese	Blood formation; bone structure	Whole-grains, legumes, tea, coffee, nuts, seeds, leafy vegetables
Molybdenum	Works with enzymes; metabolism of fat	Not completely known

ally nothing takes place in the body without water playing a vital role.

While variations may be great, the average adult's body weight is generally 50 to 60 percent water—enough, if it were bottled, to fill 40 to 50 quarts. For example, in a 150-pound man, water accounts for about 90 pounds, fat about 30 pounds, with protein, carbohydrates, vitamins, and minerals making up the balance. Men generally contain more water than women, a lean person more than an obese person.

The body uses water for virtually all its functions—for digestion, absorption, circulation, excretion, transporting nutrients, building tissue, and maintaining temperature. Almost all of the body's cells need and depend on water to perform their functions. Water carries nutrients to the cells and carries away waste materials to the kidney. Water is needed in each step of the process of converting food into energy and tissue. Water serves as an important part of lubricants, helping to cushion the joints and internal organs, keeping body tissues such as the eyes, lungs, and air passages moist, and surrounding and protecting the fetus during pregnancy.

Many adults take in and excrete between 8 and 10 cups of fluid daily. Besides drinking fluid, nearly all foods have some water. Milk, for example, is about 87 percent water, eggs about 75 percent, meat between 40 percent and 75 percent, vegetables from 70 percent to 95 percent, cereals from 8 percent to 20 percent, and bread, around 35 percent.

If normal and healthy, the body maintains water at a constant level. A number of mechanisms, including the sensation of thirst, operate to keep body water content within narrow limits. You feel thirsty when the blood starts to become too concentrated. Unfortunately, by the time you feel thirsty, you are already much in need of extra fluid, but this can be easily remedied by drinking promptly. It is therefore very important not to ignore feelings of thirst, a concern that is particularly appropriate for the elderly. For healthy individuals, it is not possible to drink too much water; it will simply be excreted.

RECOMMENDED DIETARY ALLOWANCES

The **Recommended Dietary Allowances** (Appendix A) have been prepared by the Food and Nutrition Board of the National Academy of Sciences/National Research Council in Washington, D.C. since 1941. They include recommendations on nutrient intakes for Americans (Canada has its own set of recommendations) and are revised about every five years to keep them up to date. RDAs are defined as follows: "The levels of intake of essential nutrients that, on the basis of scientific knowledge, are judged by the Food and Nutrition Board to be adequate to meet the known nutrient needs of practically all healthy persons in the United

States" (*Recommended Dietary Allowances*, 10th ed. National Research Council, 1989). Individuals with special nutritional needs and/or medical problems are not covered by the RDAs.

There are RDAs set for protein, 11 vitamins, and seven minerals, and these are outlined in Table 5. No RDA is set for either carbohydrate or fat because individuals who are meeting both the calorie and protein RDA and eating a variety of foods are assumed to be meeting these needs. The RDAs are not minimal requirements (except for sodium, potassium, and chloride), average requirements, or optimal requirements. They are safe and adequate levels with ample margins of safety designed to meet the needs of practically all of the healthy population and also to provide enough so the body can endure periods of deficient intake.

The RDAs for energy were set differently than those for the nutrients. If the energy RDAs had an ample safety margin, this could lead to obesity over time. Therefore, the energy RDAs are not padded; they represent the **average** needs of individuals.

Different RDAs have been set for separate groups of people: infants, children, men, women, pregnant women, and lactating women. Most groups (infants, children, men, and women) are further divided by age. In this manner you can look up your own RDAs by sex and age group. When you do so, you will notice that a height and weight is given for each category. This is the height and weight of the Reference Individual on which the RDAs are based. For example, the Reference Woman for females (ages 25–50 years) is 5 foot 4 inches, weighs 138 pounds, and is normally active. The heights and weights used are not ideal figures but are the actual midpoints of Americans within the given age bracket.

Although designed primarily for planning and evaluating diets and menus for groups of people (such as nursing home residents), individuals can use RDAs to examine their own diets. This is possible if intake is averaged over a long enough period of time. RDAs are also used to evaluate the quality of the national food supply and develop guidelines for good eating for the public.

❖ Table 5 Recommended Dietary Allowances (RDA) ❖

RDAs Are Set For:
Energy
Protein
Vitamins: A, D, E, K, C, thiamin, riboflavin, niacin, B-6, folate, and B-12
Minerals: calcium, phosphorus, magnesium, iron, zinc, iodine, and selenium

Estimated Safe and Adequate Daily Dietary Intakes Are Given For:
Vitamins: biotin and pantothenic acid
Minerals: chromium, molybdenum, copper, manganese, and fluoride

Estimated Minimum Requirements Are Given For:
Minerals: sodium, chloride, and potassium

When there was not enough scientific evidence to develop an RDA, the Food and Nutrition Board established a table of estimated safe and adequate daily dietary intakes. This table includes two vitamins and five minerals with ranges of intake that will meet nutritional needs and avert toxic doses. Upper levels in the safe and adequate range for these minerals (chromium, molybdenum, copper, manganese, and fluoride) should not be regularly exceeded because the toxic level may be only several times the usual intake.

Needs for sodium, chloride, and potassium are found in a separate table that estimates minimum requirements. The minimum requirement is based on what you need for growth and for replacement of normal daily losses (through sweating, urine, etc.). Dietary deficiency of these three minerals in healthy individuals is unlikely. In the case of sodium and chloride, there is no evidence that higher intakes are beneficial. In fact, for some individuals a high sodium intake aggravates problems with high blood pressure. On the other hand, higher levels of potassium may help individuals suffering from hypertension.

SO WHAT SHOULD WE BE EATING?

Dietary recommendations have been published for the healthy American public for almost 100 years. Early recommendations centered on encouraging intake of certain foods to prevent deficiencies, fight disease, and enhance growth. As the diseases of nutritional deficiency have been virtually eliminated, they have been replaced by diseases of dietary excess and imbalance—problems that now rank among the leading causes of illness and death in the United States (Table 6), touch the lives of most Americans, and generate substantial health care costs. More recent dietary guidelines have therefore centered on modifying the diet, in most cases cutting back on certain foods, to prevent lasting degenerative diseases such as heart disease.

❖ Table 6 Leading Causes of Death, ❖ United States, 1987

Rank	Cause of Death
1*	Heart diseases
2*	Cancers
3*	Strokes
4	Unintentional injuries, such as motor vehicle accidents
5	Chronic obstructive lung diseases
6	Pneumonia and influenza
7*	Diabetes mellitus
8	Suicide
9	Chronic liver disease and cirrhosis
10*	Atherosclerosis

Causes of death in which diet plays a part.
Source: The Surgeon General's Report on Nutrition and Health: Summary and Recommendations, *U.S. Department of Health and Human Services, 1988, DHHS Publication No. 88-50211.*

Dietary recommendations are quite different from RDAs. Whereas RDAs deal with specific nutrients, dietary recommendations discuss specific foods and food groups. RDAs also tend to be written in a technical style. Dietary recommendations are usually written in easy-to-understand terms.

Table 7 summarizes recent dietary recommendations. The most recent set of U.S. dietary recommendations are the *Dietary Guidelines for Americans* (third edition) which were published in 1990. These guidelines are for healthy Americans ages 2 years and over—not for younger children and infants, whose dietary needs differ. They reflect recommendations of nutrition authorities who agree that enough is known about diet's effect on health to encourage certain dietary practices.

1. Eat a variety of foods.
2. Maintain healthy weight.
3. Choose a diet low in fat, saturated fat, and cholesterol.
4. Choose a diet with plenty of vegetables, fruits, and grain products.
5. Use sugars only in moderation.
6. Use salt and sodium only in moderation.
7. If you drink alcoholic beverages, do so in moderation.

Of these seven recommendations, if you follow point 3 (eat less fat, saturated fat, and cholesterol), most of the other recommendations will fall into place. In other words, the less meat, cookies, and other fatty foods you eat, the more fruits, vegeta-

❖ **Table 7   Recent Federal Dietary Recommendations for the General Public** ❖

			Recommendation							
Year	Agency	Publication	Variety	Maintain Ideal Body Weight	Include Starch and Fiber	Limit Sugar	Limit Fat	Limit Cholesterol	Limit Salt	Limit Alcohol
1987	Department of Health and Human Services/ National Heart, Lung, and Blood Institute	National Cholesterol Education Program Guidelines	+	+	+		+	+		+
1988	Department of Health and Human Services/ National Cancer Institute	Dietary Guidelines for Cancer Prevention	+	+	+		+		+	+
1989	Department of Health and Human Services	The Surgeon General's Report on Nutrition and Health	+	+	+	+	+	+	+	+
1990	U.S. Department of Agriculture/ Department of Health and Human Services	Dietary Guidelines for Americans, 3rd ed.	+	+	+	+	+	+	+	+

bles, and grains (sources of natural sugar, starch, and fiber) you will have to consume to take their place. With less fat, your intake of sugar will probably be lower, as well as your caloric intake, enhancing the possibility of maintaining a healthy weight. Of course, you will still need to eat a variety of foods and use sodium and alcohol in moderation. Chapters 2 and 3 give specific tips to increase your intake of carbohydrates and decrease your intake of fat, saturated fat, and cholesterol. Chapter 4 gives guidelines for developing nutritious menus.

❖ ❖ ❖

CHAPTER TWO

EATING THE HIGH-CARBOHYDRATE WAY

Carbohydrate is the primary source of energy for your body. Sugar, starch, and fiber are the main forms of carbohydrate in the foods we eat. Carbohydrate-rich foods include nutritious foods such as breads and cereals, fruits and vegetables, and dried beans and peas, as well as not-so-nutritious foods such as cupcakes and soft drinks. To better understand carbohydrates, let's take a closer look at sugar, starch, and fiber.

SUGARS

When the word sugar is used in conversation, most people think of refined sugar. There are actually two types of sugars: natural and refined. Natural sugars, such as glucose and fructose, occur in fruits; whereas refined sugar, such as table sugar, is added to many of the foods we buy. Whether natural or refined, sugars are commonly referred to as **simple carbohydrates** because their structure is relatively simple compared to starch and fiber, which are called **complex carbohydrates.**

Glucose, also called dextrose or blood sugar, is found in sweet fruits such as grapes and berries, certain vegetables such as carrots, and honey. In the body, glucose is called "blood sugar" because it circulates in our blood at a relatively constant level. Blood sugar is extremely important because it provides most of the energy that will be burned by the millions of cells in your body. Although glucose appears in certain foods, it is not the major source of glucose in the body. Instead, starch and most other sugars turn into glucose in the body once eaten.

Fructose, also called fruit sugar (fruct means fruit), is found in ripe fruits and honey. Fructose is a very sweet sugar. **Lactose** is a natural sugar found in milk, although it is not very sweet.

Sucrose is the chemical name for what we know as table sugar, a refined sugar. It is composed of two single sugars: glucose and fructose. Table sugar is made from sugar cane or sugar beets and is used to sweeten many foods such as soft drinks and candies.

Table 8 lists a number of refined sugars commonly found in foods. Sucrose and corn sweeteners are the most frequently used sugars. Refined sugars are used to sweeten soft drinks, breakfast cereals, candy, baked goods such as cakes and pies, syrups, canned fruits (unless packed in juice), jams and jellies. One-quarter of the sugar consumed in the United States is in soft drinks. Table 9 lists the sugar content of various foods.

Sugar and Health

Refined sugar is an unusual food in that it is pure carbohydrate and contains no vitamins, minerals, protein, or fat. Almost all other food sources contain some combination of essential nutrients. The U.S. per person consumption of sugar is over 100 pounds a year, a substantial increase over the consumption prior to this century. The increase is related to our increased consumption of soft drinks, cakes and other bakery products, candies, syrup, jams, and jellies.

Foods high in refined sugar contribute calories without providing much in the way of other nutri-

❖ Table 8 Common Forms of Refined Sugars ❖

Form of Sugar	Description	Form of Sugar	Description
Table sugar (granulated sugar, sucrose)	Made from cane and beets. Is about 99.9 percent pure and is sold in granulated or powdered form.		sweetness is equal to that of sucrose. Used in soft drinks, baked goods, jelly, syrups, fruits, and desserts.
Corn sweeteners	Corn syrup and other sugars made from corn.	Brown sugar	Sugar crystals contained in a molasses syrup with natural flavor and color. 91 percent to 96 percent sucrose.
Corn syrup	Made from cornstarch. Mostly glucose. Only 75 percent as sweet as sucrose. Less expensive than sucrose. Used extensively in baked goods. Also used in canned goods.	Molasses	Thick syrup left over after making sugar from sugar cane. Brown in color with a high sugar concentration.
High fructose corn syrup	Corn syrup treated with an enzyme that converts glucose to fructose, which results in a sweeter product. Most common form used is 42 percent fructose because at this level its	Turbinado sugar	Sometimes viewed incorrectly as raw sugar. Produced by separating raw sugar crystals and washing them with steam to remove impurities.

❖ Table 9 Sugar Content of Foods ❖

Food/Portion	Sugar (grams)	Food/Portion	Sugar (grams)
Dairy Group		**Vegetables**	
Milk, 1 cup	12	Broccoli, ½ cup	0.7
Plain yogurt, 1 cup	12	Carrot, 1 medium raw	4
Low-fat yogurt, strawberry, 1 cup	35	Corn, ½ cup	3
Cheddar cheese, 1 oz	0.5	Winter squash, ¼ squash	4
Ice cream, soft serve, 1 cone	21		
		Beverages	
Meat, Poultry, Fish		Lemonade, from powder, 8 oz	13
Meat, poultry, and fish	—	Fruit punch drink, 8 oz	27
		Cola soft drink, 12 oz	38
Eggs			
Eggs	—	**Cakes, Cookies, Candies, Pies, and Puddings**	
		Cheesecake, ⅛ cheesecake	28
Grains		Animal crackers, 10 pieces	6
White bread, 1 slice	1	Chocolate wafers, 5 cookies	11
English muffin, 1	2	Milk chocolate, 1 oz	15
Cheerios, 1¼ cups	1	Hard candy, 1 oz	19
Honey-nut Cheerios, ¾ cup	10	Apple pie, 1 snack pie	28
Cornflakes, 1 oz	2	Vanilla pudding, ½ cup	22
Sugar Smacks, ¾ cup	16		
Rice, white, 1 cup	trace	**Sweeteners**	
		White sugar, 1 tablespoon	12
Fruits		Honey, 1 tablespoon	17
Apple, 1 medium	18	High-fructose corn syrup, 1 tablespoon	16
Banana, 1 medium	18	Pancake syrup, 1 oz	23
Orange, 1 medium	12	Molasses, 1 tablespoon	12
Apple juice, 8 oz	27		
Orange juice, 8 oz	26		

HOW TO EAT LESS REFINED SUGAR

GENERAL

1. Instead of regular soft drinks or powdered drink mixes, choose diet soft drinks, bottled waters such as seltzer, or iced tea made without added sugar or with sugar substitutes.
2. Use less refined sugars in coffee, tea, cereals, etc., or use sugar substitutes.

MEALTIME

3. Choose 100 percent pure fruit juices. Products labeled as fruit drinks, fruit beverages, or flavored drinks usually contain only small amounts of fruit juice and much refined sugar.
4. Choose unsweetened breakfast cereals. For each four grams listed under "Sucrose and Other Sugars" on a cereal box label, there is one teaspoon of sugar. For less sugar, choose cereals with less than four grams of sugar per serving, unless the sugar comes from a dried fruit such as raisins. Top cereals with fresh fruit.
5. Jams, jellies, and pancake syrup contain much refined sugar. For less (or no) refined sugar, select fruit spreads (products sweetened with fruit juice concentrates) and pancake syrup labeled reduced calorie. Other toppings for toast or pancakes are chopped fresh fruit, applesauce, apple (or other fruit) butter, or part-skim ricotta cheese and fruit.
6. Many fruited yogurts contain much sugar. For less sugar, mix fresh fruit or canned fruit (packed in its own juice) into plain yogurt.

SNACKS

7. Enjoy a fresh apple or banana instead of a candy bar if you want something sweet.
8. Buy a cookie that uses less refined sugar, such as graham crackers, vanilla wafers, ginger snaps, and fig bars.
9. Instead of sweetened pastries such as danish, try a bagel, English muffin, or fruited muffin.

DESSERTS AND BAKING

10. Instead of sweet desserts such as cake, emphasize fruits as desserts. Fresh fruit can be baked (baked apples), poached (poached pears), broiled, or made into compote. Try
    - baked pears or baked apples with a sprinkle of cinnamon or
    - broiled peach or grapefruit half with a sprinkle of nutmeg.
11. Select unsweetened frozen fruits or canned fruits packed in juice rather than fruits packed in light or heavy syrup. One-half cup of fruit canned in heavy syrup contains approximately 4 teaspoons of sugar.
12. Select gelatin and pudding mixes without sugar.
13. When baking from scratch, you can decrease the sugar in many of your recipes by about one-fourth to one-third of the original amount without any significant difference in quality. Following are guidelines for different types of baked goods.
    - You can decrease the sugar in cake recipes to ½ cup per cup of flour. Cakes with less sugar may be more like a quick bread than a cake.
    - You can decrease the sugar in muffin and quick bread recipes to 1 tablespoon sugar per cup of flour.
    - Yeast bread recipes only require 1 teaspoon sugar per cup of flour.
    - To cut down on sugar in fruit pies, use 6 tablespoons or less sugar for a regular pie and use sweet fruits.
14. Add a small amount of vanilla, cinnamon, or nutmeg to sweet baked products to enhance flavor when you reduce sugars.
15. Select baking recipes that use fruit to sweeten.
16. Use a fruit sauce (see Chapter 16 for recipe) or a sprinkling of powdered sugar in place of frosting on cake.

ents. In addition, many are high in fat, contribute excessive calories to the diet, and are sometimes consumed at the expense of foods that provide essential vitamins, minerals, and protein. Although excessive sugar consumption does not cause obesity, it can contribute to obesity.

The major health problem caused by eating sugar is **tooth decay**. The more often these foods—even small amounts—are eaten and the longer they are in the mouth before teeth are brushed, the greater the risk for tooth decay. This is because every time you eat something sweet, the bacteria that naturally live on your teeth produce acid for 20 to 30 minutes. This acid eats away at your teeth, and cavities (also referred to as dental caries) may eventually develop. Eating sugary foods as frequent between-meal snacks may be more harmful to teeth than having them at meals. To prevent dental caries, you should brush your teeth often, floss your teeth once a day, and try to limit sweets to mealtime.

Sugar Consumption Recommendations

Carbohydrates should provide approximately 55 percent of our daily calories, with sugars limited to 10 percent. The average American consumes closer to 47 percent of daily calories from carbohydrates and 18 percent from refined sugars. Foods containing large amounts of refined sugar should be eaten in moderation by most healthy people and sparingly by people with low calorie needs. For very active people with high calorie needs, sugars can be an additional source of calories. See the list of tips on how to reduce your refined sugar consumption.

STARCH

Starch is actually a long chain of glucose units that are linked together. Grains are rich sources of starch. Examples of grains include wheat, corn, rice, rye, barley, and oats. Wheat and other grains consist of three parts: the starchy endosperm, the vitamin-rich germ, and the bran, the protective outer coat that contains the fiber. The diagram of rice grain composition shows this separation of parts. Grains are used to make breads, breakfast

cereals, and pastas. Potatoes, vegetables, and dried beans and peas are also good sources of starch.

Starch and Health

Starchy foods, once avoided by dieters as fattening, are actually good choices for those who want to lose weight. Many people think that starchy foods such as bread and potatoes are high in fat and calories. They aren't—until the bread is thickly buttered and the potatoes generously topped with sour cream.

What's more, a diet high in carbohydrates just may be more slimming than a diet of comparable calories that is high in fat. Studies are still preliminary, but a research report published in the January 1989 *American Journal of Clinical Nutrition* suggested that a diet high in carbohydrates may decrease the incidence of obesity. The researcher found that when participants switched to a diet high in complex carbohydrates (starch and fiber occur together quite often), they became full more quickly (fiber fills you up) and unconsciously decreased their caloric intake (because they ate less fat).

Starch Consumption Recommendations

Carbohydrates should provide approximately 55 percent of our daily calories, with 45 percent coming from the complex carbohydrates: starch and fiber. Most people could benefit from eating more starchy foods.

FIBER

Fiber is not a single substance, but a variety. Like starch, most fibers are chains of glucose units bonded together, but what's different is that the chains can't be broken down or digested in your digestive tract. In other words, most fiber passes through the stomach and intestines unchanged and is excreted. Fiber was called roughage a few generations ago.

Fiber is found only in plant foods where it supports the plant's stems, leaves, and seeds. Like starch, fiber is found abundantly in plants, especially in the outer layers of cereal grains and the fibrous parts (like the skin and seeds) of fruits,

Rice Grain Composition

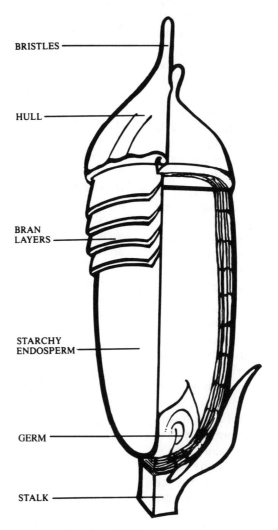

BRISTLES

HULL

BRAN
LAYERS

STARCHY
ENDOSPERM

GERM

STALK

Courtesy: Rice Council of America

legumes (dried beans and peas), and vegetables (Table 10). Fiber is not found in animal products such as meat, poultry, fish, dairy products, and eggs.

As a general rule, unrefined foods contain more fiber than refined foods because fiber is usually removed in processing. For example, raw apples contain much fiber in the skin but the skin is removed to make applesauce or canned sliced apples. Also, the milling of whole wheat in the United States to produce white flour (or wheat flour—it's the same thing) removes the germ and fiber-rich bran, leaving behind mostly starch. Whenever the bran and germ are left on the grain, the grain is called whole grain. Examples of whole grains include whole wheat, whole rye, bulgur (whole wheat grains that have been steamed and dried), oatmeal, whole cornmeal, whole hulled barley, popcorn, and brown rice. They are all good sources of fiber.

❖ *Table 10   Fiber Content of Selected Foods* ❖

Food	Serving Size	Fiber per Serving (grams)	Calories per Serving	Food	Serving Size	Fiber per Serving (grams)	Calories per Serving
Breakfast Cereals				**Vegetables**			
All-Bran	⅓ cup, 1 oz	8.5	71	Cooked broccoli	½ cup	2.2	20
Corn Bran	⅔ cup, 1 oz	5.4	98	Cooked carrots	½ cup	2.3	24
40% Bran-type	¾ cup, 1 oz	4.0	93	Cooked peas	½ cup	3.6	57
100% Bran	½ cup, 1 oz	8.4	76	Cooked potato with skin	1 medium	2.5	106
Raisin Bran-type	¾ cup, 1 oz	4.0	115	Cooked zucchini	½ cup	1.8	11
Shredded wheat	⅔ cup, 1 oz	2.6	102	Raw cucumber	½ cup	0.4	8
Cheerios-type	1¼ cup, 1 oz	1.1	111	Lettuce, sliced	1 cup	0.9	7
Cornflakes	1¼ cup, 1 oz	0.3	110	Raw tomato	1 medium	1.5	20
Nutri-Grain, wheat	¾ cup, 1 oz	1.8	102	Raw spinach	1 cup	1.2	8
Rice Krispies	1 cup, 1 oz	0.1	112	**Breads, Pastas, and Flours**			
Sugar Smacks	¾ cup, 1 oz	0.4	106	White bread	1 slice	0.4	78
Wheaties	1 cup, 1 oz	2.0	99	Whole wheat bread	1 slice	1.4	61
Dried Beans and Peas				French bread	1 slice	0.7	102
Baked beans	½ cup	8.8	155	Bran muffin	1	2.5	104
Dried peas, cooked	½ cup	4.7	115	Bagel	1	0.6	145
Kidney beans, cooked	½ cup	7.3	110	Spaghetti, regular	1 cup	1.1	155
Lima beans, cooked	½ cup	4.5	64	Spaghetti, whole wheat	1 cup	3.9	155
Navy beans, cooked	½ cup	6.0	112	Rice, polished	½ cup	0.2	82
Fruits				Rice, brown	½ cup	1.0	97
Apple, no skin	1 medium	2.7	72	Flour, white	100 grams (3½ oz)	2.9	333
Apple, with skin	1 medium	3.5	81	Flour, whole wheat	100 grams (3½ oz)	7.3	327
Banana	1 medium	2.4	105				
Orange	1	2.6	62	**Nuts**			
Apple juice	4 ounces	0.4	56	Almonds	10 nuts	1.1	79
Vegetables				Peanuts	10 nuts	1.4	105
Cooked green string beans	½ cup	1.6	16				

Source: Lanza, Elaine, and Ritva R. Butrum, 1986. *A critical review of food fiber analysis.* Journal of the American Dietetic Association 86(6): 732–43.

There are two major types of fiber—**insoluble** and **soluble**. Soluble fiber simply means that it dissolves in water, forming a gellike consistency; whereas insoluble fiber does not dissolve in water. The characteristics of each type help explain the different effects each has on health (to be discussed further). The amount of fiber in a plant varies from one kind of plant to another and may vary within a species or variety depending on growing conditions and maturity of the plant at the time of harvest.

The following foods contain soluble fibers:

- Beans and peas, such as kidney beans, pinto beans, chick-peas, split peas, and lentils
- Some cereal grains, such as oats and barley
- Some fruits and vegetables, such as apples, grapes, citrus fruits, and carrots

Insoluble fiber includes the structural parts of plants such as skins and the outer layer of the wheat kernel. You have seen insoluble fiber in the skin of whole kernel corn and the strings of celery. It is also found in:

- wheat bran
- whole grains such as whole wheat and brown rice, and products made with whole grains such as whole wheat or rye bread
- many vegetables, such as potatoes, green beans, and cabbage
- seeds

Most foods contain **both** soluble and insoluble fibers.

Fiber and Health

Fiber provides your body with the following benefits:

- Since insoluble fiber holds water, stools produced by a high fiber diet tend to be bulkier and softer and pass more quickly and more easily through the intestines.
- A diet high in insoluble fiber helps prevent hemorrhoids and diverticulosis, a disease of the large intestine that causes the intestinal walls to weaken and bulge out into pockets.
- Insoluble fibers may help reduce the risk of colon and breast cancer.
- Studies indicate that soluble fibers may help reduce the level of cholesterol in the blood. In particular, studies of people eating oats, oat bran, and beans show that these foods seem to help lower blood cholesterol levels. At the same time, these people were consuming a diet with much less fat, so this certainly influenced the outcome as well. Eating more soluble fiber may help lower your blood cholesterol when combined with an overall health plan that includes eating less fat, less cholesterol, and exercising.
- Soluble fiber helps diabetics maintain control of their blood sugar levels.
- Fiber-rich foods usually require more chewing and provide an increased sense of fullness or satiety, so they are excellent choices when trying to lose weight.

Fiber Consumption Recommendations

The Food and Nutrition Board of the National Academy of Sciences has not set a Recommended Dietary Allowance for fiber. However, the importance of fiber has been stressed by several health organizations and the federal government. The National Cancer Institute recommends 20 to 30 grams of fiber per day with an upper limit of 35 grams. Unfortunately, the average American only takes in about 10 to 11 grams of fiber a day. The accompanying list contains tips on how to increase your fiber intake.

HOW TO EAT MORE COMPLEX CARBOHYDRATES

You can increase the complex carbohydrates in your diet by choosing more foods high in starch and fiber, as listed below.

Good Sources of Starch
  Breads, both whole grain and white
  Breakfast cereals, cooked and ready-to-eat
  Flours, whole grain and white
  Pastas, such as macaroni and spaghetti
  Grains, such as barley and rice
  Legumes, such as dried peas, beans, and
    lentils
  Starchy vegetables, such as potatoes, corn,
    sweet peas, and lima beans

Good Sources of Fiber
  Legumes, such as kidney beans, lima
    beans, and split peas
  Whole grains, such as brown rice (Refined
    products have the same amount of
    starch, but little of the fiber)
  Whole grain breads, other grain bakery
    products
  Whole grain cereals, cooked and ready-to-
    eat
  Fruits, especially the skins and edible
    seeds
  Vegetables
  Nuts (in moderation—they're high in fat)
    and seeds

Table 11 will help you determine how much complex carbohydrate (and sugar) you need (based on 45 percent of total calories).

❖ *Table 11   How Much Carbohydrate* ❖
You Need Daily

If You Need This Level of Calories:	You Need:*
1200	165 grams total carbohydrate
	135 grams complex carbohydrate
	30 grams sugar
1500	206 grams total carbohydrate
	168 grams complex carbohydrate
	38 grams sugar
1800	248 grams total carbohydrate
	203 grams complex carbohydrate
	45 grams sugar
2000	275 grams total carbohydrate
	225 grams complex carbohydrate
	50 grams sugar
2200	303 grams total carbohydrate
	248 grams complex carbohydrate
	55 grams sugar
2400	330 grams total carbohydrate
	270 grams complex carbohydrate
	60 grams sugar
2600	358 grams total carbohydrate
	293 grams complex carbohydrate
	65 grams sugar
2800	385 grams total carbohydrate
	315 grams complex carbohydrate
	70 grams sugar
3000	413 grams total carbohydrate
	338 grams complex carbohydrate
	75 grams sugar

The amount of total carbohydrate is calculated as 55 percent of total calories, complex carbohydrate as 45 percent of total calories, and sugar as 10 percent of total calories. Although it is desirable to eat higher levels of complex carbohydrate than indicated here, sugar intake should be limited to these levels, with emphasis being on natural rather than refined sugars.

When increasing your fiber intake, do so slowly to avoid problems with cramps, diarrhea, and excessive gas. Also, chew foods well and be sure to drink at least 8 to 10 glasses of water each day (this includes the water in drinks like tea and juice) because fiber takes water out of the body with it. Fiber-rich foods are not recommended for acute diseases of the gastrointestinal tract such as diverticulitis, ulcerative colitis, and inflammatory bowel disease.

The following are tips to increase the complex carbohydrate in your diet.

1. Start each day with a breakfast cereal containing at least four grams of fiber.
2. Eat a muffin in the morning instead of sweetened pastries. For more fiber, eat a wheat bran muffin or an oat bran muffin.
3. Eat at least 6 to 11 servings of breads, cereals, pasta, and other starches daily. As much as possible choose whole grain products, such as brown rice rather than white rice, popcorn rather than potato chips, whole wheat crackers rather than refined crackers. Choose whole grain breads, such as whole wheat, over refined breads such as white bread, and, for more fiber, check that the bread contains at least two grams of fiber per slice.
4. Eat between three to five servings of vegetables each day. One serving is ½ cup cooked or 1 cup raw vegetable. Eat salad **and** one or two vegetables with your dinner each night. Avoid mashing or grinding vegetables (this decreases the fiber content).
5. Eat two to four servings of fruits each day. One serving is ½ cup of juice or canned fruit, 1 piece of fresh fruit, or 1 cup grapes, berries, or melon. Choose whole fruit rather than fruit juice, and raw fruit, such as an apple, rather than applesauce. Eat fruit between meals and as dessert.
6. Eat beans and peas at least two to three times each week. Try split pea or lentil soup for lunch, beans on salads, baked beans as a side dish, or canned or cooked beans as a filling in taco and tortilla shells. To avoid getting gas from beans, always cook them thoroughly and discard the soaking water before cooking them. Lima beans, split peas, and lentils are the most easily digested.

TIPS TO INCREASE FIBER

GENERAL

1. The majority of breads and baked goods available are made with white flour, a poor source of fiber. For more fiber, choose whole grain breads and baked goods, such as whole wheat and rye bread, and items made with bran, such as bran muffins. The term "wheat bread" on a food label does not mean whole wheat, and color is not a good indication because colorings can be added to make a product look more like whole wheat. Look for whole wheat bread (made with 100 percent whole wheat flour) or another whole grain listed first on the ingredient label. Other whole grain ingredients include cracked wheat, oatmeal, whole cornmeal, and whole rye.

2. Eat fruits, preferably in their whole form, at any meal or for snacks, at least two times, ideally four times each day.

BREAKFAST

3. Choose whole grain and bran cereals for good fiber sources and make sure the cereal contains at least four grams of dietary fiber per serving.

4. Whole fruits have more fiber than fruit juice so include whole fruits with your breakfast along with juice.

5. Bran muffins are a high-fiber breakfast food.

LUNCH AND DINNER

6. Select soups rich in split peas, beans, lentils, and vegetables. Use barley to thicken vegetable soups.

7. Use whole wheat or other whole grain pasta instead of refined pasta products. For example, make macaroni salad with whole wheat macaroni for added fiber and flavor, or serve whole wheat spaghetti with homemade tomato sauce.

8. Top casseroles with wheat germ.

9. Add bran flakes to casseroles and meat loaf.

10. Use cooked or canned dry beans and peas in main dishes, side dishes, and salads. For example:
    - Combine black beans and rice with chili powder or other peppery seasoning for a Caribbean-style dish.
    - Try a mixture of any of these with a vinegar and oil dressing for a three- or four-bean salad: green beans, wax beans, kidney beans, lima beans, great northern beans, or chick-peas.
    - Add kidney beans or chick-peas to a lettuce or spinach salad.

11. Use brown rice instead of white rice.

12. Leave the skin on potatoes.

13. Have a bean salad or mixed green salad with plenty of vegetables such as carrots, broccoli, cauliflower. Include kidney or garbanzo beans as well.

SNACKS

14. Most commercial cookies contain little fiber, unless made with whole grains, such as oats, or dried fruits, such as raisins, dates, and figs.

15. Choose whole grain crackers, such as whole wheat crackers, or crackers made with bran.

16. Fresh fruits and popcorn are two high-fiber snacks.

DESSERTS AND BAKING

17. Bake or broil fruits for dessert. Try
    - baked pears or baked apples with a sprinkle of cinnamon
    - broiled peach or grapefruit half with a sprinkle of nutmeg

18. Use fresh, frozen, canned, or dried fruits when baking muffins, pancakes, or quick breads. Dried apricots, raisins, bananas, blueberries, or apples add extra fiber and variety in flavor.

19. White flour, and baking mixes using white flour, contain little fiber. For more fiber,

choose whole grain flours, such as whole wheat, and mixes using whole grain flour. Substitute half the white flour called for in a recipe with whole wheat flour.

20. For puddings, try rice (use brown rice), tapioca, and bread (use whole wheat bread).

❖ ❖ ❖

CHAPTER THREE

101 WAYS TO EAT LESS FAT AND CHOLESTEROL

In recent years there has been much discussion about how much fat and cholesterol we eat, what kind of fat we eat, and the relationship between fats (and cholesterol) and cardiovascular (heart and artery) disease. A high level of blood cholesterol has been identified as one of the major risk factors for having a heart attack or a stroke in which the heart or brain may become damaged. This finding is important because your diet, particularly your fat intake, affects your blood cholesterol level. This chapter will explore the nature of fat and cholesterol, the relationship between fats and health, and what you can do to lower your risk of cardiovascular disease.

FAT

Fat has a variety of functions in the body and in food. It provides a concentrated source of energy: one gram of fat provides 9 calories, while one gram of carbohydrate or protein provides 4 calories. This means that foods rich in fat add much to the caloric content of the diet.

About 15–20 percent of the weight of healthy normal-weight men is fat (about 18–25 percent for women). At least half of your fat deposits are located just beneath the skin where it helps to cushion body organs (acting like shock absorbers) and provide insulation (so you maintain a constant body temperature). Fats are also an important component of cells, including the outer layer of the cell.

Because fats slow digestion and the emptying of the stomach, they delay the onset of hunger and make you feel full longer. In addition to creating a feeling of fullness, fats increase the palatability of foods by enhancing their aroma, taste, flavor, juiciness, and tenderness.

The bulk of your body's fat is in the form of triglycerides, and 90 percent of the fat in foods is also in the form of triglycerides. A triglyceride is made of three fatty acids attached to a unit of glycerol. Fatty acids may be one of three different types:

- Saturated
- Monounsaturated
- Polyunsaturated

Fat in Foods

All fat in foods is made up of mixtures of the three types of fatty acids. If a food contains mostly saturated fatty acids, it is considered a saturated fat; if it contains mostly polyunsaturated fatty acids, it is a polyunsaturated fat. Animal fats are generally more saturated than the liquid vegetable oils. Table 12 shows the proportions of different fatty acids in fats and oils.

Saturated fat raises your blood cholesterol more than anything else in your diet, so let's take a look at the foods in which it is found. Animal products are a major source of saturated fat in the typical American diet. The fat in whole milk dairy products (like butter, cheese, whole milk, ice cream, and cream) contains high amounts of saturated fat. Skim milk and skim milk products contain less fat and saturated fat.

Saturated fat is also concentrated in the fat that surrounds meat and in the white streaks of

❖ Table 12 Fatty Acids in Fats and Oils ❖

Fats and Oils (1 tablespoon)	Saturated Fatty Acids (grams)	Monounsaturated Fatty Acids (grams)	Polyunsaturated Fatty Acids (grams)
Fats with large amounts of saturated fatty acids include:			
Coconut oil	11.8	0.8	0.2
Palm kernel oil	11.1	1.5	0.2
Cocoa butter	8.1	4.5	0.4
Butter	7.1	3.3	0.4
Palm oil	6.7	5.0	1.3
Lard	5.0	5.8	1.4
Fats with large amounts of monounsaturated fatty acids include:			
Olive oil	1.8	9.9	1.1
Canola oil	0.9	7.6	4.5
Peanut oil	2.3	6.2	4.3
Fats with large amounts of polyunsaturated fatty acids include:			
Safflower oil	1.2	1.6	10.1
Corn oil	1.7	3.3	8.0
Soybean oil	2.0	3.2	7.9
Cottonseed oil	3.5	2.4	7.1
Sunflower oil	1.4	6.2	5.5
Margarine, liquid	1.8	3.9	5.1
Margarine, soft tub	1.8	4.8	3.9

fat in the muscle of meat (marbling). Well-trimmed cuts from certain sections of the animal, such as the round, are lower in saturated fat than well-marbled untrimmed meat. In general, poultry is lower in saturated fat than meat, especially when the skin is removed. Fish is generally lower in saturated fat than poultry and meat.

A few vegetable fats—coconut oil, palm kernel oil, and palm oil—are high in saturated fat. Although recently the food industry has largely discontinued the use of these fats in many foods, they may be used for commercial deep fat frying and in foods such as cookies and crackers, whipped toppings, coffee creamers, cake mixes, and even frozen dinners.

Polyunsaturated fats are found in greatest amounts in safflower, corn, soybean, cottonseed, sesame, and sunflower oils, which are commonly used in salad dressings and for cooking oils. Nuts and seeds also contain polyunsaturated fats, enough to make nuts and seeds a rather high calorie snack food depending on serving size. Another type of polyunsaturated fat is found in the oils of fish and shellfish. The omega-3 fatty acids

found in fish oil may be beneficial in preventing heart disease.

Fats high in monounsaturated fats are liquid at room temperatures but become hard when refrigerated. Examples of monounsaturated fats include olive oil, peanut oil, and canola oil. Like other vegetable oils, these are used in salad dressings and for cooking oils.

Both monounsaturated and polyunsaturated fats tend to reduce blood cholesterol levels. Table 13 summarizes the food sources of the different types of fat.

When looking at fat in foods, it is also important to distinguish between two different concepts: the percentage of fat **by weight** in a food and the percentage of **calories from fat** in a food. Claims such as "80 percent fat free" refer to the percentage of fat by weight. This percentage is based on the weight of the product, not the calories the product provides. Therefore, a product that touts itself as being "80 percent fat free" could still derive most of its calories from fat. For example, one ounce of cheddar cheese contains 9 grams of fat and 110 calories. Although it is

❖ **Table 13   Food Sources of** ❖
Saturated Fat, Monounsaturated Fat,
Polyunsaturated Fat, and Cholesterol

	Food Sources
Saturated Fat	Meat, poultry, fish, dairy products, butter, lard, palm oil, palm kernel oil, coconut oil
Monounsaturated Fat	Olive, canola, peanut, avocado, and nut oils
Polyunsaturated Fat	Safflower, sunflower, soybean, corn, cottonseed, and sesame oils, fish oils
Cholesterol	Egg yolk, liver and other organ meats, whole milk and whole milk cheeses, cream, ice cream, butter, meat, poultry, fish, certain shellfish

approximately 65 percent fat free, 74 percent of its calories are from fat.

CHOLESTEROL

Cholesterol is a fat-like substance found in foods of animal origin. Cholesterol does not appear in any plant foods. Pure cholesterol is an odorless, white, waxy, powdery substance. You cannot taste it or see it in the foods you eat.

Cholesterol is found only in animal foods: egg yolks (it's not in the whites), meat, poultry, fish, milk, and milk products. Egg yolk and organ meats (liver, kidney, sweetbread, brain) are the main sources of cholesterol in most diets—one egg yolk contains about 10 times as much cholesterol as one ounce of meat, poultry, or fish. Both the lean and fat of meat and the meat and skin of poultry contain cholesterol. In milk products, cholesterol is mostly in the fat, so lower fat products contain less cholesterol. Egg whites and foods that come from plants, like fruits, nuts, vegetables, grains, cereals, and seeds, have no cholesterol. Table 14 lists the cholesterol content of common foods.

Your body needs cholesterol to function normally. It is present in every cell in all parts of the body, including the brain and nervous system, muscle, skin, liver, intestines, heart, and skeleton. Cholesterol is used by the body to make bile,

which allows us to digest fats, and to form cell membranes, sex hormones, and vitamin D.

Cholesterol is supplied through animal foods but your liver makes enough to meet your body's needs, even if you didn't eat any! The human body manufactures about 1 to 2 grams each day.

Cholesterol is carried throughout the body in the blood. High levels of blood cholesterol have been found to increase your risk for heart disease. Your blood cholesterol level becomes elevated due to a variety of factors including high intakes of fat, saturated fat, and dietary cholesterol and excess calories leading to overweight. The main food factor connected to high blood cholesterol is a high fat (especially saturated fat) intake, **not** your cholesterol intake. If you are overweight or have a high fat intake (they usually go hand in hand), you can do something about it. Other factors affecting blood cholesterol levels are not so controllable. They include the following.

• Genetic factors affect your blood cholesterol level and can determine how much you can lower your level by diet. Some people have high

❖ **Table 14   Cholesterol in Foods** ❖

Food and Portion	Cholesterol (milligrams)
Liver, braised, 3 ounces	331
Egg, whole, 1	274
Beef, short ribs, braised, 3 ounces	93
Beef, ground, lean, broiled medium, 3 ounces	74
Beef, top round, broiled, 3 ounces	84
Chicken, roasted, without skin, light meat, 3 ounces	72
Haddock, baked, 3 ounces	63
Mackerel, baked, 3 ounces	64
Swordfish, baked, 3 ounces	43
Milk, whole, 8 ounces	33
Milk, 2% fat, 8 ounces	18
Milk, 1% fat, 8 ounces	10
Skim milk, 8 ounces	4
Cheddar cheese, 1 ounce	30
American processed cheese, 1 ounce	27
Cottage cheese, low-fat, 1 ounce	2

Source: *United States Department of Agriculture*

blood cholesterol levels regardless of what they eat.

- Age and sex also influence blood cholesterol levels. In the United States blood cholesterol levels in men and women start to rise at about age 20. Women's blood cholesterol levels prior to menopause are lower than those of men of the same age. After menopause, however, the cholesterol level of women usually increases to a level higher than that of men. In men, blood cholesterol generally levels off or declines slightly around age 50.

FAT, CHOLESTEROL, AND YOUR HEALTH

As stated in the 1989 National Research Council's report entitled *Diet and Health: Implications for Reducing Chronic Disease Risk* (National Academy Press):

There is clear evidence that the total amounts and types of fats in the diet influence the risk of cardiovascular diseases, certain forms of cancer, and obesity. While it is evident that dietary patterns are important factors to the cause of several major diseases, dietary modification can reduce such risks.

In this section we will discuss in more detail the relationship between fat and cardiovascular disease, cancer, and obesity.

Heart disease is the number one killer in the United States. More than 6 million Americans have symptoms of **coronary heart disease**, a disease of the arteries that supply blood to the heart muscle. Most coronary heart disease is due to blockages in the arteries themselves. Cholesterol and fat, circulating in the blood, build up in the walls of these arteries. This buildup narrows the arteries and can slow or block the flow of blood. This process is known as **atherosclerosis**. Atherosclerosis is a slow progressive disease that may start very early in life, yet might not produce symptoms for many years. Most heart attacks are caused by a clot forming at a narrow part of an artery which supplies blood to the heart muscle.

Blood carries a constant supply of oxygen to the heart. If the flow of blood is slowed or blocked, the oxygen supply may be reduced or cut off. Without enough oxygen to the heart muscle, there may be chest pain (called **angina**), and if the oxygen is cut off, there is heart muscle injury and a heart attack.

Elevated blood cholesterol is one of the three major controllable risk factors for coronary heart disease; the following is a list of these factors.

Risk Factors for Coronary Heart Disease
- High blood cholesterol
- Cigarette smoking
- High blood pressure
- Obesity
- Diabetes
- Being a male
- Family history of heart disease before the age of 55

Of these, none is more important than high blood cholesterol. Without cholesterol building up in the arteries, heart attacks would not happen. The higher your cholesterol level the greater your chance of getting heart disease, especially at levels of 200 mg/dL or more (see the accompanying list). Your total, or serum, cholesterol level refers to the amount of cholesterol, measured in milligrams, in 100 milliliters of blood. More than half the adults 20 years of age or older in the United

❖ **Risk Classifications** ❖
of Cholesterol Levels

Total Cholesterol

Desirable: Less than 200 mg/dL
Borderline–High: 200–239
High: 240 or more

LDL Cholesterol

Desirable: Less than 130 mg/dL
Borderline–High: 130–159
High: 160 or more

HDL Cholesterol

Not at risk: More than 35 mg/dL
At risk: Less than 35

States have total blood cholesterol levels of 200 mg/dL or more. About one out of every four adults has a blood cholesterol level considered high (240 mg/dL or more).

To adequately measure the risk of heart disease, it's important to know not only how much cholesterol is in the bloodstream, but also the level of two lipoproteins (these are substances in the body that transport triglycerides and cholesterol around): **low-density lipoproteins (LDL)** and **high-density lipoproteins (HDL)**. Both carry triglycerides, cholesterol, and protein in varying proportions around the body.

LDLs carry most of the cholesterol (60–70%) found in the blood and transport fat from the liver to other parts of the body. If the LDL level is elevated, cholesterol and fat can build up in the arteries and contribute to heart and artery disease (the arteries supplying the brain or heart may become obstructed). This is why LDL cholesterol is often called "bad cholesterol."

HDLs carry less fat than LDLs and contain only a small amount of cholesterol, about 20–25 percent of blood cholesterol. It is thought that HDLs carry cholesterol back to the liver for disposal. Thus, HDLs help remove cholesterol from the blood, preventing the buildup of cholesterol in the walls of arteries. HDL cholesterol is often called "good cholesterol" because the more you have, the more you are protected from heart disease.

LDL and HDL cholesterol levels more accurately predict your risk of cardiovascular disease than a total cholesterol level alone. A high LDL cholesterol level or a low HDL cholesterol level increases your risk and can be equally dangerous.

So how do you lower your blood cholesterol level and LDLs, and increase your HDLs? Here are some recommendations.

- If you are overweight, lose weight. Most overweight people with elevated blood cholesterol can help lower their cholesterol levels and increase their HDLs by losing the excess weight.
- Regular physical activity may help control your weight and is associated with a reduced risk of heart disease and lower blood pressure. Exercise is one of the best ways to increase HDLs.

- The National Cholesterol Education Program recommends that all healthy Americans change their eating patterns to lower their blood cholesterol levels. The accompanying chart lists the recommended guidelines. To implement these guidelines, you will probably need to eat fewer foods high in fat and saturated fat (to be discussed). Reducing the amount of dietary fat and saturated fat is the most effective way to lower LDLs (except by medication). By substituting (partially) monounsaturated and polyunsaturated fats for saturated fats, you can lower your LDLs.
- Although many health groups suggest restricting cholesterol intake to 300 milligrams per day, there is not total agreement on this issue. Some experts argue that it is more important to watch your fat and saturated fat intake because reducing the saturated fat content of your diet has about a threefold greater effect in reducing blood cholesterol levels than reducing the cholesterol content of your diet. Also, cholesterol appears in many nutritious foods such as eggs and whole milk, whereas many foods that are high in fat (like french fries and cupcakes), offer little in the way of nutrition and could be easily omitted from the diet.

Besides affecting the development of heart disease, fat also affects the development of cancer. Cancer is the second leading cause of death in the United States. There is a direct relationship between dietary fat and the risk of certain kinds of cancer, such as cancer of the colon and rectum. Some studies of breast and prostate cancer have shown especially strong associations of cancer risk with the intake of saturated fatty acids and with dietary fat from animal sources.

High fat intake may also be associated with the development of obesity in humans. Studies have shown that a significant reduction in fat calories is associated with weight loss. Calories from fat are more troublesome for your body than calories from starches, sugars, proteins, and even alcohol. A hundred calories of fat counts more than a hundred calories from these other nutrients. This is because the body is more efficient at converting

NATIONAL CHOLESTEROL EDUCATION PROGRAM DIETARY GUIDELINES

1. Eat less than 30 percent of your total daily calories from fat.
   - Less than 10 percent of your calories should come from saturated fat.
   - No more than 10 percent of your calories should come from polyunsaturated fat.
   - 10–15 percent of your calories should come from monounsaturated fat.

2. Eat less than 300 milligrams of cholesterol each day.
3. Eat 50–60 percent of your daily calories from carbohydrates.
4. Adjust your caloric intake to achieve or maintain a desirable weight.

---

fat calories into body fat. When people significantly reduce the fat in their diets, they tend to replace the fat with more grains, fruits, and vegetables. When this happens, the intake of fiber, vitamin C, the B vitamins, potassium, calcium, magnesium, phosphorus, iron, zinc, and copper increases.

High intake of polyunsaturated fats has been directly linked to cancer in laboratory animals and possibly to cancer in humans. Although we like to think of polyunsaturated fat as the good fat, it should still be eaten in moderation.

RECOMMENDATIONS FOR FAT AND CHOLESTEROL CONSUMPTION

Most Americans get at least 37 percent of their calories from fat and more than 10 percent from saturated fat. By comparison, in 1910, fat made up just 27 percent of calories. There is no RDA for fat; guidelines generally recommend that no more than 30 percent of daily calories should come from fat. Since there are 9 calories in a gram of fat, that means you are entitled to 50 grams of fat if you eat 1500 calories a day (Table 15). It is also recommended that you decrease the amount of saturated fat in your diet to no more than 10 percent of total calories and increase polyunsaturated fats to 10 percent of total calories.

Remember when you are using these recommendations that not everything you eat must have fewer than 30 percent calories from fat. You should balance foods with a slightly higher fat content with foods that have a much lower fat content so your total fat calories are less than 30 percent.

Like fat, there is no RDA for cholesterol. Guidelines generally recommend that cholesterol intake should be less than 300 milligrams daily, about twice what the average American diet normally provides. Some cholesterol is necessary in the infant's diet, and cholesterol restriction before two years of age is not recommended.

❖ Table 15 Recommended Fat ❖ and Saturated Fat Intake

If Your Total Daily Calories Are:	Total Fat* (grams)	Saturated Fat* (grams)
1,200	40	13
1,500	50	17
1,800	60	20
2,000	67	22
2,200	73	24
2,400	80	27
2,600	86	29
2,800	93	31
3,000	100	33

Total fat is 30 percent of total calories. Saturated fat is 10 percent of total calories.

BEFORE-AND-AFTER MODIFIED RECIPE

BEEF STROGANOFF—ORIGINAL RECIPE

1 pound beef round steak, cut in strips,
   2" × ½ "
2 ounces flour
1 teaspoon salt
¼ teaspoon pepper
4 tablespoons butter
¼ cup onion, chopped finely
½ cup mushrooms
8 oz. beef stock, hot
6 oz. sour cream

1. Dredge meat in flour, salt and pepper.
2. Brown meat in butter. Add onion and mushroom and saute.
3. Pour in beef stock and simmer 1-½ hours until meat is tender.
4. Turn off heat and stir in sour cream until thickened. Serve over noodles.

Yield: 4 servings

BEEF STROGANOFF—REVISED RECIPE

12 oz. beef round steak, cut into bite-size strips
1 tablespoon cooking oil
2 cups mushrooms, sliced fresh
½ cup onions, chopped
4 oz. defatted beef stock
1 tablespoon tomato paste
8 oz. plain, lowfat yogurt
4 teaspoons cornstarch

1 teaspoon sugar
½ teaspoon salt
Dash pepper
2 tablespoons white wine

1. Stir-fry meat in hot oil till brown, 2–3 minutes.
2. Add vegetables and stir-fry 3–4 minutes.
3. Stir in stock and tomato paste.
4. Add rest of ingredients except wine. Cook and stir until thickened and bubbly.
5. Cook two minutes more and stir in wine. Serve over noodles.

The following changes took place in the revised recipe.

1. Less meat was used.
2. The dredging of the meat was skipped as it added both salt and calories.
3. Less oil was used to brown the meat because of a different technique, stir-frying. The meat was also cut smaller to allow it to be stir-fried and cooked more quickly.
4. More fresh vegetables were used for flavor and body.
5. Defatted stock and tomato paste were used to decrease fat and calories and increase flavor.
6. Instead of sour cream, plain yogurt stabilized with cornstarch and flavored with wine was used.

101 WAYS TO EAT LESS FAT AND CHOLESTEROL

General

1. Table 16 gives substitutions for modifying recipes. See above for an example of a modified recipe.
2. Eat smaller servings of meat, poultry, and fish. Plan 2 to 3 ounces of meat, poultry, or fish at a meal. The illustration on page 48 shows the size of a 3-ounce cooked serving of ground meat, a pork chop, and a chicken quarter. Make complex carbohydrates an important part of meals, as they contain little fat (such as grains, dried beans and peas, and pasta).
3. Cook soups, stews, and any braised foods one day ahead, refrigerate, and remove the congealed (solid) fat.
4. Drink skim or 1% milk. Whole milk contains 3.25 percent fat by weight, 2% milk contains 2 percent fat, 1% milk contains 1 percent fat, and skim milk contains almost no fat. Both 1% and skim milk provide the same nutrients as whole milk or 2% milk, while providing much less saturated fat and cholesterol and fewer calories. See Table

❖ **Table 16 Recipe Substitutions to Reduce Fat, Saturated Fat, and/or Cholesterol** ❖

Instead of:	Use:	Instead of:	Use:
1 whole egg	Egg substitutes	1 cup shortening	⅔ cup vegetable oil
In baking:		1 cup sour cream	1 cup reduced-fat sour cream or
1 whole egg	2 egg whites		1 cup low-fat yogurt; in
2 whole eggs	1 whole egg plus 1 egg white or		cooking, substitute 1 cup
	3 egg whites		plain low-fat yogurt plus 1
1 cup regular milk	1 cup skim or 1% milk		tablespoon of cornstarch or
1 cup heavy cream	1 cup evaporated skim milk		flour (to prevent separation
1 cup light cream	1 cup plain low-fat yogurt		or curdling during cooking—
1 cup whipped cream	Whip ⅓ cup heavy cream and		mix together while cold)
	add ⅔ cup plain nonfat	1 tablespoon cream	1 tablespoon Baker's cheese or
	yogurt	cheese	Neufchatel cheese or
	Whip well-chilled evaporated		reduced-fat cream cheese
	skim milk flavored with	1 ounce regular	1 ounce part-skim cheese
	vanilla	cheese	
1 tablespoon butter	1 tablespoon stick margarine	1 ounce baking	3 tablespoons cocoa and 1
or lard		chocolate	tablespoon vegetable oil

17 for a nutritional comparison of these products.

5. Use skim or 1% milk in your coffee, tea, and other hot beverages.

6. Most breads and bread products are low in fat with only 1 to 2 grams of fat per serving. Choose in moderation those that are relatively high in fat (see Table 18) such as some dinner rolls, and all croissants and biscuits. A 4-inch croissant may have as much as 4 teaspoons of butter in it! A biscuit made from rolled dough in cans may have as much as 9 grams of fat!

7. For less fat, saturated fat, and cholesterol, choose a cheese made from skim milk or low-fat milk with 4 grams of fat or less per ounce and/or use less of it! (By comparison, many fresh meats have 5 grams of fat per ounce.) Table 19 is a guide to fat in cheeses. Get more mileage out of hard cheese by grating rather than slicing when cooking.

8. Eat only 3 egg yolks each week. Count most baked goods as containing ½ egg serving.

9. Choose vegetable oils high in polyunsaturated fats (corn oil, safflower oil, soybean, cottonseed, and sunflower oil), or monoun-

❖ **Table 17 Fat and Cholesterol in Milk** ❖

Nutrition Information per Serving	Whole Milk	2% Milk	Skim Milk
Serving Size	1 cup	1 cup	1 cup
Calories	150	121	86
Protein	8 g	8 g	8 g
Carbohydrates	11 g	12 g	12 g
Fat	8 g	5 g	less than 1 g
Polyunsaturates	less than 1 g	less than 1 g	0 g
Saturates	5 g	3 g	less than 1 g
Cholesterol	33 mg	18 mg	4 mg

Source: Eating to Lower Your High Blood Cholesterol, *National Institutes of Health, 1989 (NIH Publication No. 89-2920).*

Guide to 3-Ounce Cooked Serving Sizes

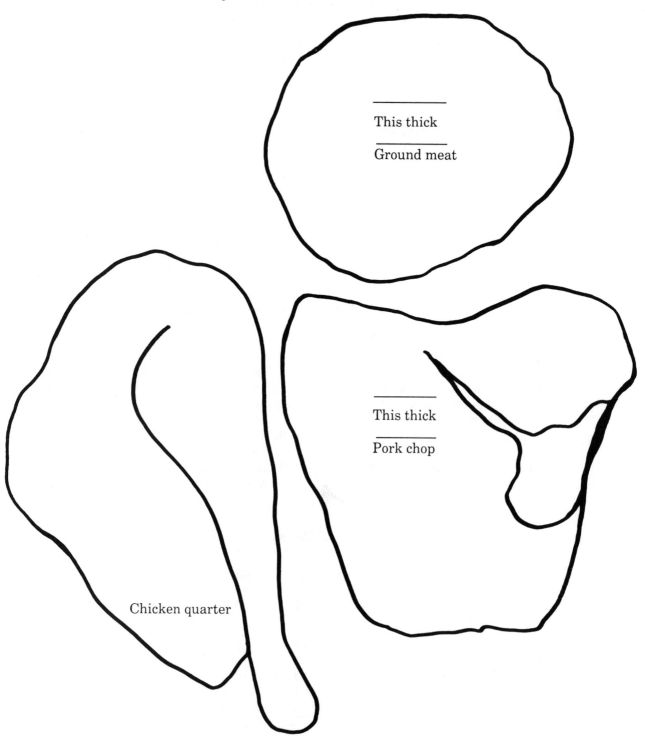

This thick

Ground meat

This thick

Pork chop

Chicken quarter

Courtesy: National Live Stock and Meat Board

❖ *Table 18   Comparison of Fat in Breads* ❖

Breads Made with Little Fat (2 grams of fat or less per serving)	Higher-in-Fat Breads
Bagel	Biscuit
Bread sticks	Brioche
Cracked wheat bread	Cheese bread
Dinner/pan roll	Cornbread
English muffin	Crescent roll or
French bread	croissant
French roll	Popover
Hamburger roll	
Hot dog roll	
Italian bread	
Kaiser roll	
Oatmeal bread	
Pita pocket	
Pumpernickel bread	
Raisin bread	
Rice cakes	
Roman meal bread	
Rye bread	
Tortilla, corn	
Tortilla, flour	
Wheat bread	
White bread	
Whole wheat bread	

saturated fats (olive, canola, and peanut oils for cooking and in salad dressings). Use sparingly.

10. Saute in nonstick pans as much as possible, as they require only a small amount of fat, if any, for cooking. If you must use fat, use as little vegetable oil as possible or vegetable oil cooking spray.

11. Saute in wine, vermouth, defatted broth, or vegetable juice.

12. Instead of sauteing vegetables, oven-roast them, whole and unpeeled to intensify the flavor before using them in a dish.

13. For less fat and saturated fat, choose a vegetable oil margarine with 6 grams or less fat and 1 gram or less saturated fat per tablespoon. Butter and other animal fats, although they contain equal amounts of fat, are high in saturated fats. Use sparingly.

Breakfast

14. To make scrambled eggs and omelets, use one whole egg and add extra egg whites to make larger servings.

15. Fill omelets with blanched vegetables such as chopped broccoli or spinach instead of regular cheese.

16. Cereal products, both cooked and dry, are low in fat—with the exception of those that contain coconut or coconut oil, like many types of granola. (Many granolas are high in fat—check the label.)

17. Instead of choosing doughnuts or danish, pick lower-in-fat foods such as bagels and toast (unless you have found a low-fat or no-fat danish such as Sara Lee Free and Light Danish).

18. The fat content of commercial muffins varies. Some are relatively low in fat, others resemble cake more than a muffin, which is a type of quickbread. Try to select a muffin with 5 grams or less of fat, or better yet make your own in large quantities and freeze. See recipes on pages 276–277.

19. Spread toast, bagels, and the like with fruit butters (they are not made of butter, but contain fruit and sugar), all-fruit spreads, part-skim ricotta mixed with plain nonfat yogurt, chopped fruit or vegetables with low-fat cottage cheese, or Neufchatel cheese.

20. The fat content of frozen breakfast foods such as pancakes and waffles varies. Try to select one with 6 grams or less of fat per 2 waffles or French toast or 3 pancakes.

21. For a breakfast meat, choose Canadian bacon or turkey bacon rather than regular bacon because it has less fat. Also, look for breakfast sausage made with turkey rather than beef or pork.

22. Make French toast with bananas and skim milk (see recipe on page 185) rather than eggs and regular milk.

Lunch

23. Yogurt can be made from regular, low-fat, or skim milk. For less fat, saturated fat,

❖ *Table 19 Guide to Fat in Cheeses* ❖

Lowfat 0–3 g fat/oz	Medium Fat 4–5 g fat/oz	High Fat 6–8 g fat/oz	Very High Fat 9–10 g fat/oz
Natural Cheeses			
*Cottage cheese (¼ cup) *Dry curd*	*Mozzarella *Part skim*	Bleu cheese	Cheddar
Cottage cheese (¼ cup) *Lowfat 1%*	*Ricotta (¼ cup) *Part skim*	*Brick	Colby
Cottage cheese (¼ cup) *Lowfat 2%*	String cheese *Part skim*	Brie	*Cream cheese (1 oz = 2 tablespoons)
Cottage cheese (¼ cup) *Creamed 4%*		Camembert	Fontina
Sap sago		Edam	*Gruyere
		Feta	Longhorn
		Gjetost	*Monterey jack
Look for special lowfat brands of mozzarella, ricotta, cheddar, and monterey jack.	*Look for reduced fat brands of cheddar, colby, monterey jack, muenster, and swiss.*	Gouda	Muenster
		*Light cream cheese (1 oz = 2 tablespoons)	Roquefort
		Limburger	
		Mozzarella, *whole milk*	
		Parmesan (1 oz = 3 tablespoons)	
		*Port du salut	
		Provolone	
		*Ricotta (¼ cup), *whole milk*	
		Romano (1 oz = 3 tablespoons)	
		*Swiss	
		Tilsit, *whole milk*	
Modified Cheeses			
Pasteurized process, imitation, and substitute cheeses with 3 grams of fat/oz or less.	Pasteurized process, imitation, and substitute cheeses with 4–5 grams of fat/oz.	Pasteurized process swiss cheese	*Some pasteurized process cheeses are found in this category—check the labels.*
		Pasteurized process swiss cheese food	
		Pasteurized process american cheese	
		Pasteurized process american cheese food	
		American cheese food cold pack	
		Imitation and substitute cheeses with 6–8 grams of fat/oz.	

Check the labels for fat and sodium content. 1 serving = 1 oz. unless otherwise stated.
*These cheeses contain 160 mg or less of sodium per 1 oz.
Reprinted with permission of American Heart Association, Nutrition Committee, Alameda County Chapter.

cholesterol, and calories, choose yogurts lowest in fat such as nonfat or low-fat yogurt.

24. Use fresh vegetables such as mushrooms, peppers, onion, and zucchini on pizza instead of high-fat toppings such as pepperoni and sausage.

Sandwiches

25. Avoid high-fat processed meats, such as many luncheon meats, because 60 percent to 80 percent of their calories come from fat—much of which is saturated. Other examples of these processed meats are bacon, bologna, salami, hot dogs, and sausage (see Table 20). In some cases these processed meats are made from turkey or chicken and may be lower in fat. Read the label for information on grams of fat per serving. Avoid those with more than 4 grams of fat per ounce. Select hot dogs with no more than 6 grams of fat each.

❖ **Table 20 Fat and Cholesterol** ❖
in Processed Meats

Product (3½ ounces)	Total Fat (grams)	Saturated Fat (grams)	Cholesterol (milligrams)
Beef			
Salami, cured, smoked	20.7	9.0	65
Bologna, cured	28.5	12.1	58
Frankfurter, cured	28.5	12.0	61
Pork			
Ham, cured	9.0	3.1	59
Fresh, Italian sausage	25.7	9.0	78
Smoked link sausage, cured, grilled	31.8	11.3	68
Bacon, fried	49.2	17.4	85

Source: Eating to Lower Your High Blood Cholesterol, *National Institutes of Health, 1989 (NIH Publication No. 89-2920).*

26. For sandwiches, try the following (2 to 3 ounces is all you need):
    • fresh-cooked turkey, chicken breast, or lean roast beef
    • water-packed tuna
    • low-fat cheese
27. Eat peanut butter sandwiches in moderation (at 16 grams of fat/2 tablespoons).
28. Eat a meatless lunch. For example, try one of the following.
    • Stuff pita bread with meatless chili, hummus with lettuce and tomato, or low-fat cottage cheese mixed with chopped apple and raisins.
    • Pita bread can also be stuffed with all kinds of fresh vegetables, chunks of skim-milk mozzarella cheese, and reduced calorie salad dressing.
29. Instead of putting butter, margarine, or mayonnaise on sandwiches, use mustard and fill them up with vegetables such as lettuce, tomato, and onion.
30. See the "Mix and Match" list on the next page for more lunch ideas.

Salads

31. Use a variety of crisp greens as the base. For salad toppings, emphasize fresh fruits and vegetables and cooked beans and peas. For protein, choose low-fat cheeses, low-fat cottage cheese and low-fat yogurt, rather than shredded cheddar cheese, chopped eggs, nuts, and seeds.
32. When preparing or buying salads as entrees, use small amounts of poultry or lean meats with lots of fresh fruits and vegetables.
33. The following are low-calorie salad dressings: lemon juice and/or tomato juice with herbs, flavored vinegars, or vinegar with vegetable or fruit purees (they function like the oil in a dressing) for a natural, flavorful dressing.
34. Make your own oil and vinegar salad dressing using a flavored vinegar such as raspberry or balsamic with fresh herbs such as basil, dill, or parsley. Use three parts vinegar to one part oil. Depending on the ingredients chosen, you may be able to decrease the amount of oil. If it's too tangy, add mustard.
35. To make a good creamy dressing, combine buttermilk with a soft, low-fat cheese.
36. Use reduced fat and fat-free versions of salad dressings and mayonnaise.
37. Use plain low-fat or nonfat yogurt, low-fat buttermilk, or whipped cottage cheese as a substitute for sour cream in salad dressings (or dips).

Dinner
Soups and Sauces

38. Clear soups, such as chicken noodle, are lower in calories and fat than cream soups, such as cream of broccoli or New England clam chowder. For less fat and calories, select soups with less than 4 grams of fat per cup, or make your own soups such as vegetable or minestrone (see recipes at end of Chapter 14).
39. Thicken soups (also sauces) with cornstarch dissolved in cold liquid or grated raw potato instead of roux (fat and flour). Vegetable soups can be thickened with barley.

MIX AND MATCH LUNCH IDEAS

On the Outside	On the Inside	Inside or Outside
Whole wheat bread	Low-fat cheese	Cherry tomatoes
Rye bread	Chick-pea spread*	Shredded lettuce
Multigrain roll	Sliced turkey or chicken	Green pepper strips
Tortilla	breast	Cucumber slices
Pita bread	Tuna fish salad*	Spinach leaves
Pumpernickel bread	Cottage cheese with chopped	Radishes
	vegetables*	Mixed salad
	Meatless chili	Carrot sticks
	Hummus	Three/four bean salad*

Other Ideas

Low-fat or skim milk yogurt with fruit
Cheese pizza with vegetable toppings

Beverages	Desserts
Skim milk	Fresh fruit
Iced tea or coffee	Fig bar
Unsweetened fruit juice	Oatmeal raisin cookie
Vegetable juice	Graham cracker
Bottled water	No fat, whole grain fruit cookie (try Health Valley)

Recipe appears in this book. Check index for page number.

40. Legumes, cooked and pureed, make great soups without cream or high-fat thickeners such as roux.
41. Use a puree of vegetables to take the place of butter in a sauce. Examples of vegetable purees include eggplant with lemon or beans pureed with roasted garlic and hot peppers.
42. You can also use vegetable purees to thicken sauces or alone as a sauce.
43. Substitute salsas for rich sauces and gravies.
44. Refrigerate meat drippings so the fat will solidify and you can remove it or use a fat separator cup (see Chapter 7).
45. Make your own vegetable stock (see recipe in Chapter 14) and use it as the basis for soups and sauces. Vegetable stock can also be used as the braising liquid and for cooking rice.
46. If you must use canned chicken broth, refrigerate first, then skim off the fat.
47. Make your own low-fat salsa by mixing diced fresh or unsalted canned tomatoes with diced onions, green peppers, and chilies.
48. To make a medium white sauce, substitute

skim milk for regular milk and use only 1 tablespoon margarine for each 2 tablespoons flour. Or use evaporated skim milk and broth, and thicken with cornstarch or arrowroot.

49. Use flavored vinegars in sauces to add zest. Use apple-cider vinegar with poultry, white wine vinegar with fish, and red wine vinegar with beef.

Entrees

50. Choose lean cuts of meat or poultry, fish, or shellfish. Lean cuts of meat are listed below. Most fish is lower in saturated fat and cholesterol than meat and poultry. Shellfish varies in cholesterol content—some is relatively high and some is low—but a serving has less cholesterol than found in 1 egg and less fat than meat and poultry.

Lean Cuts of Meat

Beef: Round (eye of round, top round, bottom round, round tip), loin (top loin), sirloin, and chuck (arm), extra lean ground beef
(Select grade beef contains less fat than choice grade, which contains less than prime grade. Most of the meat in supermarkets is choice.)

Pork: Tenderloin, center loin roasts, and chops

Veal: All trimmed cuts except commercially ground veal and veal cutlets

Lamb: Leg, loin roasts and chops, foreshank

51. No-fat or low-fat Italian (or other style) dressing makes excellent marinades for meat, poultry, and vegetables. You can also use wine-flavored vinegars, lemon juice or fruit juices mixed with herbs.

52. Ground beef is available in different forms. Although there may be variation from store to store, ground beef is usually higher in fat than ground chuck, while ground round and ground sirloin are leaner. Some supermarkets label their ground beef regular, lean, and extra lean. Ask your supermarket meat manager about the fat content in their ground meats. Or select a sirloin steak and ask the butcher to trim it well and grind.

53. Replace half of the ground beef in a recipe with ground turkey without any noticeable taste difference. Increase spices to make up for the milder flavor of turkey. See Chapter 8 for more information on making burgers with ground turkey or chicken.

54. Organ meats, such as liver, are high in cholesterol but contain little fat and many vitamins and minerals. Eat in moderation.

55. Use less meat, poultry, or fish in main dishes and casseroles by combining them with pasta, rice, other grains, or vegetables.

56. Remove chicken skin before eating. The skin is where much of the fat is. Don't remove it before cooking, because the chicken will dry out excessively.

57. Battered frozen fish contain more fat than plain fish. Choose a plain frozen fish fillet instead and top it with whole wheat bread crumbs or wheat germ and low-fat Italian dressing.

58. Frozen convenience entrees often derive much of their calories from fat. Try to select one with 10 grams of fat or less per serving.

59. Trim visible fat from meats before cooking.

60. When cooking meats, poultry, and fish, use cooking methods that use little or no fat, such as roasting, broiling, grilling, boiling, stir frying, barbecuing, or poaching. Avoid pan-frying or deep-fat frying.

61. Place meat and poultry on a rack when roasting or broiling so that fat can drain away from the meat.

62. Use a vegetable oil spray or a small amount of oil to coat a frying pan (preferably use nonstick) when sauteing or cooking in fat.

63. If your recipe calls for cooking in butter or olive oil, you don't have to totally eliminate it from the recipe. Instead of cooking in butter or olive oil, think of these as seasoning agents and add a small amount at the final stages of cooking so the taste remains with the final product.

64. Baste meat and poultry with unsalted broth (season with herbs and spices), unsalted to-

mato juice, table wine, or fresh lemon juice instead of fatty drippings.

65. After browning ground meat or poultry, strain in a colander lined with paper towels to remove fat.

66. Do not substitute cheese for meat ounce for ounce. Often, when people cut back on meat, they replace it with cheese, thinking they are cutting back on their saturated fat and cholesterol. They couldn't be more wrong! Because regular cheeses are prepared from whole milk or cream, they are also high in saturated fat and cholesterol. Ounce for ounce, meat, poultry, and most regular cheeses have about the same amount of cholesterol. But cheeses have much more saturated fat.

67. Use cooked or canned dry beans and peas in main dishes, side dishes, and salads. For example:
   - Combine black beans and rice with chili powder or other peppery seasoning for a Caribbean-style dish.
   - Try a mixture of any of these with a vinegar and oil dressing for a three- or four-bean salad: green beans, wax beans, kidney beans, lima beans, great northern beans, or chick-peas.
   - Add kidney beans or chick-peas to a lettuce or spinach salad.

68. Have at least two meatless meals each week using, for instance, pasta, dry beans and peas, and/or grains. If you use any cheese, use small amounts of low-fat ones. See recipes at the end of Chapters 11 and 13. Try:
   - Whole wheat spaghetti with fresh tomato sauce
   - Whole wheat macaroni and chick-pea stew in tomato sauce
   - Eggplant Parmesan made with broiled eggplant, tomato sauce, and Parmesan cheese

69. Serve pasta with:
   - Marinara sauce (a spicy tomato sauce) on pasta and top it with one tablespoon Parmesan cheese.
   - Make your own light tomato sauce (see recipe on page 242).
   - Make a sauce from garlic or shallots sauteed in a small amount of olive oil, then deglaze the pan with vinegar (to dissolve the food particles in the bottom of the pan), add the other ingredients (other vegetables, seafood, or whatever the recipe calls for) and enough wine or broth to make a sauce, simmer until tender, and toss with pasta.
   - Substitute evaporated skim milk in pasta recipes that call for cream.
   - Pasta doesn't have to be served just with a sauce—dress up pasta dishes with chopped, julienned, and sliced vegetables of different textures and colors. For example, add sliced mushrooms and broccoli flowerettes to your favorite tomato sauce.

70. You can cut down on calories, fat, and cholesterol in baked pasta recipes by using vegetables instead of meat. Healthy revisions include zucchini lasagne, spinach-stuffed rigatoni, or broccoli and low-fat cheese stuffed shells.

71. When cooking pasta, don't add oil to the boiling water to prevent sticking. Simply use plenty of water: 4 to 6 quarts for 1 pound of pasta.

Side Dishes

72. Include at least three servings of vegetables and grains, such as rice or pasta, at dinner every night.

73. Steam, broil, boil, bake, stir-fry, or microwave vegetables. Don't fry!

74. Instead of cooking greens, such as collards, with bacon or ham, cook in meat broth that has been refrigerated and the fat removed from the top.

75. If buying frozen fried potatoes, choose those that are bigger (they have less fat than smaller ones) and can be baked in the oven without oil. Avoid Tater Tots as they are ground potatoes that are mixed with oil before being shaped. Try to select frozen potatoes with less than 5 grams of fat per 3½-ounce serving.

76. Instead of sour cream on potatoes, use plain

low-fat (or nonfat) yogurt seasoned with herbs, whipped low-fat cottage cheese with a little lemon juice, or low-fat ranch dressing.

Snacks

77. Hard and soft pretzels are good snack choices as they are very low in fat and a good source of complex carbohydrate. Pretzels made with whole wheat flour and coated with sesame seeds (rather than salt) are more nutritious than those made with white flour and salt.

78. Most microwave popcorn contains much fat. For no fat and fewer calories, choose popcorn that can be air popped, or choose a microwave brand with 100 calories or less per one-ounce serving. If air popping popcorn, use garlic, onion, or chili powder or a small amount of grated Parmesan for seasoning.

79. To make a healthy pizza snack, use low-fat cheeses such as skim-milk mozzarella, and top with fresh vegetables like green peppers, mushrooms, and zucchini. Mini-pizzas can be made with pita bread, a little Parmesan cheese, vegetables, garlic powder, and oregano.

80. Fresh fruits and vegetables are popular snack foods. Raw vegetables with dip and fruit with low-fat cheese, such as cottage cheese, are great combinations. Or make a dip for fruit with 8 oz plain low-fat yogurt, 3 tablespoons strawberry fruit spread, and ½ teaspoon cinnamon. Use salsa or hummus (chick-pea spread) as a dip for raw vegetables.

81. Breads are great snack choices. Try whole grain breads, pita bread, bread sticks made with a minimum of oil, mini-rolls, quick breads, and muffins. You may want to spread a thin layer of peanut butter or fruit spread on breads and crackers, or you can stuff a pita pocket with lettuce, tomato, and any other vegetable and top with diet dressing.

82. Crackers contain varying amounts of fat. For less fat, choose crackers made with 3 grams or less of fat per one-half ounce, the size of a normal serving. Examples include crispbreads, matzo, melba toast, saltines, and rice cakes.

83. Nuts and seeds derive about 80 percent of their calories from fat. For less fat and saturated fat, choose them in moderation and choose those brands that are dry-roasted.

Desserts and Baking

84. Commercial cakes, pies, and cookies are often high in fat, saturated fat, and calories. In addition, some are quite high in cholesterol. There are some that are acceptable.
  * angel food cake or sponge cake—serve with fruit
  * fig bars, gingersnaps, graham crackers, animal crackers
  * baked goods specially made without fat. Try to select cakes with 5 grams or less of fat per serving and cookies with 4 grams or less of fat per ounce.

85. Bake or broil fruits for dessert. Try:
  * Baked pears or baked apples with a sprinkle of cinnamon
  * Broiled peach or grapefruit half with a sprinkle of nutmeg
  * Fruit compote

Add a little wine, liqueur, fresh herbs, or a dusting of spice to add interest and flavor.

86. Choose frozen desserts such as ices, sherbets, sorbets, ice milk, frozen juice bars, and frozen yogurt, which contain (in most cases) less saturated fat than ice cream. Ice cream has at least 12 percent fat. Ice milk has less fat and the fat content of frozen yogurt varies, but it is generally less than ice cream (avoid those with nuts). See Chapter 10 for more information. Ices and sorbets are basically fruit, sugar, and water and therefore contain no fat.

87. Great toppings for frozen yogurt or ice milk include pureed fruit sauce, crushed oatmeal cookies, wheat germ, chopped dried fruit, and fresh fruits. Choose crushed Oreos and M & Ms in moderation!

88. If making pudding from scratch or a mix, use skim or 1% milk.

89. Flavored gelatin is a tasty dessert without fat.
90. When choosing a cake or brownie mix, choose those made with less fat, such as five or fewer grams fat per serving. Angel food cake and gingerbread are moderate in fat content.
91. When baking from scratch, you can decrease the fat in many of your recipes by about one-fourth to one-third of the original amount without any significant difference in quality. Another way to reduce fat is to use half the amount of fat called for in the recipe, along with an equal amount of applesauce. Following are guidelines for different types of baked goods (see Chapter 16 for more information).
    - In recipes for **muffins, quick breads,** and **biscuits,** the minimum amount of fat is 1 to 2 tablespoons per cup of flour.
    - Some **yeast breads,** such as English muffins and French bread, can be made without any fat.
    - The minimum amount of fat in **cake** recipes is 2 tablespoons per cup of flour. You can't use vegetable oil in cakes that require creaming so use unsaturated, unsalted margarine.
    - Soft drop **cookies** generally contain less fat than crisp rolled cookies. The fat level can usually be adjusted to 2 tablespoons per cup of flour. Lowering the fat too much in rolled cookies can make a dough that is difficult to roll out.
    - Use a regular stick margarine for pie crusts, pastries, cakes, or crispy cookies. For quickbreads such as muffins and soft cookies, use a soft tub margarine, liquid margarine, or oil (they contain less saturated fat than stick margarine).
92. Substitute as described in Table 5.
93. For cake frosting, blenderize ricotta cheese and thin with juice, honey, rum, or extracts.
94. Use powdered sugar as a frosting on cakes.
95. Use fruit sauce as a topping for cakes.
96. Fill a meringue cup with fresh fruits and unsweetened fruit sauce.
97. Instead of making two-crust pies, make fruit cobblers and crisps and cut the amount of sugar used.
98. To decrease the fat in a pie crust, use one cup of flour to 3 to 4 tablespoons stick margarine and 3 tablespoons of cold water. It won't be as flaky, but it also won't be as fatty. Using oil in pie crusts does not work very satisfactorily.
99. Substitute raisins and chopped dried fruit in baking for chocolate chips.
100. Grease baking pans with vegetable oil spray.
101. Omit half the nuts called for in recipes since nuts are high in fat.

Use the summary of guidelines for fat content when shopping at the supermarket.

GUIDELINES FOR BUYING FOODS AT THE SUPERMARKET

❖　❖　❖

Food	Try to Buy One with No More Than
Soups	4 grams fat per cup
Frozen or canned entree/dinner	10 grams fat per dinner
Processed meat	4 grams fat per ounce
Hot dogs	6 grams fat each
Cheese	4 grams fat per ounce
Frozen potatoes	5 grams fat per 3½-ounce serving
Cake or pie (including mixes)	5 grams fat per serving
Cookies	4 grams fat per ounce
Crackers	3 grams fat per half ounce
Muffin	5 grams fat per medium muffin
Margarine	6 grams fat per tablespoon
Salad dressing	1 gram fat per tablespoon

❖ ❖ ❖

CHAPTER FOUR

SUPERMARKET SMARTS

PLANNING NUTRITIOUS MENUS THAT SAVE TIME AND MONEY

Many people would say they don't plan menus—at least they don't write them down in advance. But everyone plans, if only for how to stock the refrigerator. Menu planning means thinking about what foods to eat together for a meal, a day, or a week. Food choices are influenced by habit, by the occasion, by time and food available, and by what you feel like eating, as well as by your own concern for nutrition. There are many advantages to planning meals, and you don't need to be locked into a rigid schedule. Planning ahead:

- **Helps avoid too many calories, and too much fat, sugars, and sodium in your diet.** You can plan your food choices ahead of time so you will be more likely to make nutritious choices.
- **Increases variety.** You can include the different types of foods you need for nutrients and fiber. You can experiment with a new recipe, try new styles of preparation, and vary the colors, textures, flavors, and shapes of foods to make meals attractive and interesting.
- **Saves time and effort.** Needed items will be on hand, which means fewer trips to the grocery store. Planning helps you make good use of leftovers, which can decrease preparation time and food cost.
- **Saves money.** When you go to the store you will know what you need. Then you can compare prices and buy only what you can use without waste. Preplanned quick meals can re-

place more costly convenience items and restaurant meals at least some of the time.

Planning Nutritious Menus

In 1958, the U.S. Department of Agriculture published *Food for Fitness—A Daily Food Guide* that included a description of the **Basic Four Food Groups**. The four food groups include meats and meat substitutes, milk and milk products, fruits and vegetables, and grains. Each group contains foods of similar origin and nutrient content. For example, the grain group includes foods such as breads and cereals made from grains which provide thiamin, niacin, and iron. According to the Basic Four Food Groups plan, you should eat two servings daily from the meat group, two servings from the milk group, four servings of fruits and vegetables, and four servings of grains.

The Basic Four Food Groups concept is somewhat limited in its usefulness. It is certainly possible to eat the proper number of servings from each group and, at the same time, eat entirely too many calories and too much fat (by drinking whole milk, eating fatty cuts of meat, eating too much cheese, and so on). It is also possible to follow the plan and not get enough of all necessary vitamins and minerals, particularly if you choose many enriched foods (such as white bread) instead of whole foods (such as whole wheat bread). Finally, many foods do not fit into any of the food groups. Foods that are high in fat and/or sugar, such as margarine, mayonnaise, salad dressing, cakes, and cookies, do not appear in any of the food groups.

❖ *A Pattern for Daily Food Choices* ❖

Food Group	Major Dietary Contributions	Suggested Daily Servings	What Counts as a Serving?
Breads, cereals, and other grain products • Whole grain • Enriched	Provide starch, thiamin, riboflavin, niacin, and iron. Whole grains also provide fiber, folic acid, magnesium, and zinc.	**6 to 11** (Include at least several servings per day of whole grain products and eat products from a variety of grains.)	▶ 1 slice of bread ▶ ½ hamburger bun or English muffin ▶ a small roll, biscuit, or muffin ▶ 3 to 4 small or 2 large crackers ▶ ½ cup cooked cereal, rice, or pasta ▶ 1 ounce of ready-to-eat breakfast cereal
Fruits • Citrus • Other fruits	Contribute many nutrients as well as dietary fiber. Citrus fruits, melons, and berries are excellent sources of vitamin C. Deep yellow fruits are high in vitamin A. Fruits also add color, flavor, texture, and sweetness to the diet.	**2 to 4** (Have a vitamin C-rich food every day and a vitamin A-rich food every other day.)	▶ a whole fruit such as a medium apple, banana, or orange ▶ a grapefruit half ▶ a melon wedge ▶ ¾ cup of juice ▶ ½ cup of berries ▶ ½ cup cooked or canned fruit ▶ ¼ cup dried fruit
Vegetables • Dry beans and peas (legumes) • Starchy • Other vegetables	Supply fiber, some starch or protein; also provide many vitamins and minerals.	**3 to 5** (Include all types regularly; use dark green leafy vegetables, dry beans, and peas several times per week.)	▶ ½ cup of cooked vegetables ▶ ½ cup of chopped raw vegetables ▶ 1 cup of leafy raw vegetables, such as lettuce or spinach
Meat, poultry, fish, and alternates (eggs, dry beans, and peas)	Provide protein, niacin, thiamin, vitamins B_6, B_{12} (animal foods only), iron, phosphorus, and zinc.	**2 to 3** (total 5 to 7 ounces lean)	Amounts should total 5 to 7 ounces of cooked lean meat, poultry, or fish a day. Count 1 egg, ½ cup cooked beans, or 2 tablespoons peanut butter as 1 ounce of meat.

❖ *A Pattern for Daily Food Choices* ❖

Food Group	Major Dietary Contributions	Suggested Daily Servings	What Counts as a Serving?
Milk, cheese, and yogurt	As the best sources of calcium in U.S. diets, they provide protein, riboflavin, vitamins B_{12}, A, thiamin, and if fortified, vitamin D.	**2** for adults; **3** for teens and women who are pregnant or breast-feeding; **4** for teens who are pregnant or breast-feeding. (Choose low-fat milk and dairy products.)	▶ 1 cup of milk ▶ 8 ounces of yogurt ▶ 1½ ounces of natural cheese ▶ 2 ounces of process cheese
Fats, sweets, and alcohol	These foods are calorie-dense, not nutrient-dense. Fats provide 9 calories per gram; sugars, 4 calories per gram; and alcohol, 7 calories per gram.	Avoid too many fats and sweets. If you drink alcoholic beverages, do so in moderation.	

Source: *United States Department of Agriculture*

The Basic Four Food Groups concept is also becoming outdated. When the concept was developed, there were RDAs for less than 10 nutrients; in the most recent version (1989) of the RDA, there are requirements for 26 nutrients. The emphasis has switched from eating enough of different foods to prevent deficiencies, to balancing your diet to prevent diseases such as heart disease and cancer.

The most recent food group concept was featured in *Dietary Guidelines for Americans* (third edition) in 1990. According to **A Pattern for Daily Food Choices**, each day's menus should include foods from five major food groups:

1. Breads, cereals, and other grain products
2. Fruits
3. Vegetables
4. Meat, poultry, fish, and alternates (eggs, dry beans and peas, nuts, and seeds)
5. Milk, cheese, and yogurt

Foods from the sixth food group—fats, sweets, and alcoholic beverages—should be used in moderation, if at all. The Pattern for Daily Food Choices shows you the types of food to include in your daily menus. How much you serve depends on your own calorie needs and those of your family members.

The pattern suggests ranges of daily servings from most groups—three to five servings of vegetables, for example. To make sure you get the nutrients and fiber you need, plan your menus to include at least the lower number of servings from each food group each day. People with lower calorie needs will need only the lower number of servings. They'll also have to be careful about choosing small portions and lower calorie foods within each group. Young children may not need as much food, so they can have smaller amounts from all groups except milk. Other people will need more food than the lower number of servings to meet their calorie needs. These people can eat larger portions and include additional foods from the first five food groups.

Also, vary your choices of foods within each group, because specific foods differ in the kinds and amounts of nutrients they provide. For example, include in a week's menu different breads, fruits, and vegetables as well—especially dark green leafy vegetables, dry beans and peas, and

PERSONALIZED SCORECARD FOR LABEL READING

❖ ❖ ❖

Calories: _____
(Use page 20 in Chapter 1 to determine your calorie needs.)

Total Fat: _____
(Use page 45 in Chapter 3 to determine how many grams of fat you need based on fat providing 30 percent of calories.)

Saturated Fat: _____
(Use page 45 in Chapter 3 to determine how many grams of saturated fat you need based on it providing 10 percent of calories.)

Cholesterol: __300 milligrams or less__

Total Carbohydrate: _____
(Use page 37 in Chapter 2 to determine your needs for total carbohydrate, complex carbohydrate, and sugars.)

Complex Carbohydrate: _____

Sugars: _____

Dietary fiber __25–35 grams__

Sodium __2,400 milligrams or less__

Potassium __3,500 milligrams__

---

whole-grain breads and cereals. You can follow the Checklist for Healthy and Practical Menus to ensure a nutritious, well-balanced menu.

Planning Menus that Save Time

Everyone is looking to save time preparing meals. Try these tips.

- Plan to cook extra on the weekends or day off. These foods can then be reheated or prepared in another way during the week. For example, anytime you make foods such as soups, stews, chili, or spaghetti sauce, make extra and freeze in meal-size portions or refrigerate for use within a few days. Double your meat loaf recipe and freeze half the uncooked meat mixture as patties or meatballs to use later or freeze some in muffin tins to make mini-loaves. Planned leftovers cut preparation time and save food dollars.

- Evaluate recipes in terms of how much preparation and cooking time they require. The Quick Chili (page 63) is an example of this type of planning. Fish, stir-fry mixtures, and most vegetables cook quickly. Roasts, stews, and casseroles take longer.

- New recipes and food preparation methods often take longer the first time you try them. Try only one new item at a time.

❖ Lower-Cost Meat and Poultry Cuts ❖ and Fish Species

Beef	Poultry	Fish
Bottom round	Whole turkey	Alaska pollock
Chuck roll	Whole roaster	Whitefish
Flank steak	chicken	Mackerel
Stewing beef	Turkey wings	Ocean perch
Ground beef	Turkey	Shark
(choose	drumsticks	
lean or	Ground	
extra lean)	turkey	
Cube steak		

- Ask family members to take part in planning meals (and preparing them too!). Consider asking each member to plan one meal per week.

Planning Menus that Save Money

Like most people, you are probably interested in getting the best quality food without spending a bundle. Here are some helpful tips.

- Plan on using less expensive cuts of meat and poultry and fish species; see the list above for examples.

- Plan one or more meatless meals each week. Use dry beans and peas, such as kidney beans, and grains such as rice. See Chapter 11 for more information and recipes.

❖ *Checklist for Healthy and Practical Menus* ❖

If you write out your menus, select several to help you answer the questions below. Then answer the following questions.

1. Does a day's menu provide at least the lower number of servings from each of the major food groups?

	YES	NO
6 servings of grain products?	____	____
2 servings of fruit?	____	____
3 servings of vegetables?	____	____
2–3 servings of lean meat or the equivalent (totaling 5 oz per day)?	____	____
2 servings of milk, yogurt, or cheese?	____	____

2. Do the menus have several servings of whole grain breads or cereals each day? ____ ____
3. Do menus for a week include several servings of:
   Dark green leafy vegetables, such as spinach, broccoli, romaine lettuce? ____ ____
   Dry beans or peas, such as kidney beans, split peas, lentils? ____ ____
4. Do menus include some vegetables and fruits with skins and seeds (baked potatoes with skin, summer squash, berries, apples, or pears with peels)? ____ ____
5. Underline all of the foods in your menus that are high in fat, sugars, or sodium.
   Are other foods that are served with them lower in fat, sugars, or sodium? ____ ____
   Are other meals on the same day lower in fat, sugar, or sodium, so that total intake is moderate? ____ ____
6. Are the menus practical for you in time? ____ ____
7. Are the menus practical for you in cost? ____ ____
8. Are the foods acceptable in taste for your family? ____ ____

Source: Preparing Foods and Planning Menus Using the Dietary Guidelines, *U.S. Department of Agriculture, Home and Garden Bulletin No. 232-8, 1990.*

- Use less meat, poultry, or fish in recipes. Two ounces (once cooked) per serving is plenty.
- Check the store ads for sales. Plan some of your meals around what is on sale at your store this week.
- Plan meals with as few convenience foods as possible, as they are more expensive. Try to prepare as many foods yourself as time allows.
- Use planned leftovers to make use of large meat cuts and other foods that are more cost-effective. Roast a chicken or beef roast and slice some to eat while hot. Cool the rest quickly and cut into meal-size portions for use later in casseroles, stir-fry dishes, sandwiches, soups, stews, and salads. Freeze the portions you won't use within a day or two.

READING FOOD LABELS

A typical supermarket offers about 20,000 different items. Nutrition labels on supermarket foods have become scorecards for millions of health-conscious Americans. To make your own score-card to use when label reading, fill in the one provided, following the directions given. Facts found on labels tell not only what the product is, but what ingredients are in it, the company responsible for the product, and frequently nutri-

Evaluating a Recipe for Time Required and Nutrition

Quick Chili

Recipe Preparation Time
Active: 10 minutes   **Total:** 20 minutes

4 servings, about ¾ cup each

Per serving:

Calories 230	**Cholesterol** . . . . .34 milligrams
Total fat . . . . .9 grams	**Sodium** . . . . . . .390 milligrams
Saturated fatty acids . .3 grams	

Lean ground beef	½ pound
Kidney beans, drained (save liquid)	15½-ounce can
Bean liquid	⅓ cup
"No-salt-added" canned tomato puree	1 cup
Instant minced onion	1 tablespoon
Chili powder	1½ tablespoons

1. Cook beef in hot frypan until lightly browned. Drain off fat.
2. Stir in remaining ingredients.
3. Bring to a boil. Reduce heat, cover, and simmer 10 minutes.

Menu Suggestion: Serve with mixed salad greens with reduced-calorie dressing, whole-wheat rolls, and juice-pack canned pineapple chunks. (Menu preparation time including recipe: **active**, 15 minutes; **total**, 20 minutes)

This recipe is a time-saver and only requires 20 minutes to prepare because it:

- has only 6 ingredients, none of which require preparation.
- has only 3 major preparation steps. All are very simple.
- uses one pan for all steps. This saves on preparation and cleanup time.
- uses canned rather than dry beans so they cook quickly.
- uses a small amount of liquid and cooks just long enough to blend flavors and become thickened.
- can be doubled, and used at another meal. For example, it could be combined with macaroni in a skillet main dish, in chili burgers served sloppy-joe style, in taco salad, or as a potato topper.

This recipe is also a nutritious choice because:

- lean ground beef is used in place of regular ground beef.
- the amount of ground beef per serving in this dish is less than 2 ounces.
- ground beef is browned without added fat. Fat that accumulates during cooking is drained off.
- kidney beans are a good source of fiber and starch.
- "no-salt-added" tomato puree is lower in sodium than most other processed tomato products. No salt is added to the recipe as the chili powder provides much of the flavor.

tion information and the date by which it should be sold or used. Further, labels may give details about substances that you may wish to avoid, such as fat, sodium, or cholesterol. Indeed, surveys show that about four out of five people look at ingredient lists. And more than two out of three people say they're looking at labels for substances they want to avoid for health reasons.

Since 1938 the federal government has required basic information on food labels. The **Food and Drug Administration (FDA)** regulates labels on all packaged foods except for meat, poultry, and egg products, which are regulated by the **U.S. Department of Agriculture (USDA)**. The FDA is currently reviewing its labeling regulations to see how food labels can be made more "user friendly." Under current rules, the amount of information on food labels varies, but all food labels must contain at least the following.

- The name of the product
- The net contents or net weight, which includes the liquid in canned foods
- The name and place of business of the manufacturer, packer, or distributor
- A list of ingredients

For most foods, all of the ingredients must be listed on the label and must be identified by their common or usual names. The ingredient that is present in the largest amount, by weight, must be listed first. Other ingredients follow in descending order according to weight, as shown in the sample cracker label.

The FDA introduced **nutrition labeling** in 1971 and requires it on the food label when a manufacturer adds a nutrient to the product (as in enriched breads and cereals) or when a claim is made for the product, such as "low calorie." Many manufacturers also voluntarily put nutrition labeling on their products, in fact, more than half the processed foods found in stores contain nutrition labeling. By May 1993, nutrition labeling will be mandatory on most foods. In all, about 300,000 food labels will be affected and the amount of information required on the label will more than double. These and other proposed FDA regulations are outlined in the following list and are discussed in more detail here.

Summary of Proposed Food Labeling Regulations

1. Nutrition Labeling
   - Mandatory for almost all packaged foods
   - Voluntary for raw produce, fish, meat, and poultry
   - Revised list of nutrients
   - New standards for dietary intake
2. Serving Sizes
   - Standardized for over 100 food categories
   - Based on portion sizes normally consumed
   - In household measures
3. Regulated Definitions of Nutrient Content Terms
   - Free
   - Fresh
   - Light
   - More
   - Less
   - High
   - Low
   - Reduced
   - Source of
4. Regulated Definitions of Terms on Meat and Poultry Packaging
   - Lean
   - Extra lean
5. Allowable Health Claims
   - Fat and cancer
   - Fat and heart disease
   - Calcium and osteoporosis
   - Sodium and hypertension
6. Ingredient Labeling Changes
   - Listing of ingredients in standardized foods
   - Listing of all FDA-certified color additives by name
   - Declaration of sulfites and MSG on label
   - Declaration of the percentage of actual fruit or vegetable juice on the label of all juice beverages

Mandatory Nutrition Labeling

Now, nutrition information will be mandatory on processed foods that are meaningful sources of nutrients; that is to say, on virtually all packaged foods. Excluded would be most spices, small packages (generally those no larger than a package of Life Savers), and food produced by small businesses (those with food sales of less than $50,000 a year and total sales of less than $500,000 a year).

The nutrients to be listed on nutrition labeling, as shown, will be changed to keep pace with the nation's changing health concerns. Thiamin, ri-

INGREDIENT LABELING FOR CRACKERS

Ingredients: Enriched wheat flour containing niacin, reduced iron, thiamine mononitrate (Vitamin B1) and riboflavin (Vitamin B2), vegetable shortening (partially hydrogenated soybean and/or cottonseed oils), sugar, salt, corn syrup, leavening (sodium bicarbonate, sodium acid pyrophosphate, monocalcium phosphate)

boflavin, and niacin would become optional listings because the U.S. population generally does not suffer from diseases related to deficiencies of these commonly available B vitamins.

Nutrition information will be presented in

Information to Be Included on Proposed Nutrition Labels

Frozen Vegetables IN SAUCE

NUTRITION INFORMATION PER SERVING

		RECOMMENDED DAILY INTAKE*
Serving Size: ½ cup	(126g)	
Servings per container:	2	
Calories	140	1,600-2,800
Calories from fat	80	480-840

NUTRIENT	AMOUNT	RECOMMENDED DAILY INTAKE*
Total Fat	9 g	53-93 g
Saturated fat	2 g	18-31 g
Cholesterol	0 mg	300 mg
Sodium	380 mg	2,400 mg
Total Carbohydrate	14 g	240-420 g
Complex Carbohydrate	10 g	
Sugars	4 g	
Dietary Fiber	3 g	18-32 g
Protein	4 g	40-70 g

PERCENT OF DAILY VALUE

Vitamin A	10
Vitamin C	10
Calcium	2
Iron	4

*Ranges are based on recommended intakes and food consumption surveys. Advisable calorie, fat, carbohydrate, fiber, and protein intake should vary based on age, sex, height, weight, metabolism, and activity level.

quantitative amounts—for example, 4 grams of fat—and/or as percentages of certain dietary reference values. The format of the new nutrition label will be decided upon in late 1992.

Regarding nutrition labeling for raw fruits, raw vegetables, and raw fish, grocery stores are being asked to make available nutrition information on the 20 most frequently consumed items in each category. This program is voluntary and by May 1993, if at least 60 percent of stores are displaying the information, the guidelines will continue to be voluntary. If not, regulations would be written to make the display mandatory. The USDA is also developing similar arrangements for raw meat and poultry.

A modified form of nutrition labeling will be required for vitamin and mineral supplements. The label will show the quantitative amount and percentage of the daily reference value of all vitamins and minerals, and the quantitative amount of calories and foods components—such as fat, carbohydrates, or fiber—present in more than insignificant amounts.

Serving Sizes

The nutrition content on many, but not all, labels is to be based on the serving or portion size customarily consumed by an average person over the age of 4, and it must appear in household and metric measures, such as 1 cup (240 milliliters). This rule applies to 131 categories of food. Any package that contains less than 2 servings is considered a single-serving container. For example, the proposed standard serving size for a soft drink is 8 ounces. So a 12-ounce can would be considered a single serving and its nutrient content would have to be declared on the basis of the contents of the entire can. Any description such

THE PROPOSED FDA DICTIONARY
FOR DESCRIPTIVE TERMS ON FOOD LABELS

❖ ❖ ❖

Here are the definitions for nutrient content claims.

FREE AND LOW

Free: An amount that is "nutritionally trivial" and unlikely to have a physiological consequence

Calorie Free: Fewer than 5 calories per serving

Sugar Free: Less than 0.5 grams per serving

Sodium Free and Salt Free: Less than 5 milligrams of sodium per serving

Low: Would allow frequent consumption of a food "low" in a nutrient without exceeding the dietary guidelines. Per serving and per 100 grams (a little less than half a cup) of food, these amounts would be defined as:

Low Sodium: Less than 140 milligrams per serving and per 100 grams of food

Very Low Sodium: Less than 35 milligrams per serving and per 100 grams of food

Low Calorie: Less than 40 calories per serving and per 100 grams of food

A food that is normally free of or low in a nutrient may make such a claim, but the claim must indicate that the condition exists for all similar foods—for example, "fresh spinach, a low-sodium food."

HIGH AND SOURCE OF

High and Source of: Are intended to emphasize the beneficial presence of certain nutrients, not to characterize levels of nutrients that increase the risk for chronic diseases. "High" is 20 percent or more of the dietary reference values. "Source of" is 10 percent to 19 percent of these values. Any high-fiber claim for a food containing more than 3 grams of fat per serving and per 100 grams of the food must be accompanied by a declaration of total fat.

REDUCED, LIGHT, LESS, MORE

Use of these terms must be accompanied by information about the food that is the basis for comparison—the identity of the comparable food, the percentage (or fraction) by which the referenced food has been modified, and the amount of the nutrient that is the subject of the claim.

Reduced: Reduced sodium: The food contains no more than half the sodium of the comparison food.
Reduced calories: The food has reduced calories by one-third.

Less: May be used to describe nutrients if the reduction is at least 25 percent.

Light: May be used on foods that contain one-third fewer calories than a comparable product. Any other use of the term "light" must specify if it refers to the look, taste, or smell: for example, "light in color."

More: Could be used to show that a food contains more of a desirable nutrient, such as fiber or potassium, than does a comparable food. To use the term "more," a food must contain at least 10 percent more of the given nutrient than the comparable food.

DEFINITIONS RELATED TO FAT AND CHOLESTEROL

Fat Free:	Less than 0.5 grams of fat per serving, providing that it has no added fat or oil ingredient.
Low Fat:	3 grams or less of fat per serving and per 100 grams of the food.
(Percent) Fat Free	May only describe foods that meet "low fat" definition above.
Reduced Fat	No more than half the fat of an identified comparison. To avoid trivial claims, the reduction must exceed 3 grams of fat per serving.
Low in Saturated Fat	May be used to describe a food that contains 1 gram or less of saturated fat per serving, and not less than 15 percent of calories from saturated fat.
Reduced Saturated Fat	No more than 50 percent of the saturated fat than the food with which it's compared. Foods with a reduction of 25 percent or greater may have a comparative claim using the term "less." If "reduced saturated fat" or a comparative claim is used, it must indicate the percent reduction and the amount of saturated fat in the food with which it's compared. The reduction of saturated fat must exceed 1 gram.
Cholesterol Free:	Less than 2 milligrams of cholesterol per serving and 2 grams or less saturated fat per serving.

Low in Cholesterol:	20 milligrams or less per serving and per 100 grams of food, and 2 grams or less of saturated fat per serving.
Reduced Cholesterol:	50 percent or less of cholesterol per serving than its comparison food. Foods with reductions in cholesterol of 25 percent or more may bear comparative claims using the term "less," but both "reduced cholesterol" and comparative claims must be fully explained, and the reduction in cholesterol must exceed 20 milligrams per serving.

All claims of cholesterol content are prohibited when a food contains more than 2 grams of saturated fat per serving. The label of a food containing more than 11.5 grams of total fat per serving or per 100 grams of the food must disclose those levels immediately after any cholesterol claim.

FRESH

Fresh:	Can only be linked to raw foods, foods that have not been frozen, processed, or preserved. Adding approved waxes or coatings, using approved pesticides after harvest, or applying a mild chlorine wash or mild acid to raw produce would not prohibit the use of the term "fresh."
Freshly:	With a verb such as "prepared," "baked," or "roasted," may be used if the food is recently made and has not been frozen or heat processed or preserved.

as "low sodium" also would have to be based on the entire contents of the can.

Defining Nutrient Content Terms
The FDA now has a dictionary for food producers, marketers, and consumers that contains consis-

tent and uniform definitions for an expanded list of terms. There are definitions for nine core terms, called descriptors or nutrient content claims, that could be used to describe a food if the food meets that definition. These nine are free, low, high, source of, reduced, light or lite, less, more, and fresh. These nine terms have also been given specific definitions when used with certain nutrients, such as low sodium. The FDA dictionary list gives more information on each descriptor.

If a food is labeled with a descriptor for a certain nutrient but that food contains other nutrients at levels known to be less healthy, the label would have to bring that to consumers' attention. For example, if a food making a low-sodium claim is also high in fat, the label must state "see back panel for information about fat and other nutrients."

Health Claims

The Nutrition Labeling and Education Act of 1990 provided, for the first time, the specific statutory authority to allow food labels to carry claims about the relationship between the food and specific diseases or health conditions. This was a major shift in labeling philosophy. Until 1984, a food product making such a claim on its label was treated as a drug and considered misbranded unless the claim was backed up by an approved new drug application.

The FDA has examined the scientific evidence on 10 relationships between nutrients and the risks of certain diseases. Of the relationships considered, these four are currently supported and would be allowed on labels:

1. calcium and osteoporosis
2. sodium and hypertension
3. fat and cardiovascular disease
4. fat and cancer

Two other claims—fiber and heart disease, and fiber and cancer—are being reviewed further. The following claims are not allowed: omega-3 fatty acids with heart disease, folic acid with neural tube defects, antioxidant vitamins (such as C and E) with cancer, or zinc with immune function in the elderly.

Proposals for the general requirements for health claims set forth a number of definitions to clarify their meanings. One of the most significant defines the nutrient levels that would disqualify a health claim. Disqualified are those foods that contain more than 11.5 grams of fat, 4 grams of

saturated fat, 45 milligrams of cholesterol, or 360 milligrams of sodium per amount commonly consumed, per labeled serving size, and per 100 grams (about 3½ ounces).

Ingredient Labeling

The FDA has always required the ingredients of packaged foods to be listed on the labels. But certain common foods such as mayonnaise, macaroni, and bread, made according to "standard" recipes set by the FDA, have been exempt from the requirement to list all their ingredients. The FDA now considers listing of all ingredients necessary even for standardized foods, mainly because many of today's consumers, unlike their parents or grandparents, don't know what these foods are made of. The FDA will also require:

- the listing of all FDA-certified color additives by name
- an explanation on the label that the list of ingredients is in descending order of predominance by weight
- the listing of all sweeteners together in the ingredient list, under the collective term "sweeteners," when more than one sweetener is used in a product. Following the collective term, each sweetener would be listed in parentheses in descending order of predominance by weight.
- identification of caseinate as a milk derivative when used in foods that claim to be nondairy, such as coffee whiteners, because some people with milk allergies use nondairy products
- declaration of sulfites used in standardized foods because some people are allergic to these preservatives
- declaration of protein hydrolysates, used in many foods as flavors and flavor enhancers. Most important, for consumers with religious or cultural dietary requirements, the food source of the additive would have to be identified.
- declaration of monosodium glutamate (MSG), a flavor enhancer, on the label whether it is added as a separate ingredient or as a component of protein hydrolysates
- declaration of the percentage of actual fruit or vegetable juice on the label of all juice bever-

ages, whether full strength or diluted. Beverages made from several juices that identify individual juices on the labels must declare the percentage of each of the identified juices.

SMART-SHOPPING TIPS

Probably the biggest decision to make about shopping is where to shop. Check prices in nearby stores for several foods you buy on a regular basis. Then decide which store offers reasonable prices and other features important to you, such as convenient location, variety and good quality of foods, parking, check cashing, and so on.

You may choose a chain or large independent store because it offers more variety, more shopping convenience, and better prices than smaller stores. Warehouse stores generally offer excellent prices but not always the widest variety. For certain foods, you may prefer a specialty shop like a bakery, vegetable stand, or natural food store. Natural food stores often offer bulk foods such as rolled oats, rice, grains, and nuts at cheaper prices than supermarkets. They are also sometimes the only place to buy whole grain flours, whole grain cookies, and whole grain pasta. Local food co-ops, when available, often offer good prices and quality.

Wherever you decide to shop, it's usually best to pick a convenient, reasonably priced store and stay with it. Store-hopping for advertised specials or to redeem coupons can be pennywise, but un-

less the stores are close together it can be costly in gasoline or bus fare, and time.

Before shopping:
- Plan menus to include a variety of foods from each of the major food groups with moderate amounts of fat, sodium, and sugar.
- Consider how much money you have to spend on food.
- Make a shopping list, checking what foods are on hand. Keep a piece of paper near the refrigerator at all times and jot down items as you need them. Use it as the basis for your shopping list. Also read your recipes carefully to be sure you will have all the ingredients on hand when you need them.
- Organize your shopping list according to where they are found in your supermarket. For instance, group all fresh fruits and vegetables together.
- Check store ads for specials and write on your shopping list those you want to take advantage of. Don't buy specials that you don't need or can't store. A bargain is no bargain if you don't need it.
- If you use coupons, go through them and pull out those you can use. Use coupons for products you normally buy. They do not always represent a savings when used on products you don't ordinarily buy.
- Go to the store when it is not too crowded and when you have time to select with care. Also,

Unit Pricing

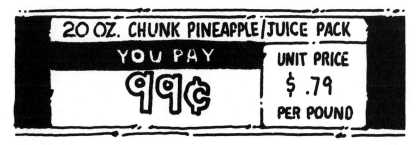

Many supermarkets provide a quick and easy way to compare prices. It's called unit pricing. The unit price label shows both the retail price, the total price you pay, and the price per pound, ounce, quart, or other unit. Comparing the unit price among brands and container sizes of a product can help you find the best buys. Unit pricing information is usually located on the shelf edge directly below or above the item.

GUIDELINES FOR CHECKING FOOD QUALITY

❖ ❖ ❖

Product	Signs of Good Quality	Signs of Poor Quality*
Fresh Meat	Beef: bright cherry red Pork: pale pink Lamb: pink Veal: pinkish white	Sour smell Slimy to the touch Odd color such as brown or green (indicates mold or bacteria)
Fresh Poultry*	Smooth, clean, firm flesh No odor No blood present No discolorations	Soft, flabby flesh Distinct smell Blemishes, bruises, blood Purple or green colors
Fresh Whole Fish	Fresh and pleasant smell Firm, elastic, clear flesh Bulging, clear eyes	Fishy smell Soft, bruised flesh Sunken, dull eyes
Fresh Fish Fillets or Steaks	Moist flesh Translucent sheen	Dried out flesh Separating flesh Fishy smell
Fresh Shellfish	No odor Alive in shell Shell is closed (clams, oysters, etc.)	Fishy smell If in shell, shell is partly open
Milk	Appropriate date Cold—less than 45°F	Outdated Warm—over 45°F
Fresh Eggs	Clean No cracks	Dirty Cracked shells (Old eggs float in water.)
Produce	Appropriate color, size, and shape	Bruises, blemishes, cracks Decay Insects Mold
Frozen Foods	Frozen—less than 10°F No signs of having been thawed and refrozen	Thawed Large ice crystals (indicates product has thawed and refrozen) Water stain on box (indicates product has thawed and refrozen)

Canned Foods	Undamaged	Leaking, rusty, dented cans
	Normal appearance	Swollen cans
Other Dry Goods (such as flour)	Intact packaging	Tears, punctures in packaging
	Dry	Damp
	No evidence of mold or bugs	Moldy, bugs evident

In most cases, these signs indicate spoilage and/or contamination, so do not purchase these foods.

try to avoid shopping when you're hungry or tired, as you tend to buy more and not pay as much attention.

While shopping:
- Read ingredient labels.
- Use nutrition labels to help select food products.
- Use open dating information to assure quality and freshness (see Table 21). Also visually check foods for quality so you avoid buying foods that are contaminated or spoiled; use the guidelines provided.
- The sample unit pricing label shows how you can compare prices; these are not always available. Large packages, store brands, and sale items are often, but not always, cheaper than other brands or container sizes.
- Buy store brands and generic items when their taste and quality suit your needs.
- Stock up on store specials in reasonable amounts. Don't buy more than you can store and use in an appropriate time.
- Avoid overbuying, particularly perishables, to minimize food waste.
- To save time, ask family members to help in the shopping and ask them to pick up certain items.
- Pack cold foods together to keep them cold and for ease in finding and putting away first once at home.

After shopping:
- Minimize time foods are in the car. Keep perishables out of direct sunlight. Make food shopping the last errand you do so you can go directly home.

❖ **Table 21   Open Dating** ❖

Types of Open Dates	Description
Pull-By or Sell-By Date	The last date the product should be sold. The Pull-By date allows enough time to use the product at home under proper storage conditions. Commonly used on milk, cheese, and packaged meats.
Freshness or Best If Used By Date	This date is the last day the product can be expected to be at its peak quality. Commonly used on bakery goods and packaged cereals.
Expiration or Use-By Date	The last date the food should be used. Commonly used on refrigerated doughs and yeasts. If egg cartons include an expiration date, the eggs should be sold by the date marked.
Pack Date	The date the food was manufactured or processed and packaged. This type of dating is used mainly for foods that have a long shelf life, liked canned goods.

- Store foods promptly and properly to maintain their nutritive value and quality. Put the refrigerated foods away first—they are usually the most perishable. Next put away the frozen foods, and last, the dry goods. To check on how to store a specific food, look up the food in the index.
- Place newer foods in the back of the refrigerator, freezer, and cabinet shelves, so older foods will be used first.

❖ ❖ ❖

CHAPTER FIVE

KITCHEN BASICS

COOKING METHODS

There are many different methods for cooking, and they can be separated into three groups based on the cooking medium: liquid, dry heat, or fat. Cooking in liquids includes those methods in which heat is provided by water or other liquids such as stock or steam. Examples include boiling, simmering, poaching, steaming, and braising. These methods are usually associated with less tender cuts of meat, vegetables, and other foods. Dry heat cooking includes those methods in which the heat is dry, not moist, such as hot air. Examples include roasting, baking, barbecuing, broiling, pan-broiling, and grilling. These methods are associated with poultry, fish, tender cuts of meat, and some vegetables. Cooking in fat includes sauteing, stir-frying, deep-frying, and pan-frying. A discussion of each cooking method follows.

Cooking in Liquid

Boiling is cooking in a boiling liquid (at 212°F) or cooking the liquid itself at a boil. Boiling is not often used for cooking foods because of the intense agitation and bubbling. It is used to cook pasta, lobsters, crabs, and starchy or root vegetables such as potatoes, corn on the cob, lima beans, and turnips.

Boiling Tips

1. The liquid left after boiling can become a tasty broth or base of a sauce.
2. Watch carefully so the liquid does not boil over.

Simmering is cooking in a liquid that is just below boiling and has bubbles floating slowly to the surface. Examples of simmered foods include soups, sauces, and stews.

Simmering Tips

1. First, bring the liquid to a boil, then reduce to simmer.
2. Watch closely so that it doesn't boil.
3. Stir frequently for even cooking.

Poaching is cooking in a hot liquid that is bubbling on the bottom of the pot but is otherwise calm. The poaching liquid may be fish or vegetable stock, dry white wine, or seasoned water, depending on its use. Examples of poached foods include poached eggs and poached fish.

Poaching Tips

1. Never let the liquid boil.
2. The liquid should just cover the food.
3. The poaching pot or pan should be partially uncovered so the steam can escape and the liquid does not simmer or boil.

Steaming means cooking with steam, either with or without pressure. Steam cooks quicker than boiling water because it contains nine times more heat. When steam is under pressure, the temperature increases to 250°F and the cooking is even more rapid. Steaming vegetables is an excellent way to retain color, flavor, and nutrients, and not use any fat!

Steaming Tips

1. Place steamer basket in pot with a little boiling water and cover. Cook until the vegetables are just tender.
2. Watch the cooking time carefully to prevent overcooking foods.

Braising is cooking food in a small amount of liquid in a covered container at a low heat (300°–325°F). It is used mainly for meats that need longer cooking times to become tender. The amount of liquid will vary, but it often covers from one-third to two-thirds of the food. The liquid is usually served with the food. The part of the food that is uncovered is cooked by the hot, steamy air in the covered container.

You can braise foods in a covered container placed on the range or in the oven. Oven braising tends to cook more evenly. Examples of braised foods include pot roast, stew, and braised vegetables.

Braising Tips

1. Braised meats are usually seared or browned first. Brown in a small amount of oil or its own fat.
2. For more flavor, simmer meat in meat or poultry broth, cider, wine, or a combination of these for added flavor. Add vegetables and herbs for an aromatic blend of flavors without salt.
3. The longer the food cooks, the more tender it will be.
4. Stir frequently.
5. If you are braising meat or poultry, do it one day before it is served, so you can refrigerate it overnight and then remove the fat that has congealed (become solid white).

Cooking in Dry Heat

Dry heat cooking methods are excellent choices when considering nutrition. Fat does not have to be used during cooking, and fat from meat and poultry can easily drip away during the cooking process.

Roasting or baking is cooking uncovered with heated air in an enclosed space. Roasting normally refers to meats and poultry, while baking refers to fish, baked products, and casseroles. Vegetables can be cooked in the oven as well. Examples include potatoes, sweet potatoes, winter squashes, and onions.

Roasting/Baking Tips

1. When using the oven for roasting or baking, preheat it, leave space for air circulation, keep the door closed as much as possible, rotate the food, and use an oven thermometer. All these measures are important to promote even cooking.
2. Place meat and poultry on a rack to drain fat, prevent the bottom from cooking in the pan juices, and allow heat to circulate around the meat.
3. If basting the food, use lemon juice, fruit juice, broth, or wine for flavor without adding fat.
4. To bake vegetables, wash, prick skins, and place on a baking sheet in the oven.

Grilling is done on an open grid over a heat source which may be an electric or gas element, hot coals, or burning wood. Grilling is commonly used to prepare meat, poultry, fish, and even vegetables, and is a low-fat way to cook, as the fat drips away from the food. Just be sure to baste the food, or marinate it, without fat. Chapter 8 has more information on these topics.

Grilling Tips

1. Trim fat from meat and use lean meat to prevent flare-up of flames and to reduce calories.
2. Baste the food as it cooks to prevent drying out. Use lemon juice, fruit juice, broth, low-fat Italian dressing, or wine for flavor.
3. If you use charcoal briquettes, choose those with the least amount of filler, chemicals, or coal because they may flavor your grilled foods.
4. The best grilling temperature is when the charcoal has been burning for 30–45 minutes and is gray in color.
5. Sprinkle aromatic herbs such as thyme, rosemary, or sage over the coals as they add light flavor to grilled foods.
6. Clean the grill after cooking with a wire brush and apply a coating of vegetable oil. Don't let black residue build up on your grill.

Broiling is cooking with direct heat from above. Broilers may be gas or electric. It is a high-heat cooking method that does not require fat and cooks foods quickly. Steaks, chicken, fish, and certain vegetables (such as onions, zucchini, and tomatoes) are all foods that are commonly broiled.

Broiling Tips

1. Always preheat the broiler.
2. Use a broiling pan or rack set in a shallow pan to allow fat to drain away.
3. Marinate tender meats for 30 minutes, tougher cuts for up to 24 hours. Marinate fish fillets or steaks for only 30 minutes.
4. Thinner foods and foods to be cooked rare can be placed closer to the heat than thicker foods and foods to be cooked well done. If thicker foods or foods to be cooked well done are placed too close to the heat, the outside will be done before the inside is at the proper degree of doneness.
5. Turn thick foods once for more even cooking. Fish less than 1-inch thick, shellfish, and similar thin foods don't need to be turned.
6. Watch foods carefully.
7. The side turned to the heat last cooks in much less time (about half) than the first side.

Pan-broiling is cooking uncovered in a saute pan or skillet without adding any fat or liquid. Fat is drained off as it accumulates. Bacon and hamburgers are two examples of foods that can be pan-broiled.

Pan-broiling Tips

1. Don't use too high a temperature.
2. Drain off the fat to avoid frying the food.

Cooking in Fats

Cooking in fats has a major nutritional drawback: the food being cooked always absorbs some fat. This problem can be overcome when sauteing and stir-frying by doing two things: use a nonstick pan, and use only a small amount (a tablespoon or less) of oil or vegetable cooking spray. Also, sauteing does not have to be done in oil; it can be done using wine, vermouth, defatted broth, or vegetable juice.

Sauteing is cooking food quickly over high heat in a small amount of fat. Examples include sau-teed chicken and sauteed vegetables such as onion and green peppers.

Sauteing Tips

1. Use just enough fat to prevent sticking. A non-stick pan works best.
2. Dust meats before sauteing to prevent sticking to the pan and to get even browning.
3. The pan must be preheated before adding the food so the food does not simmer.
4. Do not overfill the pan to avoid lowering the temperature.
5. Flip the food during cooking for even cooking.

Stir-frying is cooking small-sized foods over high heat in a small amount of oil. The high heat and the constant movement of the food keep it from sticking and burning. Stir-frying preserves the crisp texture and bright color of vegetables. Stir-frying cooks foods quickly. Chicken and vegetables are often stir-fried.

Stir-frying Tips

1. Cut up thin strips or diced portions of meat, poultry, fish, vegetables, or any combination. Avoid watery ingredients because they make the fat splatter.
2. Coat the cooking surface with a thin layer of oil.
3. Preheat equipment to high temperature.
4. Stir food rapidly during cooking and don't overfill the pan or wok.
5. When meat is almost done, add small pieces of vegetables such as broccoli, cauliflower, zucchini, sprouts, carrots, mushrooms, tomatoes, or green onions, as they cook quickly.

Deep-frying means to cook food completely covered in hot fat. Fried foods cook quickly and small-sized tender foods are best to ensure a fully cooked tender product. The goals of deep-frying are a crisp surface, golden color, good flavor, and a minimum of fat absorption by the food. Examples of deep-fried items include french fries, fried chicken, and fried fish.

Deep-frying Tips

1. Always fry at appropriate temperatures—usually 325°–375°F. Periodically check the temperature against the thermostat setting with a

COOKING TERMS

Baste. To moisten the surface of a food item with a liquid, such as meat drippings or juice, during the cooking process.

Batter. A mixture of flour, eggs, and a liquid used to coat foods prior to frying.

Blanch. To dip a raw food into boiling water for a few seconds to kill surface bacteria, set the color, or partially cook the food item.

Blend. The process of mixing two or more ingredients thoroughly until uniform.

Bread. To coat a food item with flour, then an egg wash consisting of eggs and a liquid (milk, water), and finally with bread crumbs prior to cooking.

Cream. To mix fat and sugar until it is light and fluffy.

Cut In. A method of mixing used in the preparation of pie dough that requires cutting fat into flour to form small pea shapes or other desired size. Cutting in can be accomplished with the use of a special pastry blender, two butter knives, a fork, or the use of a special attachment on an electric countertop mixer.

Deglazing. After a food is sauteed, put wine or stock into the same pan to dissolve (or deglaze) browned bits of food.

Dredge. A process of gently dragging a moistened food item through a dry seasoned ingredient so the coating will stick to the surface.

Flute. To make a grooved pattern on the edge of pie crust, fruits, or vegetables.

Fold In. A delicate process of using a gentle over-under motion to mix two ingredients without an appreciable loss in volume.

Glaze. To give a glossy appearance to the surface of a food by applying a sauce.

Knead. A continuous process of working bread dough either by hand or in a mixer to develop the gluten and mix the ingredients.

Marinate. To soak a food in a seasoned liquid to develop flavor and, in the case of tough meats, to soften the meat. The marinade usually contains an acidic ingredient, such as citrus fruit juices, vinegar, tomato juice, or alcohol. These ingredients tenderize. A marinade often includes some oil and seasonings.

Mix. To combine two or more ingredients by stirring or blending.

Reduce. Simmering or boiling a liquid until its volume is decreased. At this point its flavors will be quite concentrated.

Sear. To brown a food (usually meat) at high temperatures briefly to produce browning, which adds color and flavor to the food. This process only partially cooks foods.

Whip. To beat rapidly to incorporate air. Often done with a wire whip or whisk.

---

fat thermometer. Proper temperature is important to make sure that both the inside and outside of the food are uniformly cooked. If the temperature is too low, more fat is absorbed by the food.

2. Don't fill the frying basket more than half full to prevent the fat from losing temperature.

3. Fry just prior to serving the food as fried foods get soggy quickly.

4. When frying fish or another strong-flavored food, don't fry anything else in the same fat or the food will absorb the strong flavors. For instance, french fries will taste like fish.

5. Shake the basket occasionally to keep foods from sticking together.

6. Keep frying equipment and fat clean.

Pan-frying means cooking foods in a pan over a moderate heat in a small to moderate amount of fat. It is different from sauteing because it uses less heat and requires more fat. Fish fillets, chops, and chicken pieces can all be pan-fried.

❖ *A Nutritional Comparison* ❖
of Cooking Methods

High-Fat Cooking Methods
Pan-fry
Deep-fat fry
Saute (with more than 1 tablespoon oil)

Low-Fat Cooking Methods*
Broil
Steam
Roast/bake
Grill
Barbecue
Braise (defat the braising liquid when
    cooking is completed)
Boil
Simmer
Stir-fry (using a small amount of oil)
Saute (using a small amount of oil)
Microwave

*To be considered low-fat, baste or marinate these foods
with low-fat sauces and do not add fat during the cooking.*

Pan-frying Tips
1. Use enough fat to cover about one-half the
   thickness of the food.
2. Turn food at least once for even cooking.

The nutritional comparison provided distinguishes types of cooking methods. You should also find the list of essential cooking terms most helpful.

MICROWAVE COOKING

Microwave cooking refers to the use of a specific tool rather than to a cooking method. The top five uses of the microwave oven are, in order:

1. Reheating
2. Warming
3. Defrosting
4. Making popcorn
5. Heating frozen foods

Despite its many uses and fast speed, the microwave has in no way replaced the range and oven as primary cooking equipment. This is in part because the microwave does not brown foods and cooks unevenly, leaving cold spots and hot spots, in foods. If you have ever eaten a quiche warmed up in the microwave, you know about cold spots and hot spots. Your quiche may have been tough, overcooked, and too hot to eat in one area, while still frigid in others. These problems can be somewhat overcome by stirring and rotating foods during cooking. Newer microwaves have turntables that almost completely overcome this problem.

Though microwaves produce heat directly in the food, they really don't cook food from the inside out. With thick foods like roasts, microwaves generally cook only about an inch of the outer layers. The heat is then slowly conducted inward, cooking along the way. Microwaved foods continue to cook after they are removed from the oven because the food molecules are still vibrating. This is why "standing time" is included in microwave recipes.

Just as in conventional cooking, there are several factors that influence microwave cooking times. These include size (larger foods take longer), shape (thin foods cook quicker), density (porous foods cook quicker), type of ingredients (water and fat cook quicker), volume (as volume increases so does cooking time), and the starting temperature of the foods (warmer foods heat up quicker). An area of a food where there is increased moisture will heat more quickly than other areas. So, when heating up a jelly donut, for instance, it's a good idea to let the donut stand after cooking for a minute or two so the very hot jelly can cool off. Also, you don't need to add fat to meat, poultry, or fish, and you can use little water for vegetables. Microwaving is an excellent way to retain vitamins and color in vegetables. See the microwave cooking and safety tips for more details.

MEASURING BASICS

We measure ingredients in one of three ways:
- Number, such as two apples or one egg
- Volume, such as teaspoon or cup
- Weight, such as 2 ounces or 1 pound

When you measure ingredients by volume, you are actually measuring the amount of space of the

MICROWAVE COOKING AND SAFETY TIPS

1. Uneven distribution of microwaves in the oven's cavity can cause "hot spots" or over-cooking of foods in certain areas. This also occurs on thin edges of foods. Frequent stirring or rotation of dish can minimize this problem.

2. When you defrost food in the microwave, cook it immediately as defrosting often starts cooking the edges of the food.

3. Debone large pieces of meat before cooking because the bone shields the meat around it from thorough cooking.

4. Do not cook whole, stuffed poultry in the microwave. Cook bird and stuffing separately for even cooking.

5. Arrange smaller items or mixed foods uniformly in a covered dish so they cook evenly. Add a bit of liquid so foods do not dry out.

6. If your recipe calls for a certain size cooking container, use the exact one recommended. The size and shape of the container are important. Cooking a food in a differently shaped dish than the one recommended could cause the amount of cooking time to vary. For instance, large size dishes are usually recommended to avoid boil-overs.

7. If a dish is covered, make sure there is some room for excess steam to escape either by lifting a corner or piercing holes in plastic wrap. Do not let plastic wrap touch the food because dangerous chemicals may get into the food.

8. Use the exact cooking time recommended. Microwaves cook quickly and 15 seconds too long can mean the difference between having dinner and not having dinner!

9. Increase the cooking time if you increase the size of the recipe. A general rule to follow when increasing the size of a recipe is: when doubling a recipe, increase the cooking time to slightly less than 2 times as long and change the dish size accordingly. When cutting a recipe in half, decrease cooking time to slightly more than half and change the dish size accordingly.

10. For all foods, observe the standing time given in the recipe, usually about one-third of the cooking time. Food completes cooking during the standing time.

11. Use a meat thermometer or other thermometer to check for doneness of meat and poultry. Check in several places, avoiding fat and bone which give inaccurate readings. The internal temperature should reach 160°F for red meat, 180°F for poultry. Fish should flake.

12. Don't use the microwave to cook eggs in their shells—they will burst. Also don't use the microwave for home canning.

13. Sealed containers must not be heated in the oven. The food or liquid could expand quickly and explode.

14. To prevent a steam burn when removing lids or wrap from the cooking dish, lift cover slowly, tilting it so the steam is released away from you.

15. Use potholders to remove heated food from the oven.

16. Do not heat baby formula in nursers with disposable plastic inserts. Hot spots in milk heated in these bottles may weaken the seams, causing the plastic to burst and spill hot milk on the baby.

17. You can warm formula in hard plastic and glass baby bottles by removing the cap and nipple first. For 8 ounces of milk or formula at refrigerator temperature, microwave on high 30 seconds. Let stand for a minute. Shake well and test the temperature by shaking some of the liquid on top of your hand.

18. Do not microwave solid baby foods in the jars. Transfer to a microwave-safe dish and cook 4 ounces of solid food for about 15 seconds on high power. Always stir, let stand 30 seconds, and taste-test before using. Food that's ready should feel lukewarm to you.

COMMON UNITS OF MEASURE

❖ ❖ ❖

1 tablespoon = 3 teaspoons	1 pint = 16 fluid ounces
1 fluid ounce = 2 tablespoons	1 quart = 2 pints
1 cup = 16 tablespoons	1 quart = 4 cups
1 cup = 8 fluid ounces	1 quart = 32 fluid ounces
1 pint = 2 cups	1 gallon = 4 quarts

ingredients, such as in 1 tablespoon, 1 cup, 1 fluid ounce, 1 quart, and 1 gallon. The list of common units of measure shows common volume measurements and their equivalents.

To measure a dry ingredient, such as flour, overfill the volume measure with the dry ingredient before leveling it off. The term "level" refers to leveling the top of the volume measure with a straight edge (i.e., spatula)—and please, not your finger!

To measure a wet ingredient, such as water, put the volume measure on a flat surface and fill to the proper line.

You can also measure many ingredients by weight using a scale, as follows:

1. Weigh the empty container that will hold the ingredient and set the scale to zero.
2. Place the ingredient on the scale until the scale reads the desired weight.

There is a common misconception in the use of the liquid measurement cup and its use as a conversion for dry measurements. For example, when 8 fluid ounces of a liquid such as water (or a liquid of the same density) is needed in a recipe, it would be alright to measure water in a 1 cup liquid measurement container. If that same recipe calls for 8 ounces of all-purpose flour, it would be incorrect to pour the all-purpose flour in an 8-ounce liquid measurement container because all-purpose flour has a different density than water. (One cup of all-purpose flour weighs 4 ounces— one cup of water weighs 8 ounces.)

USING KNIVES

It is important to understand a number of safety tips before using knives, so be sure to read the Rules of Knife Safety.

Basic Slicing and Dicing (and more)

Knives are used to cuts foods into uniform shapes and sizes so they have an attractive appearance and cook evenly. Some basic cuts and shapes are described and illustrated below.

1. Slice—to cut into uniform slices or cross cuts
2. Dice—to cut into uniform cubes
   - small dice: ¼-inch cube
   - medium dice: ½-inch cube
   - large dice: ¾-inch cube
3. Chop—to cut into irregularly shaped pieces
4. Mince—to chop very fine
5. Shred—to cut into thin strips
6. Julienne—to cut into small, thin strips, about ⅛ inch by ⅛ inch by 2½ inches long

Following are instructions on how to handle a chef's knife, as well as slice, dice, chop, and mince.

How to Handle a Chef's Knife

1. To hold the knife, grasp the heel of the blade with part of your thumb on one side and part of your forefinger on the other, as the illustration shows. The remaining fingers fit under the handle. Your grip should be secure but relaxed. This grip gives you the most control and force.
2. Your other hand holds the item being cut with

RULES OF KNIFE SAFETY

USING KNIVES SAFELY

1. Cut away from the body.
2. Cut away from anyone near you.
3. Use a cutting board and put a damp cloth under it to keep the board from slipping.
4. Use the right knife for the job. Don't use a lightweight knife for a heavy-duty job.
5. Keep knives sharp. Since a dull knife requires more pressure to cut, it is more dangerous than a sharp knife.
6. Always pick up a knife by its handle.
7. Don't use knives to cut string, open cans or bottles, or as a screwdriver.

CARRYING KNIVES SAFELY

1. Carry the knife beside you, point down, and cutting edge back and away from you.

2. If a knife falls, do not try to catch it. Get out of the way.

CLEANING KNIVES SAFELY

1. Do not put a knife in a sink full of water; instead, put on the drainboard to avoid cuts.
2. Wipe from dull to sharp edge.
3. Do not put knives in the dishwasher. The heat and bouncing around may harm the blade.

STORING KNIVES SAFELY

1. Never put a knife loosely in a drawer. This practice is not only unsafe but the knife blade will become dull from sliding against the drawer. Use a rack, a case, or a magnetized board so the blade is protected.
2. Don't leave knives near the edge of a table because they can be easily knocked off.

Basic Cuts and Shapes

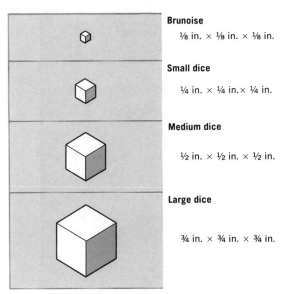

Brunoise

⅛ in. × ⅛ in. × ⅛ in.

Small dice

¼ in. × ¼ in.× ¼ in.

Medium dice

½ in. × ½ in. × ½ in.

Large dice

¾ in. × ¾ in. × ¾ in.

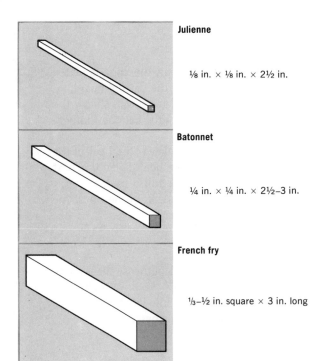

Julienne

⅛ in. × ⅛ in. × 2½ in.

Batonnet

¼ in. × ¼ in. × 2½–3 in.

French fry

⅓–½ in. square × 3 in. long

How to Handle a Chef's Knife

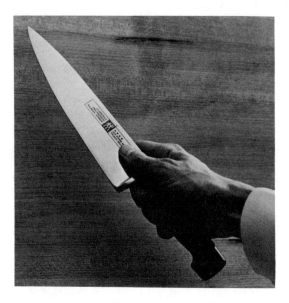

How to Slice

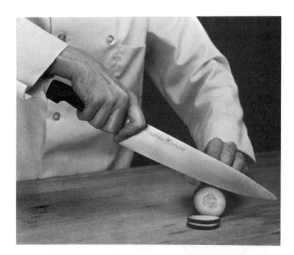

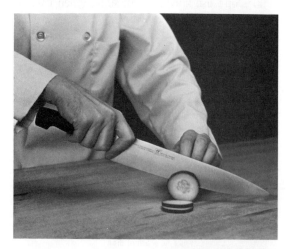

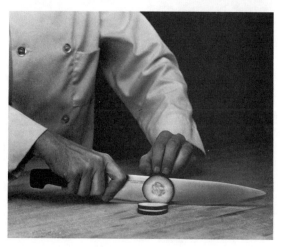

your fingertips curled under and your knuckles guiding the blade. Fingertips are always curled under to protect them from cuts.
3. Use the tip of the blade for cutting small items, the center of the blade for most work, and the heel of the blade for heavy or coarse work.

How to Slice

1. As depicted in the photos, the knife is placed at a 45-degree angle to the cutting board.
2. Move the knife forward and down, slicing the items to the desired width. Let the knife do the work.
3. When the slice is completed, the heel of the knife is on the cutting board. For the next slice, raise the heel and pull it back.
4. When cutting thin foods, keep the tip of the knife on the cutting board.

How to Dice

1. First, cut the item into lengthwise slices of the appropriate thickness (¼, ½, or ¾ inch).
2. Stack the slices and cut into lengthwise strips, again to the desired thickness.
3. Placing the strips in a pile, cut them crosswise into the dice of desired size.

How to Chop

1. While holding the tip of the knife against the cutting board with 3 to 4 fingers of one hand, rock the knife up and down at a quick pace.
2. At the same time, swivel the knife gradually around the board to evenly distribute the chopping action across all of the items being cut.
3. After making several passes with your knife, redistribute the pile.
4. Wipe the blade with a clean and dry cloth when it has excessive food clinging to it.

How to Mince

1. Use the same procedure as chopping and chop into fine pieces.

Sharpening Knives

In most instances, sharpening a knife can be easily done by adapters that are built into most countertop can openers. A few strokes on each side of the knife may provide a satisfactory cutting edge. A mobile knife sharpener that can be moved from one location to another is available in both home and commercial versions. An electric, moderately priced knife sharpener is best for home use. Some versions have one grooved area for presharpening the knife and another area for honing a smooth edge on the knife.

Professional cooks use two pieces of equipment to sharpen their knives: a sharpening stone and a steel. A sharpening stone can do the sharpening, while a steel can true a blade so as to perfect the edge and maintain a sharp edge.

How to Sharpen a Knife Blade Using a Sharpening Stone

1. You may want to lubricate the stone by thoroughly rubbing in a tablespoon of oil.

Using a Sharpening Stone

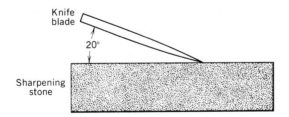

2. Hold the knife firmly with one hand on the top and the other hand gripping the handle.
3. As shown in the illustration, hold the knife blade at a 20-degree angle to the stone, place the tip at one end of the stone, and slowly draw the knife across the stone while pressing gently on the blade.
4. Draw the knife smoothly across the stone to the heel of the blade.
5. Make the same number of strokes on each side of the blade (5 is common). Only a few strokes should be necessary unless the knife has been mishandled. Make sure strokes are even and go in one direction only.

How to True a Knife Blade Using a Steel

1. Hold the steel in one hand, away from your body at a 45-degree angle.
2. Hold the knife vertically in your other hand, with the blade at a 20-degree angle to the steel. Touch the steel with the heel of the blade.
3. Draw the knife lightly along the steel, using an even and regular stroke.
4. Repeat this motion on the other side of the steel for the other side of the knife. Five or six strokes for each side is sufficient. Too much steeling can make the blade dull.

FOOD STORAGE RULES

The first rule of food storage in the home is to refrigerate or freeze perishables right away. Refrigerator temperature should be 40 to 45 °F, and the freezer should be zero. Check both "fridge" and freezer periodically with a good thermometer.

Poultry and meat heading for the refrigerator may be stored as purchased in the plastic wrap for a day or two. If only part of the meat or poultry is going to be used right away, it can be wrapped loosely for refrigerator storage. Just make sure juices can't escape to contaminate other foods. Leftovers should be stored in air-tight containers. Store eggs in their carton rather than on the door, where the temperature is warmer. Seafood should always be kept in the refrigerator or freezer until preparation time. Tightly wrap foods destined for the freezer.

Don't crowd the refrigerator or freezer so tightly that air can't circulate. Check the leftovers in covered dishes and storage bags daily for spoilage. Anything that looks or smells suspicious should be thrown out. A sure sign of spoilage is the presence of mold, which can grow even under refrigeration. While not a major health threat, mold can make food unappetizing. Mold is deceptive in that only a small part is visible. The larger part extends below the surface of the food. See page 101 for guidelines that explain when you can simply cut out the mold and when it is necessary to throw out the whole food.

Many items besides fresh meats, most vegetables, and dairy products need to be kept cold. For instance, mayonnaise and ketchup should go in the refrigerator after opening. Some spices keep best when refrigerated. Always check the labels on cans or jars to determine how the contents should be stored. If you've neglected to refrigerate items, it is best to throw them out.

For foods that can be stored at room temperature, some precautions will help make sure they remain safe. Potatoes and onions should not be stored under the sink, because leakage from the pipes can damage the food. Potatoes don't belong in the refrigerator either. Store them in a cool, dry place. Don't store any foods near household cleaning products or chemicals because of the danger of accidental contamination.

When you're putting canned goods away, move the older ones to the front of the shelf and put the new cans in the back row so you'll be sure to use the older ones first. Check all cans to see if any are sticky on the outside. This may indicate a leak. Cans that appear to be leaking may contain a deadly bacteria that causes botulism (see Chapter 6 for more information) and should be returned to the store.

If you are freezing foods, do the following to ensure that the high-quality food you put into the freezer is still high-quality when it comes out:

1. Freeze foods at their peak quality. Don't wait until they are at or near the end of their useful life.
2. Use appropriate packaging to prevent freezer burn and protect flavors. Freezer burn appears as grayish-brown leathery spots on frozen food. It occurs when air reaches its surface.

Although undesirable, freezer burn does not make the food unsafe, merely dry in spots. Cut it away either before or after cooking the food. Supermarket meat wraps, while safe for freezing, are permeable to air. Over time, this contributes to freezer burn and rancidity, when fats and oils develop an off-taste and odor. Overwrap these packages with airtight heavy-duty foil, plastic wrap and bags, or freezer paper as you would any food to be frozen. Do not rely on waxed paper. Freeze unopened vacuum packages as is. When freezing food in plastic bags, push all the air out before sealing. Residual air can change into ice crystals and cause fats to go bad.

3. Freeze food as fast as possible to maintain its quality. Ideally, a food 2 inches thick should freeze completely in about 2 hours. If your home freezer has a "quick-freeze" shelf, use it. And, regardless, arrange packages in one layer until frozen. Rapid freezing prevents undesirable large ice crystals from forming.

While freezing does keep food safe to eat, it does affect quality. To maximize the tenderness, flavor, aroma, juiciness, and color of frozen foods, be sure to follow the previous guidelines.

PRESERVING NUTRIENTS IN STORAGE AND COOKING

Five factors are responsible for most nutrient loss of food: high temperature, long cooking, baking soda, exposure to the air, and dissolving in water (such as the water-soluble vitamins). Because the fat-soluble vitamins (A, D, E, and K) are insoluble in water, they are fairly stable in cooking. The water-soluble vitamins (and minerals) easily leach out of foods during washing or cooking. Here are tips to retain nutrients in foods.

1. Buy food that is fresh and of high quality. Examine fresh fruits and vegetables thoroughly for appropriate color, size, and shape.
2. Store fruits and vegetables in the refrigerator (except green bananas, potatoes, and onions) because they contain enzymes that make fruits and vegetables age and lose nutrients.

The enzymes are more active at warm temperatures.

3. Store canned foods in a cool, dry place and limit the time they are in storage. In general, the longer the storage period and the higher the storage temperature, the greater the loss of nutrients.

4. Freezing offers a good way of retaining nutrients when foods are properly packaged, frozen at peak quality, and kept below 0°F.

5. Foods should be used as quickly as possible because vitamins are often lost in storage.

6. When washing vegetables, do so quickly and do not soak them. Avoid bruising vegetables—this causes vitamin loss.

7. To retain vitamins when cooking vegetables, steaming, microwaving, and stir-frying work well because the cooking is done quickly. If boiling vegetables, the longer they are cooked, the higher the nutrient loss. Cook vegetables just until tender and use as little water as possible.

8. Potatoes and other vegetables that are boiled or baked without being peeled retain many more nutrients than if peeled and cut. In general, the smaller the pieces into which you cut vegetables before cooking them, the higher the vitamin loss. Leaching and oxidation are increased by having created more exposed surfaces. Vegetables (and fruits) should not be cut more than necessary.

9. Frying's high temperature can destroy vitamins in vegetables. For instance, french-fried potatoes lose much of their vitamin C.

10. Never use baking soda with vegetables as it will cause nutrient loss.

11. After broiling and roasting meats and poultry, you can skim off the fat and use the remaining drippings in gravies or pour them directly over the meat. In this way, you recover some of the water-soluble B vitamins.

12. Use the cooking water from vegetables to prepare soup.

13. Do not wash white rice before cooking as it washes off vitamins and iron.

14. Don't make foods too far ahead of when they will be served.

Factors that destroy vitamins and minerals often spoil the color, flavor, and texture of food as well.

COLD STORAGE GUIDELINES

❖ ❖ ❖

These short but safe time limits will help keep refrigerated food from spoiling or becoming dangerous to eat, and will keep frozen food at top quality.

Product	Refrigerator (40°F)	Freezer (0°F)
Eggs		
Fresh, in shell	3 weeks	Don't freeze
Raw yolks, whites	2–4 days	1 year
Hard-cooked	1 week	Don't freeze well
Liquid pasteurized eggs or egg substitutes, opened	3 days	Don't freeze
unopened	10 days	1 year
Mayonnaise, commercial		
Refrigerate after opening	2 months	Don't freeze
TV Dinners, Frozen Casseroles		
Keep frozen until ready to serve		3–4 months
Deli and Vacuum-Packed Products		
Store-prepared (or homemade) egg, chicken, tuna, ham, macaroni salads	3–5 days	
Prestuffed pork and lamb chops, chicken breasts stuffed with dressing	1 day	These products don't freeze well.
Store-cooked convenience meals	1–2 days	
Commercial brand vacuum-packed dinners with USDA seal	2 weeks, unopened	
Soups and Stews		
Vegetable or meat-added	3–4 days	2–3 months
Hamburger, Ground, and Stew Meats		
Hamburger and stew meats	1–2 days	3–4 months
Ground turkey, veal, pork, lamb, and mixtures of them	1–2 days	3–4 months
Hot Dogs and Lunch Meats		
Hot dogs, opened package	1 week	In freezer wrap, 1–2 months
unopened package	2 weeks	
Lunch meats, opened	3–5 days	
unopened	2 weeks	

Bacon and Sausage

Bacon	7 days	1 month
Sausage, raw from pork, beef, turkey	1–2 days	1–2 months
Smoked breakfast links, patties	7 days	1–2 months
Hard sausage—pepperoni, jerky sticks	2–3 weeks	1–2 months

Ham, Corned Beef

Corned beef		Drained, wrapped
In pouch with pickling juices	5–7 days	1 month
Ham, canned		
Label says keep refrigerated	6–9 months	Don't freeze
Ham, fully cooked—whole	7 days	1–2 months
Ham, fully cooked—half	3–5 days	1–2 months
Ham, fully cooked—slices	3–4 days	1–2 months

Fresh Meat

Steaks, beef	3–5 days	6–12 months
Chops, pork	3–5 days	4–6 months
Chops, lamb	3–5 days	6–9 months
Roasts, beef	3–5 days	6–12 months
Roasts, lamb	3–5 days	6–9 months
Roasts, pork and veal	3–5 days	4–6 months
Variety meats—tongue, brain, kidneys, liver, heart, chitterlings	1–2 days	3–4 months

Meat Leftovers

Cooked meat and meat dishes	3–4 days	2–3 months
Gravy and meat broth	1–2 days	2–3 months

Fresh Poultry

Chicken or turkey, whole	1–2 days	1 year
Chicken or turkey pieces	1–2 days	9 months
Giblets	1–2 days	3–4 months

Cooked Poultry, Leftover

Fried chicken	3–4 days	4 months
Cooked poultry dishes	3–4 days	4–6 months
Pieces, plain	3–4 days	4 months
Pieces covered with broth, gravy	1–2 days	6 months
Chicken nuggets, patties	1–2 days	1–3 months

Fish

Lean (such as cod)	1–2 days	Up to 6 months
Fatty (such as salmon)	1–2 days	2–3 months

Milk — 5 days — 1 month

Cheese		
Swiss, brick, processed	3–4 weeks	Not recommended
Cheddar	4–8 weeks	6 months

GUIDELINES FOR SAVING FOOD AFTER THE REFRIGERATOR STOPS WORKING

REFRIGERATOR FOOD—WHEN TO SAVE AND WHEN TO THROW IT OUT

❖ ❖ ❖

	Food Still Cold, Held at 40°F or Above Under 2 Hours	Held Above 40°F for Over 2 Hours
Dairy		
Milk, cream, sour cream, buttermilk, evaporated milk, yogurt	Safe	Discard
Butter, margarine	Safe	Safe
Baby formula, opened	Safe	Discard
Eggs		
Eggs, fresh	Safe	Safe
Hard-cooked in shell	Safe	Discard
Egg dishes	Safe	Discard
Custards and puddings	Safe	Discard
Cheese		
Hard cheeses, processed cheeses	Safe	Safe
Soft cheeses, cottage cheese	Safe	Discard
Fruits		
Fruit juices, opened	Safe	Safe
Canned fruits, opened	Safe	Safe
Fresh fruits, coconut, raisins, dried fruits, candied fruits, dates	Safe	Safe
Vegetables		
Vegetables, cooked	Safe	Discard after 6 hours
Vegetable juice, opened	Safe	Discard after 6 hours

Baked potatoes	Safe	Discard
Fresh mushrooms, herbs and spices	Safe	Safe
Garlic, chopped in oil or butter	Safe	Discard
Casseroles, soups, stews	Safe	Discard
Meat, Poultry, Seafood		
Fresh or leftover meat, poultry, fish, or seafood	Safe	Discard
Thawing meat or poultry	Safe	Discard if warmer than refrigerator temperatures
Meat, tuna, shrimp, chicken, egg salad	Safe	Discard
Gravy, stuffing	Safe	Discard
Lunch meats, hot dogs, bacon, sausage, dried beef	Safe	Discard
Pizza—meat topped	Safe	Discard
Canned meats (NOT labeled "Keep Refrigerated") but refrigerated after opening	Safe	Discard
Canned hams labeled "Keep Refrigerated"	Safe	Discard
Pies, Pastry		
Pastries, cream filled	Safe	Discard
Pies—custard, cheese-filled, or chiffons	Safe	Discard
Pies, fruit	Safe	Safe
Bread, Cakes, Cookies, Pasta		
Bread, rolls, cakes, muffins, quick breads	Safe	Safe
Refrigerator biscuits, rolls, cookie dough	Safe	Discard
Cooked pasta, spaghetti	Safe	Discard
Pasta salads with mayonnaise or vinegar base	Safe	Discard
Sauces, Spreads, Jams		
Mayonnaise, tartar sauce, horseradish	Safe	Discard if above 50°F for over 8 hours
Peanut butter	Safe	Safe
Opened salad dressing, jelly, relish, taco and barbeque sauce, mustard, catsup, olives	Safe	Safe

FROZEN FOOD—WHEN TO SAVE AND WHEN TO THROW IT OUT

❖ ❖ ❖

	Still Contains Ice Crystals and Feels as Cold as if Refrigerated	Thawed. Held Above 40°F for Over 2 Hours
Meat, Poultry, Seafood		
Beef, veal, lamb, pork, and ground meats	Refreeze	Discard
Poultry and ground poultry	Refreeze	Discard
Variety meats (liver, kidney, heart, chitterlings)	Refreeze	Discard
Casseroles, stews, soups, convenience foods, pizza	Refreeze	Discard
Fish, shellfish, breaded seafood products	Refreeze. However, there will be some texture and flavor loss.	Discard
Dairy		
Milk	Refreeze. May lose some texture.	Discard
Eggs (out of shell) and egg products	Refreeze	Discard
Ice cream, frozen yogurt	Discard	Discard
Cheese (soft and semi-soft), cream cheese, ricotta	Refreeze. May lose some texture.	Discard
Hard cheeses (cheddar, Swiss, Parmesan)	Refreeze	Refreeze
Casseroles containing milk, cream, eggs, soft cheeses	Refreeze	Discard
Cheesecake	Refreeze	Discard
Fruits		
Juices	Refreeze	Refreeze. Discard if mold, yeasty smell, or sliminess develops.
Home or commercially packaged	Refreeze. Will change in texture and flavor.	Refreeze. Discard if mold, yeasty smell, or sliminess develops.
Vegetables		
Juices	Refreeze	Discard after held above 40°F for 6 hours.
Home or commercially packaged or blanched	Refreeze. May suffer texture and flavor loss.	Discard after held above 40°F for 6 hours.

Breads, Pastries

Breads, rolls, muffins, cakes (without custard fillings)	Refreeze	Refreeze
Cakes, pies, pastries with custard or cheese filling	Refreeze	Discard
Pie crusts	Refreeze	Refreeze
Commercial and homemade bread dough	Refreeze. Some quality loss may occur.	Refreeze. Considerable quality loss.

Other

Casseroles—pasta, rice based	Refreeze	Discard
Flour, cornmeal, nuts	Refreeze	Refreeze

❖ ❖ ❖

CHAPTER SIX

FOOD SAFETY

INTRODUCTION

Even if you choose a very nutritious diet, there are still dangers lurking in your food, and they seem to be reported in the media all too frequently. Perhaps salmonella, listeria, lead, and migrating chemicals are not great topics for dinner conversation, but they may be in the dinner you are eating. This chapter will examine these hot food safety topics:

- the bacteria and viruses that cause foodborne illness
- seafood safety
- pesticides and food additives
- the safety of your pots, pans, and dishes
- the safety of your microwave

FOODBORNE ILLNESS

Foodborne illness, commonly called food poisoning, is a preventable disease caused by undesirable substances in food such as bacteria, bacterial toxins, and molds. Most cases of foodborne illness are never reported to the health department because most people never think that it may be related to the food they ate. In fact, most persons attribute the illness to many other factors, for example, 24-hour flu, I ate too much, I was really stressed out that day. Can you imagine telling your mother or spouse (or worse yet, your grandmother) that you think you had gotten ill from their food!

Common symptoms of foodborne illness include diarrhea, abdominal cramping, fever, sometimes blood or pus in the stool, headache, vomiting, and severe exhaustion. However, symptoms will vary according to the type of bacteria and by the amount of contaminants eaten. Symptoms may come on as early as a half hour after eating the contaminated food or they may not develop for several days or weeks. They usually last only a day or two, but in some cases can persist a week to ten days.

Your susceptibility to and the severity of the disease depend on many factors: what the nature of the organism is, how old you are, what physical condition you are in, and even your genetic makeup. Unfortunately the individuals to whom foodborne diseases poses the most serious threat are those with a weak immune system—pregnant women, very young children, the elderly, people with chronic diseases, and people with AIDS and cancer.

The prime causes of foodborne illness are a collection of bacteria with tongue-twisting names: Salmonella, Staphylococcus aureus, and Listeria monocytogenes, as examples. Bacteria (and viruses) are so small that they cannot be seen by the naked eye. They are one-celled organisms that grow rapidly in food (they double in number every 20 minutes, as the diagram of bacterial reproduction illustrates) when given adequate time and temperature. Bacteria cause foodborne illness when they multiply in food to the point that when the food is eaten, you become sick. Luckily, only a small number of bacteria cause foodborne illness. Table 22 lists major foodborne diseases of bacterial origin.

Where are bacteria? To be short and sweet about it: everywhere! They are:

Bacterial Reproduction

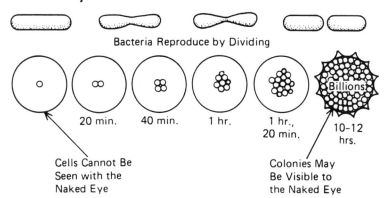

Bacteria Reproduce by Dividing

20 min. 40 min. 1 hr. 1 hr., 20 min. 10–12 hrs.

Cells Cannot Be
Seen with the
Naked Eye

Colonies May
Be Visible to
the Naked Eye

Reprinted with permission from Applied Foodservice Sanitation, *Fourth Edition. Copyright © 1992 by the Educational Foundation of the National Restaurant Association.*

- On your skin
- On your face
- In your nose, mouth, and throat
- In coughs and sneezes
- In hair
- On your hands, under your fingernails, and around and in rings and watches
- In cuts, boils, pimples, burns, infected eyes and ears

As you can see, there are bacteria all around and on us!

Bacteria also exist in some of the foods we purchase at the store, such as fresh eggs and poultry. A few years ago you could tell a potentially contaminated egg by its broken or dirty shell. Now a perfectly fine-looking egg may contain the disease-causing bacteria *Salmonella enteritidis*. Salmonella is passed into the egg by an infected hen before the shell is formed, so it's impossible to know by its appearance if an egg is contaminated. Perhaps 1 in 200 eggs is affected by salmonella. Follow the precautions listed when using eggs and poultry to prevent foodborne illness.

❖ *Table 22   Organisms That Can Bug You* ❖

Disease and Organism That Causes It	Source of Illness	Symptoms
Bacteria		
Botulism Botulinum toxin (produced by *Clostridium botulinum* bacteria)	Spores of these bacteria are widespread. But these bacteria produce toxin only in an anaerobic (oxygenless) environment of little acidity. Found in a considerable variety of canned foods, such as corn, green beans, soups, beets, asparagus, mushrooms, tuna, and liver paté. Also in luncheon meats, ham, sausage, stuffed eggplant, lobster, and smoked and salted fish.	Onset: Generally 4–36 hours after eating. Neurotoxic symptoms, including double vision, inability to swallow, speech difficulty, and progressive paralysis of the respiratory system. **Get medical help immediately. Botulism can be fatal.**
Campylobacteriosis *Campylobacter jejuni*	Bacteria on poultry, cattle, and sheep can contaminate meat and milk of these animals. Chief food sources: raw poultry, meat, and unpasteurized milk.	Onset: Generally 2–5 days after eating. Diarrhea, abdominal cramping, fever, and sometimes bloody stools. Lasts 7–10 days.

Disease and Organism That Causes It	Source of Illness	Symptoms
Bacteria		
Listeriosis *Listeria monocytogenes*	Found in soft cheese, unpasteurized milk, imported seafood products, frozen cooked crab meat, cooked shrimp, and cooked surimi (imitation shellfish). The *Listeria* bacteria resist heat, salt, nitrite, and acidity better than many other microorganisms. They survive and grow at low temperatures.	Onset: From 7–30 days after eating, but most symptoms have been reported 48–72 hours after consumption of contaminated food. Fever, headache, nausea, and vomiting. Primarily affects pregnant women and their fetuses, newborns, the elderly, people with cancer, and those with impaired immune systems. Can cause fetal and infant death.
Perfringens food poisoning *Clostridium perfringens*	In most instances, caused by failure to keep food hot. A few organisms are often present after cooking and multiply to toxic levels during cool down and storage of prepared foods. Meats and meat products are the foods most frequently implicated. These organisms grow better than other bacteria between 120–130°F. So gravies and stuffing must be kept above 140°F.	Onset: Generally 8–12 hours after eating. Abdominal pain and diarrhea, and sometimes nausea and vomiting. Symptoms last a day or less and are usually mild. Can be more serious in older or debilitated people.
Salmonellosis *Salmonella* bacteria	Raw meats, poultry, milk and other dairy products, shrimp, frog legs, yeast, coconut, pasta, and chocolate are most frequently involved.	Onset: Generally 6–48 hours after eating. Nausea, abdominal cramps, diarrhea, fever, and headache. All age groups are susceptible, but symptoms are most severe for elderly, infants, and infirm.
Shigellosis (bacillary dysentery) *Shigella* bacteria	Found in milk and dairy products, poultry, and potato salad. Food becomes contaminated when a human carrier does not wash hands and then handles liquid or moist food that is not cooked thoroughly afterwards. Organisms multiply in food left at room temperature.	Onset: 1–7 days after eating. Abdominal cramps, diarrhea, fever, sometimes vomiting, and blood, pus, or mucus in stools.
Staphylococcal food poisoning Staphylococcal enterotoxin (produced by *Staphyloccus aureus* bacteria)	Toxin produced when food contaminated with the bacteria is left too long at room temperature. Meats, poultry, egg products, tuna, potato and macaroni salads, and cream-filled pastries are good environments for these bacteria to produce toxin.	Onset: Generally 30 minutes–8 hours after eating. Diarrhea, vomiting, nausea, abdominal pain, cramps, and prostration. Lasts 24–48 hours. Rarely fatal.
Vibrio infection *Vibrio vulnificus*	The bacteria live in coastal waters and can infect humans either through open wounds or through consumption of contaminated seafood. The bacteria are most numerous in warm weather.	Onset: Abrupt. Chills, fever, and/or prostration. At high risk are people with liver conditions, low gastric (stomach) acid, and weakened immune systems.

❖ Table 22 Continued ❖

Disease and Organism That Causes It	Source of Illness	Symptoms
Protozoa		
Amebiasis *Entamoeba histolytica*	Exist in the intestinal tract of humans and are expelled in feces. Polluted water and vegetables grown in polluted soil spread the infection.	Onset: 3–10 days after exposure. Severe crampy pain, tenderness over the colon or liver, loose morning stools, recurrent diarrhea, loss of weight, fatigue, and sometimes anemia.
Giardiasis *Giardia lamblia*	Most frequently associated with consumption of contaminated water. May be transmitted by uncooked foods that become contaminated while growing or after cooking by infected food handlers. Cool, moist conditions favor organism's survival.	Onset: 1–3 days. Sudden onset of explosive watery stools, abdominal cramps, anorexia, nausea, and vomiting. Especially infects hikers, children, travelers, and institutionalized patients.
Virus		
Hepatitis A virus	Mollusks (oysters, clams, mussels, scallops, and cockles) become carriers when their beds are polluted by untreated sewage. Raw shellfish are especially potent carriers, although cooking does not always kill the virus.	Onset: Begins with malaise, appetite loss, nausea, vomiting, and fever. After 3–10 days patient develops jaundice with darkened urine. Severe cases can cause liver damage and death.

The problem with bacteria is that once they are in food, or once we introduce them into food (by dirty hands, contaminated equipment, etc.), they grow readily under these three conditions.

1. **In a food that contains some protein.** Foods that bacteria love include the following:
   - Meat and meat products
   - Poultry and poultry products
   - Fish and shellfish
   - Milk and milk products
   - Gravies and sauces (unless acidic)
   - Eggs—cooked and raw—and egg products
   - Cooked or heated vegetables and plant products, such as:
        Potatoes (baked or mashed)
        Tofu
        Beans, cooked
        Winter squash, cooked
        Rice, cooked
   - Potato and protein salads
2. **A temperature between 45°F and 140°F** (as noted in the list of food temperatures for control of bacteria). Refrigeration is normally at or below 45°F, so bacterial growth subsequently slows down in the refrigerator and slows substantially in the freezer (usually kept at or below 0°F). Freezing does not kill bacteria. However, room temperature is normally around 70°F—a great temperature for bacteria to grow.
3. **At least two hours in this temperature zone.**

The diagram shows the steps resulting in foodborne illness caused by bacteria. In some, but not all, cases, adequate cooking of the contaminated food (to 165°F) will prevent problems. However, cooking does not kill all forms of bacteria, and in many cases the contaminated food may not even be cooked.

Viruses also cause foodborne illness. They are organisms smaller than bacteria that must live inside another living cell in order to stay alive. Viruses cause diseases such as the common cold, measles, chicken pox, herpes, flu, and infectious hepatitis. AIDS is caused by a virus, but this virus is not spread by food. Viruses don't multiply in foods, as do bacteria, but they use food (any food)

THE UNWELCOME DINNER GUEST

❖ ❖ ❖

Many cases of salmonella are caused by the cross-contamination of poultry. The following is an example.

Henry decided to make a meal for his loving wife, Angie. It was their anniversary and he decided to cook supper (one time per year—what a sport!). Well, Henry started the meal about 4 hours before serving time, although a 2-hour preparation period was all that was needed. He removed the chicken from the refrigerator, placed it on the cutting board, and left it there for about 1 hour. After handling the chicken, he wiped his hands on his pants (he didn't wear an apron), did not wash his hands, and proceeded directly to set the dining room table using the finest china, flatware, and linens.

After setting up the dining room, he cut up the chicken on the cutting board and started to prepare his favorite recipe. He merely wiped off the board with his "all-purpose" towel draped over his shoulder. While the chicken was cooking, he de-cided to make the salad. He placed the head of iceberg lettuce on top of the board and proceeded to cut it up with the unwashed poultry knife, unwashed hands, and unwashed cutting board. All of a sudden, the phone rang—it was his boss contacting him about a very important matter. After 15 minutes on the telephone, he placed the salad in a bowl and placed it on the dining room table. Once everything was ready, Henry's wife joined him for supper.

Approximately 6 hours after the meal, the agony began. It seems that the cause of the salmonella came from the lettuce that came in contact with the unwashed cutting board used to butcher the chicken. Fever, chills, diarrhea, and vomiting took place—Henry and Angie were very ill and recovered within a few days.

This scenario is not unusual. It can happen and accounts for a substantial number of foodborne illness outbreaks. Some of the simplest things, such as washing hands and kitchen equipment, are so crucial to preventing sickness.

to get to their next victim. The best way to prevent foodborne illness caused by viruses is to keep viruses out of food by practicing good personal hygiene such as washing hands frequently and not sneezing into the food.

Foodborne illness can be one of three types.

1. A **foodborne infection** results from eating food containing harmful living organisms such as bacteria and viruses.
2. A **foodborne intoxication** results from eating food containing toxins (or poisons) produced by bacteria as they grow. Ingestion of these toxins is what makes you sick—the bacteria may even be dead! Unfortunately the toxins are odorless and tasteless and can't be detected in food. In the case of one bacteria, Staphylococcus, these toxins are heat-stable, so heating up food does not destroy them.

3. A **foodborne toxin-mediated infection** results from eating food that contains harmful living organisms that, once in your intestine, produce toxins that make you sick.

Common causes of foodborne illness, both in the home and in restaurants, are:

- Inadequate cooling
- Inadequate cooking
- Contaminated equipment
- Purchase of unsafe food

Ways to Prevent Foodborne Illness
To prevent foodborne illness do the following.

1. Keep hot foods hot and cold foods cold. For example:
   - Thaw foods in refrigerator or microwave (use immediately after microwaving). Never thaw at room temperature because thawing

PRECAUTIONS WHEN USING EGGS AND POULTRY

EGGS

Purchasing

1. Check the expiration date on the carton.
2. Make sure the carton is clean and each egg is not cracked.
3. Make sure the eggs have been under refrigeration.

Storage

4. Refrigerate at or below 45°F.
5. Store eggs properly:
   Fresh—refrigerate for up to 3–5 weeks
   Hard-cooked—refrigerate for up to 1 week
6. Store newer eggs behind older eggs.

Preparation/Cooking

7. Don't use cracked eggs—throw out!
8. Cook both yolk and white until firm. Avoid soft- or medium-cooked eggs, soft omelets, runny scrambled eggs, and coddled eggs.
9. Do not use raw eggs in recipes that don't require further cooking, such as mayonnaise, Caesar salad, mousses, homemade eggnog, and hollandaise sauce.
10. Do not reuse a container after it has had raw egg mixture in it until it is washed thoroughly.
11. Eat egg dishes right away; otherwise refrigerate them promptly.

POULTRY

Purchasing

1. Wrap poultry in a plastic bag at the store and have it bagged separately at the cash register. Poultry bought at the supermarket often leaks juices that could be contaminated.
2. Leave the chicken wrapped and get it into the refrigerator as soon as you get home.

Storage

3. Store raw poultry in the refrigerator for no more than one to two days before cooking or freezing. Store whole birds in the freezer for up to 1 year, parts up to 9 months, and giblets 3 to 4 months.
4. Refrigerate leftovers within 1–2 hours after cooking.
5. Always remove stuffing from the bird before refrigerating.

Preparation

6. Before cooking poultry, throw away packaging and rinse product under cool running water. Cut on a nonporous (such as plastic) cutting board that can be cleaned well.
7. Always stuff poultry just before cooking or cook the stuffing separately (this is preferable).
8. For less fat and less possible contamination, remove skin before cooking.
9. Set oven temperature no lower than 325°F. For doneness, cook breasts to an internal temperature of 170°F and dark meat or whole birds to 180°F or until juices run clear and flesh is tender. Always check temperature in the thickest part of the bird.
10. Wash board, utensils, and counter immediately with detergent and hot water.
11. After marinating poultry, boil the marinade before using to baste the poultry or serving.

proceeds from the outside in so surface bacteria can multiply to disease-causing levels before food is thawed all the way through.

• To cool down hot foods before refrigerating, use shallow pans and/or an ice bath. Shallow pans allow more refrigerated air to circulate around the food, enabling cold temperatures to reach the center so bacteria can't easily grow there. To make an ice bath, place the container holding the hot food into a larger container filled with ice and cold water. Stir hot foods to remove heat. Cut large pieces

Temperature of Food for the Control of Bacteria

°F		°C
250		121.1
	Canning temperatures for low-acid vegetables, meat, and poultry in pressure canner.	
240		115.5
	Canning temperatures for fruits, tomatoes, and pickles in water-bath canner.	
212		100.0
	Cooking temperatures destroy vegetative forms of most bacteria. Time required to kill bacteria decreases as temperature is increased.	
165		73.8
	Hot-holding temperatures prevent growth of bacteria.	
140		60
130	Some bacterial growth may occur. Many bacteria survive.	55
120		48.8
	Temperatures in this zone allow rapid growth of bacteria and production of toxins by some bacteria.	
60		15.5
	Some growth of food-poisoning bacteria may occur.	
45		7.2
40		4.4
32	Cold temperatures permit slow growth of some bacteria that cause spoilage and illness.	0
14		−10
	Freezing temperatures stop growth of bacteria, but allow many bacteria to survive.	
0		−17.7

How Bacteria Cause Foodborne Illness

1. Bacteria may already be in the protein-containing food or are introduced into the food by:
   - Poor food handling or personal hygiene practices (such as dirty hands or cooked foods contaminated with juices from raw poultry)
   - Dirty dishes or equipment that harbor bacteria
2. The food is given the proper time (over 2 hours) and temperature (45–140°F) for bacteria to grow.
3. Foodborne illness often results.

of meat, etc., into smaller pieces to allow heat loss.
- Promptly refrigerate or freeze leftovers. Don't cover too tightly when you first put them in the refrigerator so the heat can escape. Cover tightly within 2 hours.
- Always remove stuffing from poultry or other stuffed meats and refrigerate in separate containers.
- Always marinate foods in the refrigerator.

2. Inspect foods thoroughly when buying and before cooking and serving, for freshness and wholesomeness. For example:
   - Check canned goods for rusted, dented, and bulging cans. They may indicate the growth of a bacteria in the can which causes botulism. Also check for leaking.
   - Check that foods are not outdated.
   - Do not use eggs that are cracked because they may contain significant amounts of a bacteria that can cause foodborne illness.
   - **When in doubt, throw it out.**

3. Store foods properly. For example:
   - Cover foods in storage.
   - Do not store food in open cans.
   - Store new foods behind old.
   - Reseal packages tightly after opening. When appropriate, store foods in airtight containers.
   - Keep thermometers in both the refrigerator and freezer and check frequently. Keep refrigerators below 45°F (preferably around 40°F, and keep freezers below 0°F.
   - Defrost freezers as necessary. Frost buildup causes freezers to get warmer.
   - Store canned goods and other shelf-stable products in a cool, dry place. Do not store in a garage or cabin where the temperature may drop below 32°F or above 85°F.

- Keep storage areas clean.
- Store chemicals and pesticides separately from food to avoid contamination.
- See the food storage charts at the end of Chapter 6 for guidelines for specific foods and what to do if the refrigerator/freezer stops working.

4. Keep it clean! For example:
   - Clean all equipment, tools, tables, dishes, and so on after each use.
   - Wash kitchen towels and dishcloths frequently. Replace sponges every few weeks. Bacteria can live in each of these.
   - Store equipment, tools, and the like so they do not collect dust.
   - Use plastic cutting boards rather than wooden ones where bacteria can hide in grooves that you can't keep clean.
   - Clean off the lids of cans and soft drinks before opening.
   - Wash your can opener after each use.

5. Avoid letting the microorganisms from one food contaminate another food. For example:
   - Use clean dishes and utensils to serve food, not those used in preparation (they may be contaminated with bacteria). Serve grilled food on a clean plate too, not one that held raw meat, poultry, or fish.
   - Never mix leftovers with fresh food.
   - Store fresh raw meats, poultry, and fish on lowest refrigerator shelves so they don't drip into cooked foods.
   - Use a different spoon for stirring raw foods, such as meat that is being browned, and cooked foods.

6. Observe good hygiene practices.
   - Always wash your hands before preparing food and again after contact with raw meat and poultry (they may carry bacteria). Hands

carry amazing numbers of bacteria so keep them clean and scrub them for at least 20 seconds before rinsing.

- Do not use your apron as a hand towel because the apron will become contaminated and possibly transfer bacteria to food.
- Don't touch your face or any other part of your body while handling food because bacteria on your skin can then be introduced into food.
- Don't use your fingers to taste food. Use a spoon.
- Cover all cuts, burns, and boils with a bandage and plastic glove. Bacteria run rampant in cuts, burns, and boils, and proper bandaging is necessary to keep them out of your food.
- Use utensils such as tongs and spoons to handle food so bacteria from your hands will not contaminate the food.

7. Cook foods to adequate temperatures to kill bacteria, as described in the accompanying chart.
   - Use a thermometer to test the temperature of cooked foods. Place the thermometer into the center, or thickest, part of the food and make sure it is immersed up to the dimple on the stem in order to get an accurate reading. If using a microwave, insert the thermometer in several spots.

8. Dispose of garbage often.

SEAFOOD SAFETY

Recent studies done on the safety of seafood have made the American public aware of the fact that seafood is not subject to mandatory federal inspection, as is meat and poultry. Less than half of the nation's seafood processing plants are inspected by the Food and Drug Administration. States and localities carry most of the inspection load.

The problems with unsafe seafood include the following:

- Chemical contamination (pollutants) found in the water from which the seafood was taken is a real concern. They may include pesticides, toxic metals such as lead or mercury, or in-

dustrial chemicals such as PCBs, which are carcinogenic.

- **Bacteria and viruses** are sometimes found in seafood that came from waters contaminated with raw sewage. Seafood may also be contaminated with bacteria and viruses when they are not handled in a safe manner once harvested.
- **Natural toxins** occur in seafood that eat certain microorganisms or toxins are produced as the fish spoils.
- Some raw seafood contain **parasites** (they are not a problem as long as you cook the fish).

What can you do to prevent foodborne illness caused by seafood? Plenty, and by practicing some simple precautions you can continue to eat this low-fat source of protein.

1. Buy seafood from a reputable fish dealer. Don't buy it from a street vendor or anywhere that fish is not handled properly. Fish should not be piled high in displays, but should be displayed in individual pans with lots of ice. Raw seafood should also be kept separate from cooked.

2. When buying fresh fish, look for firm and shiny flesh in either whole fish or fillets. Press the fish with a finger; if it leaves an indentation, it's not the freshest. Dull flesh may also mean that the fish is old. If you're still uncertain about how fresh the fish is, ask to have it rinsed under cold water and then smell it. Fresh fish should have no fishy or ammonia smell.

   The shells of hard clams, mussels, or oysters should be closed, or should close when their shells are tapped. The necks of steamer clams should twitch when their shells are tapped. Crabs should move when touched. Lobsters' tails should curl under their bodies when picked up.

   When buying frozen fish, select packages that are not open, torn, or crushed on the edges. Avoid packages that are above the frost line in the store's freezer. If the package has a transparent cover, look for signs of frost or ice crystals; crystals could mean that the fish has either been stored for a long period or

COOKING FOODS SAFELY

For safe cooking, never use an oven temperature below 300°F. When testing for doneness, insert meat thermometer or microwave temperature probe into the thickest part of meat or poultry away from bone or fat. Temperature-check microwaved foods after the standing time that completes their cooking.

	Cook to This Internal Temperature	Visual Checks
Fresh Meats		
Ground Meats (Veal, beef, lamb, pork)	160°F	No longer pink
Fresh Beef		
Rare (some bacterial risk)	140°F	Red center
Medium	160°F	Pale pink center
Well Done	170°F	Gray or brown throughout
Fresh Lamb, Pork, and Veal		
Medium	160°F	Pale pink center
Well Done	170°F	Not pink
Leftover cooked meats (to reheat)	165°F	Steaming hot
Poultry		
Chicken, Turkey, Duck, and Geese, whole	180°F	Juices run clear, leg moves easily, tender
Poultry breasts, roasts	170°F	Clear juice, fork tender
Poultry thighs, wings		Cook until juices run clear
Fully cooked poultry; leftovers	Safe to eat cold if properly stored	
(to reheat)	165°F	Steaming hot
Fish and Shellfish		
Fish, filleted and whole	160°F	Flesh is opaque, flakes easily
Shellfish	160°F	Opaque, steaming hot
Eggs		
Fresh		Both yolk and white firm
Egg-based sauces and custards	160°F	Sauces coat spoon, custards are firm
Pasteurized egg substitutes	Safe uncooked	Cook as desired

thawed and refrozen. Nor should there be evidence of drying out, such as white or dark spots, discoloration, or fading of red or pink flesh. This may also indicate that the fish has been thawed and refrozen.

3. The guidelines for choosing the safest fish outline how to choose safe fish that are less likely to be contaminated. To avoid natural toxins (they can't be killed by cooking), be very cautious when buying snapper and grou-

CHOOSING THE SAFEST FISH

❖ ❖ ❖

The following chart lists some of the most popular fish, according to whether they are freshwater, near-shore, or offshore varieties, and in order according to fat content. The safest bets are the fish in the upper left corner—note the exceptions, though.

Offshore	Near-shore	Freshwater
cod	★ striped bass	yellow perch
haddock	✔ pink salmon	freshwater bass
pollock	★ bluefish	white perch
yellowfin tuna	✔ chum salmon	brook trout
flounder, sole	✔ sockeye salmon	rainbow trout
ocean perch	sardines	★ catfish
★ swordfish	herring	★ carp
Pacific halibut		lake whitefish
albacore tuna		lake trout

★ *These species probably have high levels of contaminants.* **Swordfish** *frequently exceed allowable levels of methyl mercury. Migratory fish such as* **striped bass** *and* **bluefish** *are frequently tainted with PCBs, even if they're caught offshore.* **Catfish** *and* **carp** *are bottom feeders, and are particularly vulnerable to contamination from tainted sediments. Most commercially harvested catfish is farm-raised, and relatively uncontaminated with pesticides, but drug residues from aquaculture might be a problem.*
✔ *Despite their high fat content,* **salmon** *(except those caught from the Great Lakes) tend to be relatively free of chemical contaminants.*
Source: *Reprinted with permission from* Safe Food: Eating Wisely in a Risky World, *by Michael F. Jacobson, Ph.D., Lisa Y. Lefferts, and Anne Witte Garland; Living Planet Press, 1991.*

per species in Florida, as well as mahimahi, tuna, and bluefish (also warm water species). Buy only from a trusted dealer and use quickly.

4. Eat a variety of seafood so no one species dominates.
5. Seafood should be stored at 30°F to 32°F— about 10 degrees cooler than most refrigerators. Put it in the coldest spot in your refrigerator and cook within one day. Store live shellfish, lobsters, and crabs in the refrigerator in ventilated containers.
6. Pay special attention to avoid contaminating kitchen counters and other surfaces with seafood. Wash all surfaces and utensils touched by seafood during preparation.
7. Before cooking, scrub shellfish well in several changes of water to prevent the meat from becoming contaminated when they open during cooking. Don't cook shellfish that have died—as evidenced by open shells.
8. Cook fish thoroughly, until it is firm, turns white, and it flakes or starts to separate. This takes about 10 minutes per inch of thickness.
9. Cook shellfish thoroughly (see Chapter 9).
10. Don't eat raw seafood—they may contain harmful bacteria, viruses (such as hepatitis), and parasites.

MOLDS

Ever notice a little bluish-green piece of fuzz growing on your tomatoes? Sure, you probably knew it was just a mold, but wondered, like everyone else, if you should just cut around it or throw out the tomato. Use the following list as your

❖ *Removing Molds* ❖

Throw These Foods Out	*Cut Out the Mold on These Foods (and at least an inch of food around and under it)*
Cucumbers	Bell peppers
Tomatoes	Broccoli
Spinach, lettuce, other leafy greens	Cauliflower
Bananas, peaches, melons	Cabbage
Berries	Carrots
Breads, cakes, rolls, flour	Garlic, onions
Soft cheeses like Brie or mozzarella	Potatoes
Luncheon meat and cheese (slices)	Turnips
Yogurt, cottage cheese, cream cheese	Zucchini, winter squash
Canned foods	Apples, pears
Peanut butter	Hard cheeses like cheddar or Swiss
Juices	
Most cooked leftovers	

Source: Nutrition Action Health Letter (Nov. 1991), Center for Science in the Public Interest. Reprinted with permission.

guide to dealing with funny little molds growing on your food.

Molds cause spoilage of foods (quite often fruits and bread), musty odors, and off flavors. Molds also grow on vegetables, meats, and cheese that have been exposed to the air. Although molds will be killed by most cooking, the toxins they produce will not, so you are better off removing the mold or throwing out the food.

The most hazardous molds that produce dangerous toxins do not grow in our refrigerators, but rather down on the farm. Aflatoxin is a hazardous mold found in foods stored under warm, humid conditions. It is the strongest carcinogen known to affect the rat's liver. Most commonly found in peanuts, corn, and cottonseed, and possibly wheat and rice, its levels in foods in the United States are very low and monitored regularly. Because aflatoxin does occur in peanut butter, it is best to buy national brands, which tend to be lowest in aflatoxin levels. Also, throw out any moldy peanuts, peanut butter, cornmeal, or other corn products.

PESTICIDES

Pesticides are chemicals used to control insects, diseases, weeds, fungi, mold, and other pests on plants, vegetables, fruits, and animals. Examples include insecticides (designed to kill insects) and fungicides (designed to kill fungi). Pesticides are normally applied to crops as a spray, fog, or dust to protect the crops from damage and increase their yields. The Environmental Protection Agency (EPA) is responsible for setting safety levels and for approving pesticides and other chemicals used in growing food. The Food and Drug Administration (FDA) then monitors for compliance with EPA tolerance levels for most foods. The FDA tests thousands of shipments of all foods (domestic and imported) except meat and poultry each year for pesticide residues.

The EPA over the years has banned the use of a wide variety of pesticides that were carcinogenic, and it continues to study others to determine their safety. For pesticides that it determines safe to use, it establishes minimum exposure standards or tolerances that have a built-in level of safety.

To decrease your exposure to pesticides, you can do the following.

- Buy certified organically grown produce when possible.
- Remove outer leaves of leafy vegetables such as lettuce.
- Wash produce carefully, using a brush, as washing will remove some (but not all) residues. Although pesticides are often found on the surface of a piece of fruit, such as an apple, some pesticides do concentrate in the interior of fruits and vegetables.
- Peel carrots, waxed cucumbers, apples, peaches, and pears because these foods are more likely to have hazardous pesticide residues.
- Buy less imported produce as it often has more pesticides. Buy local produce from a farmer's

market as it is probably treated with less pesticide than produce traveling from California to New York.

- Trim fat and skin from meat, poultry, and fish. Pesticides in animal feed can concentrate in animal fat. Skim fat from pan drippings, broths, sauces, and soups.
- Eat a varied diet so no one food dominates.
- The green color found under the skin of the potato is not due to pesticides, but is a natural toxin that is not destroyed during cooking. It is toxic so it is best to cut it out of the potato. This toxin is less likely to develop if potatoes are stored in a cool, dark place.

ADDITIVES

There has been much public concern about the safety of man-made additives, particularly in relationship to cancer. There are two types of additives, direct and indirect. Direct (or intentional) additives are added to food to perform a functional purpose such as adding or enhancing flavor, improving nutritional value, or preventing spoilage. About 0.5 percent of our food supply consists of intentional additives. There are about 2,800 direct additives, and the vast majority are spices and flavors such as salt, pepper, and sugar. In fact, sugar, salt, corn syrup, and dextrose account for 93 percent of all direct additives used in the United States. Indirect additives are normally present in trace amounts and result from contact of food with agricultural chemicals, processing equipment, or food containers. They are also subject to regulation. There are approximately 10,000 indirect additives, but only a small fraction actually end up in food.

The 1958 Food Additives Amendment to the Food, Drug, and Cosmetic Act provided the first specific regulation of food additives. Approval of new food additives was required before they could be marketed, and the responsibility for proving their safety was placed on the manufacturer. To use or market a substance, a company must file a petition with the FDA showing that tests prove the substance is safe. If the substance is approved as an additive, FDA prescribes the types of food in which it can be used and labeling directions, and

may also prescribe the maximum quantity that can be used.

The Food Additives Amendment exempted two groups of additives from the testing and approval process. The first is the list of substances which experts have classified "generally recognized as safe" (GRAS). This list includes substances such as flavorings and spices which are considered harmless because past extensive use has produced no known harmful effects. Also exempted from testing were "prior sanctioned substances" which FDA or USDA had approved for use in food prior to passage of the 1958 Food Additives Amendment. Additives can be removed from the lists, however, if tests indicate the substances are not safe for human consumption. All substances previously listed as GRAS are being reviewed to assure that they meet current food safety standards. Eventually all the substances will either be affirmed as GRAS or removed from GRAS status.

The 1960 Color Additive Amendments brought all colors, natural and synthetic, under the Food, Drug, and Cosmetic Act. Color additives may not be used to deceive consumers or to conceal blemishes or inferiorities in food.

The Food Additives Amendment and the Color Additives Amendments include the so-called Delaney Clause, which prohibits the approval of an additive if it is found to induce cancer when ingested by people or animals at any dosage. When the Delaney Clause was written, it was impossible to detect minute levels of carcinogens in foods as can be done now. Therefore, it was deemed necessary to eliminate from the food supply any and all carcinogens. Some people feel it is time to eliminate or modify this regulation to take into account levels of risk at smaller doses. Although the Delaney Clause is law, it is not always invoked.

Although the majority of additives used are safe, there is evidence to suggest that some are not safe and should be avoided; these are listed below.

1. Acesulfame-K—an artificial sweetener currently approved only for tabletop use, causes cancer in animals
2. Aspartame—an artificial sweetener used in soft drinks, in drink mixes, in pud-

ding and gelatin mixes, and as a tabletop sweetener; needs more testing

3. Artificial colors—much of our food is colored with synthetic colors; more artificial colors are being required to be listed on ingredient labels

4 & 5. BHA and BHT—preservatives and antioxidants that are possibly carcinogenic

6. Caffeine—a stimulant which is mildly addictive that is added to many soft drinks

7. Monosodium glutamate (MSG)—causes adverse reaction in some individuals—headaches, chest tightness; used for flavoring

8. Nitrites—used in curing of cold cuts, hot dogs, bacon, and other cured meats; nitrites are converted into nitrosamines (known to cause cancer) in the mouth, stomach, and colon

9. Saccharin—artificial nonnutritive sweetener used in many foods, known to cause cancer in animals

10. Sulfites—a preservative used to prevent discoloration of certain foods, causes severe allergic reactions in some asthmatics

CERAMIC COOKWARE AND DISHWARE

Most ceramic glaze contains lead which, if properly fired and sealed, is not cause for concern. However, some ceramic cookware (and dishware) from both outside and inside the United States has been found to leach lead in dangerous amounts into food. Ceramic items in your home may include fine china, stoneware, earthenware, and ironstone. Lead is quite toxic; consistent exposure to it can damage the nervous system and is particularly dangerous for children. Unfortunately, there is no way of telling whether a ceramic piece has an unsafe amount of lead unless you do a test using a lead-testing kit (see below). Lead also leaches from lead crystal, and it can leach into any liquid, not just alcohol. Here are

precautions to follow to lessen your chances of lead poisoning.

1. Don't store foods in ceramic cookware or dishes unless you are sure they are lead-free.

2. Avoid using ceramic dishes to serve acidic foods and beverages because they cause more lead to be leached out. Examples of acidic foods include citrus juices, apple juice, tomato products, cola-flavored soft drinks, coffee, or tea.

3. Heat also causes more lead to be leached out, so don't use ceramic cookware or dishes that you are not sure of in cooking, including microwave cooking.

4. Do not use, and perhaps dispose of, any china on which the glaze is corroded or has a chalky gray residue when dry.

5. Be cautious about using very old china and handcrafted china that is highly decorated.

6. If buying new ceramic cookware or dishes, select a manufacturer, such as Corning, that has lead-free glazes available.

7. Do not use lead crystal every day and never use it to store food or beverages.

8. If in doubt, check it out: buy a lead-testing kit. They run from $20 and up. Two sources you can check are:

> Leadcheck Swabs
> Hybrivet Systems
> P.O. Box 1210
> Framingham, Mass. 01701
> (800) 262-5323
>
> Frandon Lead Alert Kit
> Frandon Enterprises
> 511 N. 48th St.
> Seattle, Washington 98103

The safety of other cookware, such as aluminum or nonstick coatings, is discussed in Chapter 7. At this time it does not seem that aluminum, stainless steel, cast iron, copper (if it's lined with another metal), or nonstick coatings cause a health concern.

MICROWAVE SAFETY

Although the initial concern about using microwaves centered around radiation leakage, current concerns revolve around these areas.

- The use of improper containers and wraps that may leach chemicals into the food as it cooks. Government research has shown that chemicals from some plastic wraps may leach into the food as it cooks. Containers used to microwave food may also cause problems. For example, the use of margarine tubs may cause the plastic to melt.
- The use of heat susceptors in microwave packages of foods (such as popcorn and french fries) that, when heated, cause unwanted chemicals to migrate, or seep, into the food. Heat susceptors are plastic strips or metal disks found in containers and other packaging that brown and crisp foods. They were developed to improve the taste and appearance of foods such as pizza, fish sticks, popcorn, french fries, and waffles.
- The danger of children using the microwave improperly and unsafely. Severe burns can and do occur from improper microwave use. Special packaging for kids' favorite foods like popcorn, pizza, and french fries can get too hot for kids to handle. Steam from popcorn bags can burn the eyes, face, arms, and hands. Jelly donuts, pastries, hot dogs, and other foods can reach scalding temperatures in seconds. If you allow your child to use the microwave, start by reviewing the points listed below. It is generally recommended that your child be at least 10 before he or she is allowed to use the microwave unsupervised. Children should also be tall enough to see what they are doing when they remove foods from the microwave to avoid dangerous spills.

Here are tips to avoid each of these problems.

Choosing Containers and Wraps for the Microwave

1. Buy containers for the microwave that say "Microwave Safe" on the label.
2. As a rule, it's not good to use metal pans made for conventional ovens or aluminum foil because the microwaves will be reflected and could damage the oven. However, some new metal cookware is specially made for use in microwave ovens. Also avoid metal-trimmed cookware or dishes.

3. Don't use butter or margarine tubs in the microwave. When the food gets hot, it may melt the plastic, causing migration of the plastic into your food.
4. Not all glass and ceramic is microwave-safe. Here's a quick test for glass. Microwave the empty container for one minute. It's unsafe for the microwave if it's warm. It's okay for reheating if it's lukewarm. It's okay for actual cooking if it's cool.
5. Don't use plastic foam containers or any plastic disposable container. They may melt in the microwave.
6. Melamine dinnerware can burn and turn brittle.
7. Brown paper bags may contain fine pieces of metal that can cause arcing.
8. Don't let plastic wrap touch the food.
9. Paper plates, paper towels, paper napkins, and paper cups can be used in the microwave.
10. Don't thaw frozen meats in the plastic wrap and foam tray in which it comes packaged. Transfer to a microwave-safe dish to prevent harmful chemicals from getting into the food.

Avoiding Microwave Foods with Heat Susceptors

1. Use care or avoid buying products (such as pizza, fish sticks, popcorn, french fries, and waffles) that have heat susceptors. Although you can check the packaging for them, they are not always visible.

Safe Microwaving Tips for Kids (And Adults!)

1. Never turn on an empty oven. This can cause the oven to break.
2. Read package directions carefully. Make sure you know how to set the microwave oven controls (for example, 10 seconds, rather than 10 minutes).
3. Use only microwave-safe cookware and keep them in a certain place.
4. Rotate food in the microwave and stir halfway through cooking if possible.
5. Use pot holders to remove items from the microwave.

MICROWAVE MAINTENANCE TIPS

- Don't use an oven if the door does not close firmly or is otherwise damaged. If you have an older model with a soft mesh door gasket, check for deterioration.
- If there are signs of rusting inside the oven, have it repaired.
- Clean the door and oven cavity—the outer edge too—with water and mild detergent. Do not use abrasives such as scouring pads or steel wool.
- Do not allow soil or cleaner residue to accumulate on sealing surfaces.
- Follow the manufacturer's instruction manual for maintenance procedures.
- The oven should not be adjusted or repaired by anyone except properly qualified service personnel.

6. If a dish is covered, make sure there is some room for excess steam to escape.
7. When taking foods out of the microwave, pull cover off foods so steam escapes away from hands and face. Steam can burn.
8. Prick foods like potatoes and hot dogs before putting into the microwave; otherwise they might explode during cooking.

Use the tips on maintaining your microwave properly to avoid radiation problems.

❖ ❖ ❖

CHAPTER SEVEN

A GUIDE TO COOKWARE
AND DINNERWARE

COOKWARE

It's twice as hard as stainless steel, it conducts heat 28 times faster than glass, and it's non-stick for life. What is this product? It's anodized aluminum, just one of the many new inventions that have revolutionized the cookware industry in the past 10 years. Whatever material is chosen, high-quality pots and pans should distribute heat evenly and uniformly so there are no hot spots, which burn food, or cold spots, which undercook foods. Two factors will determine if your pots and pans will cook evenly.

- Type of material used: Each material used to make pots and pans conducts or distributes heat a little differently.
- Thickness of the material: A thick-bottomed pot cooks more evenly than a thin-bottomed pot. Thick-bottomed cookware is of course heavier and usually more expensive.

Each type of material used to make cookware and bakeware has its own characteristics, and they are described below. Table 23 describes common cookware and bakeware.

Aluminum

More than half (52 percent) of all cookware sold today is made of aluminum. But most of these aluminum pots and pans are coated with nonstick finishes or treated using a process that alters and hardens the structure of the metal.

One reason that aluminum became popular for cookware is that it is an excellent heat conductor. Heat spreads quickly and evenly across the bottom, up the sides, and across the cover to completely surround the food. Aluminum is also lightweight, which makes it easy to handle and not too expensive. However, because aluminum is a soft metal, it can be damaged by rough treatment. Another concern with aluminum is that it reacts with some foods, particularly high acid foods, so aluminum should not be used for long cooking of high acid foods, such as tomatoes, or for storing any foods. Aluminum also discolors some foods, such as eggs.

In the 1970s, Canadian researchers reported that patients with Alzheimer's disease had abnormally high levels of aluminum in their brains. The studies stirred a controversy about whether aluminum is the cause or result of the disease. At the same time, many concerned consumers discarded their aluminum cookware. It appears that the amount of aluminum leached in food from aluminum cookware is minimal. Aluminum appears naturally in the soil, so it is found in fruits and vegetables. Aluminum is also found in baking powder, certain food additives, and in buffered aspirin and certain antacids.

Anodized Aluminum

Now cookware manufacturers have developed a process for treating aluminum that retains the heat conductivity properties of the metal, but changes aluminum in other ways. The process, called anodization, involves a series of electrochemical baths that thicken the oxide film that forms naturally on aluminum. This supplemental coating hardens the metal, making it more

❖ *Table 23 Basic Cookware and Bakeware* ❖

Name	Description	Uses
Cookware		
Saucepan	Round pot available in various sizes from 2 cups to 6 quarts May have straight or sloped walls. One handle.	All-purpose
Sauce pot	Round pot of medium depth with two handles. Sizes range from 4 to 14 quarts.	Soups, stews, sauces, any liquids
Stockpot	Large, deep pot with straight sides and two handles	Stocks, soups, liquids
Saute pan	Wide, straight-sided, and shallow. 2½ inch sides.	Sauteing, frying, browning
Skillet or frying pan	Slope-sided shallow pan. 10- or 12-inch diameter is common.	Sauteing, frying, omelets
Roasting pan	Large rectangular pan with 2-inch sides.	Roasting meat and poultry
Bakeware		
Baking pan	Rectangular pan with straight walls, ¾ inch or more. 9 × 13 is common.	Cakes and other baked goods
Muffin pan	Rectangular pan with individual cups Number of cups varies—usually 6 or 12. Size of cup varies—mini, medium, jumbo.	Muffins, cupcakes
Cookie sheet	Large rectangular tray with no sides or ½-inch sides. 12 × 16 is common. Air-cushioned cookie sheet prevents overbrowning of bottom.	Cookies
Jelly roll pan	Large rectangular tray with shallow sides. 11 × 15 × ¾ is common.	Cookies, jelly roll
Round cake pan	Round pan with straight sides. 8- or 9-inch × 1½ is common.	Layer cakes
Square cake pan	Square pan with straight sides. 8 × 8 × 2 is common.	Cakes, brownies, bar cookies
Pie pan	Round pan with sloped walls. 8- or 9-inch diameter and 1-inch deep is common. Deep-dish pans are 1½ to 2 inches deep.	Pies
Tube pan	Deep (4½ inch) round pan that has a tube that extends from bottom to top to assure even baking. Wall slants slightly outward to help remove product from pan and provide a graceful appearance. 10-inch diameter is common.	Cakes
Bundt pan	Like tube pan except that it has fluted sides and a slightly rounded bottom. Usually 10-inch diameter and 3½ inches high.	Bundt cakes
Springform pan	Round pans with straight sides you can remove after baking. 8- or 9-inch diameter is common.	Cheesecake
Bread pan or loaf pan	Rectangular pan with slanted walls. A 9 × 5 × 3 is standard and makes a one-pound loaf.	Breads, pound cake, meat loaf

scratch-resistant. Food barely sticks on the hard, smooth surface of this altered aluminum, making it easier to clean.

Commercial Aluminum Company, the manufacturer of Calphalon, a best-selling brand of anodized aluminum cookware, claims that a final stage in the anodization process "seals the aluminum," preventing any leaching into food. Anodized aluminum cookware does not react to acidic foods, so these pots and pans are top choices for cooking rhubarb and sauces with tomato, wine, and lemon juice. Calphalon cookware is satin-gray in color and its surface cannot scratch, chip, crack, or peel. You can even use wire whisks and metal spoons with it. It is, of course, more expensive than regular aluminum.

Stainless Steel

Consumers who don't buy aluminum pots and pans usually buy stainless steel. Stainless steel accounts for 43 percent of cookware sold. Stainless steel cookware and bakeware is exceptionally durable. The finish won't corrode or tarnish and its hard, tough, nonporous surface is resistant to wear. It is more durable than aluminum and does not react with acid foods.

As stainless steel does not conduct heat evenly, most stainless steel cookware is made with copper or aluminum bottoms. Manufacturers caution against allowing salty foods to remain in stainless steel for long periods, as undissolved salt may cause pitting.

Copper

Copper is an excellent conductor of heat, especially good for range cooking. Cooks often prefer copper cookware for delicate sauces and foods that must be cooked at precisely controlled temperatures. However, copper cookware must be lined with tin or stainless steel because copper is easily dissolved by some foods with which it comes in contact and, in sufficient quantities, can cause nausea, vomiting, and diarrhea. Copper is also very expensive and requires much care to maintain, as it stains and discolors readily. The green rust that develops on copper is poisonous.

Cast Iron

The all-time classic is cast iron cookware. It's been with us for nearly 3,000 years. Cast iron is strong, inexpensive, and it's an even conductor of heat for browning, frying, and baking foods. Cooking with cast iron also provides a source of an important nutrient. Some nutritionists suggest that foods cooked in unglazed cast iron contain twice or more the amount of iron they would contain otherwise.

Cast iron utensils should be handled differently from other utensils. To prevent rust damage, the inside of cast iron cookware should be coated frequently with unsalted cooking oil. It should not be washed with strong detergents or scoured, and should be wiped dry immediately after rinsing.

Glass, Earthenware, Ceramic Cookware

Glass, earthenware, and ceramic cookware are used almost exclusively for oven cooking. They should, in most cases, not be used on a range burner because they might crack. They are breakable and poor heat conductors. Some ceramic cookware may leach lead into the food you eat—see Chapter 6 for more information.

Nonstick Coatings

Before anodized aluminum made its cookware debut, nonstick coatings stirred a mini-revolution in the American kitchen. Teflon, for instance, is a trademark for a tough, nonporous material called perfluorocarbon resin that permits cooking without the use of fats. It was first discovered by chance in 1938 and then hurried into wartime production for use in radar systems, in which other less durable substances had failed.

The noncorrosive properties of this stable plastic material made it a natural for cookware. In 1960, the Food and Drug Administration approved its use for food contact surfaces, and cookware manufacturers began turning out pots and pans with a coating that cleaned quickly and easily and that required less fat for nonstick cooking. One of the first nonstick coatings to be applied to housewares, Teflon soon became a household word.

Because nonstick finishes may be scratched by sharp or rough-edged kitchen tools, manufacturers recommend using plastic or wooden utensils. Abrasive scouring pads or cleansers should not be used to clean them. While nonstick pans do abrade with hard use and particles may chip off, these particles pass unchanged through your body.

Cooking enthusiasts now are hailing Silverstone and Excalibur nonstick coatings, which are made of three layers of the same plastic used on Teflon and other perfluorocarbon resin-coated pans. This material is extremely durable, and so inert (meaning it will not migrate) that it is used in artificial arteries, hip joint replacement parts, and other surgical implants.

DINNERWARE, FLATWARE, AND GLASSWARE

Due to the huge variety of dinnerware available, making a purchasing decision can be difficult. The intelligent selection of dinnerware starts with

❖ **Table 24 Care of Common Materials** ❖
Used in Cookware

Material	Care
Aluminum	Do not heat when empty. Do not put hot pans into sink to be washed—let cool first. Use wooden tools to prevent pitting of metal. Likewise, wash with plastic scrubber and use fine steel wool pad only for heavy stains and sticky food residue. Do not soak for more than 1 hour or use for food storage.
Anodized aluminum	Wash with soap and hot water. Avoid scouring.
Cast iron	Requires seasoning before first use. To season, coat thoroughly inside and out with vegetable oil or shortening. Wipe off excess and bake in 300°F oven, upside down, for 1 hour. Cool and wipe with a paper towel. To keep clean, wash with soapy water and sponge, or brush, and dry thoroughly over heat (using the oven or range). Do not use detergents or abrasives. Re-season when the seasoned surface is scrubbed off.
Copper	Do not heat to very high temperatures. Wash with soap and hot water and dry immediately. Use nylon sponge and soak in water only briefly. Never scour. Use nylon or wood tools to avoid scratching. Do not store foods in copper.
Earthenware	If fully glazed and high-fired, it may be able to be washed in the dishwasher. If not, wash by hand with soap and hot water. Soak well to remove residue. Cannot withstand rapid changes in temperature—may crack.
Glass	To clean, soak in warm soapy water and scrub gently. Use nylon or plastic pad for scouring to avoid scratching. Wash with baking soda to remove sticky food residue. Do not subject to rapid temperature changes unless the glass has been tempered.
Stainless steel	To clean, wash with soap and water and dry. Do not scour—abrasives may mar the polished surface. Soak off any stubborn stains.

understanding the materials commonly used to make the plates, bowls, and other dishes we use, like those shown in the photo.

- **Fine china or bone china:** Fine china is the highest quality tableware, and this is reflected in its price and appearance. Because it is fired twice at high temperatures, it is very hard, durable, and has a finely glazed finish. Fine china is also distinguished by a high degree of whiteness and translucence.
- **Stoneware:** Stoneware is composed of clay containing iron and other unrefined materials, which is why it lacks the translucence and whiteness seen in china. It usually has a beige or gray tone. It is fired at high temperatures, is nonporous, and resists chipping.
- **Ironstone:** Ironstone is a strong, hard, nonporous material that lacks the translucency and white color of fine china.
- **Earthenware:** Earthenware has a porous ceramic body which is fired at relatively low temperatures. It is often glazed and lacks the strength of stoneware and china.

The successful selection of dinnerware will depend on your needs and how much money you wish to spend.

If ceramic dishes (this includes fine china, stoneware, ironstone, and earthenware) are not properly glazed, there is the possibility of lead (which is in the glaze) being leached into foods. Unfortunately there is no way of telling whether a ceramic piece has an unsafe amount of lead unless you do a test using a lead-testing kit (see page 103 for where to get them and tips on handling this problem).

There are three basic types of flatware available: sterling silver, silver-plated, and stainless steel.

- **Sterling silver** is the most expensive choice. It is elegant in appearance and opulent to the touch. The care required to properly maintain sterling silver flatware is extensive. Because tarnish builds up, sterling must be regularly detarnished and burnished.
- **Silver-plated** flatware is just what its name implies: a base metal is coated or plated with silver for sheen and the look of elegance. The

China (Courtesy: Corning)

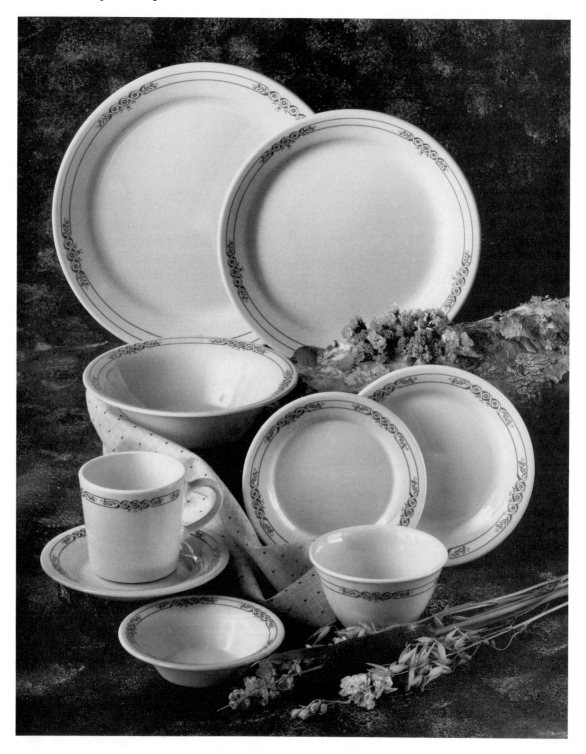

base metal may be either a brass alloy or stainless steel. Silver-plated flatware made with stainless steel costs less and is more durable than flatware made with brass alloy.

- **Stainless steel flatware** is the least expensive flatware, but there is wide variation in the price and quality of stainless steel flatware available on the market, so you really need to know what you are buying. The most durable and corrosion-resistant type of stainless steel is called "18/8" because it has 18 percent chrome and 8 percent nickel. This type of stainless steel also has a luster not seen in lesser types. Stainless steel is an excellent choice for everyday use as it is very durable, reasonably priced, easy to maintain, and comes in a wide variety of styles and patterns.

The most commonly used type of **glassware** is made of **lime glass**. Lime glassware is a combination of molten glass and soda lime. Because the natural qualities of lime impart a high level of strength to glass, lime glassware can withstand additional mechanical treatments that enhance its durability. Lime glass is reasonably priced and comes in a wide assortment of shapes and colors.

Lead glass, or crystal, is used less often to make glasses. It is made from molten glass to which lead oxide and alkalis have been added. Crystal displays a clarity and brilliance not possible in lime glassware, and the sparkle of crystal increases as the amount of lead used increases. To be classified as crystal, glassware must be at least 12 percent lead, but most fine crystal contains 24 percent. Good quality crystal should be perfectly clear. Because crystal is more expensive than lime glass and not as strong, it is generally used for special occasions and entertaining.

HAND TOOLS

Hand tools used in cooking include pancake or hamburger turners, spoons, forks, and tongs; some of these are shown in the accompanying illustrations.

- **Pancake or hamburger turners, or offset spatulas** are used for turning different foods during cooking. The blade is offset so that it slides easily under food. The blade may be slotted so that fats or liquids drain as the food is lifted. The best ones have wooden handles (they resist heat) with stainless steel blades.

- **Spoons** may be metal, wood, or plastic and are used in many ways. Because they contain cracks and crevices in which bacteria can thrive, wooden spoons are not the most sanitary. Plastic or metal are preferred. Spoons may be solid, perforated, or slotted. Perforated and slotted spoons are useful for lifting solid foods out of hot liquids. Slots drain food faster, but some small foods will slip through. The length of the handle is an important consideration. Short-handled spoons are better for mixing cold foods. Long-handled spoons are better for mixing hot foods so you don't get burned.

- **Forks** used for cooking are longer than dining forks and normally have only two or three tines so they can pierce foods easily. A **carving fork** is useful to hold the meat (or whatever is being carved) still while you cut, and it normally has a short handle. For turning foods, tongs are generally preferred because they do not pierce the food, which causes the loss of juices.

- **Tongs** come in two styles: scissor-type or spring-type. Spring-type tongs are useful for gripping small pieces of food or ice. Scissor-type tongs are larger and can grip much larger foods with more control.

Hand tools, like those shown, are used for cutting. This type includes the vegetable peeler, grater, zester, melon baller, pastry wheel, and kitchen shears.

- The **vegetable peeler** has a double blade that swivels. This feature allows it to efficiently peel fruits and vegetables with little waste. The sharp tip can be used to remove potato eyes, bruised spots, and so on. Stainless steel peelers are the best. Replace your peeler when it gets dull—it can't be sharpened.

- **Graters** are wonderful when you need to shred and grate foods such as vegetables, cheese, citrus rinds, and other foods. Metal box-style graters are easier on your knuckles than the flat graters. One side usually has smooth-edged

Offset Spatula

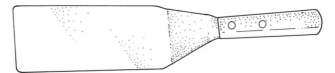

Spoons: slotted, perforated, solid

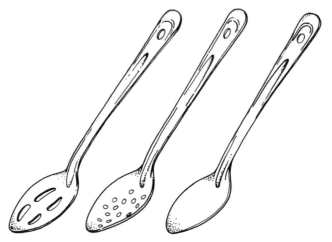

Box grater

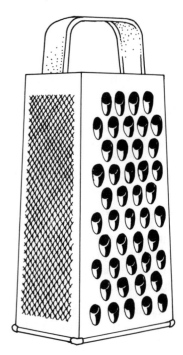

Carving fork

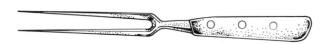

Vegetable peeler

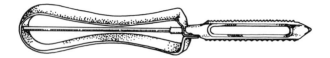

Zester

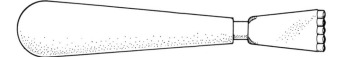

Pastry wheel

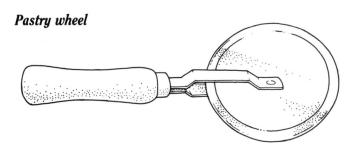

holes for grating; two sides have rough-edge punched holes for ripping foods, such as lemon peel, into small bits. The fourth side has a diagonal slit for slicing foods.

- A **zester** has tiny, sharp-edge holes that are useful for cutting orange, lemon, or lime peel. The advantage of using a zester, rather than a knife, is that the zester does not cut into the white pith attached to the peel, which is bitter.
- A **melon baller** usually has two scoops—one small and one large—that are used to scoop out melons. Stainless steel is best for a sharp edge and wooden handles are less slippery than plastic.
- The **pastry wheel** is a round, rotating blade on a handle. It is used mostly to cut pizza but can also be used to cut rolled-out dough.
- **Kitchen shears** are handy for cutting string or paper, fresh herbs, or string beans. Buy forged carbon-steel serrated blades and make sure they can be taken apart easily for cleaning.

Hand tools, such as those in the illustrations, used for mixing include whips, spatulas, and pastry blenders.

- The **wire whip** or whisk has an excellent application when preparing sauces. Great chefs have always had a wire whip available when preparing those famous sauces—stir a sauce with a wire whip and 95 percent of the time the sauce will not curdle or break down! There are heavy whips that have relatively few wires and are used for general mixing and beating, especially of heavy liquids, and there are balloon whips or piano wire whips that have many flexible wires. Balloon whips are best for whipping egg whites or cream and for mixing thinner liquids.
- **Rubber spatulas** have a rubber flap on the end that is useful for mixing thinner batters and liquids and, probably more important, for scraping out bowls to the last drop.
- The **pastry blender** looks like an arc of metal blades. The blades are attached to either a wooden or plastic handle. The pastry blender is used to evenly blend fat with flour to make pie crust and biscuits.

Other equipment include timers, thermometers, and can openers.

- A **timer** is a very simple, yet vital, piece of equipment. Get one that rings loudly and that you can take with you if you leave the kitchen. It is now possible to buy a digital timer and clock for under $20. Some can even be set to keep two or more times.
- There are several different thermometers needed in the home kitchen: a **refrigerator thermometer** that should be hung in the warmest area of your refrigerator to make sure the refrigerator stays below 45°F, a freezer ther-

Wire whips

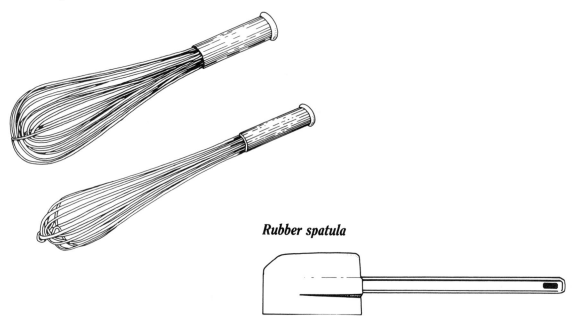

Rubber spatula

Pocket thermometer

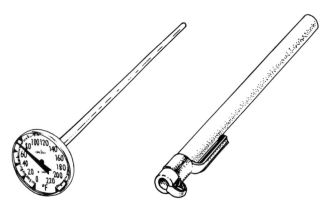

mometer that should be hung in the warmest part of your freezer to make sure it stays at or below 0°F, an **oven thermometer** that regularly tests the oven temperature in different places to make sure the thermostat is working properly, a **meat thermometer** that tests temperature of roasted meats as well as poultry and turkey, and a **pocket thermometer** or **instant read** thermometer such as the one in the pic-

ture that can be put into any food for a temperature reading within 10 seconds. Pocket thermometers usually go from 0° to 220°F and are now available with digital readout. Although they give a quicker reading, they require a new battery from time to time.

- A hand-held **can opener** takes up less space than an electric can opener, so it is recommended. There are two types of can openers:

gear-driven or a friction can opener. With the friction can opener, you spear the can to open it and then it clings tightly to the edge of the can while you wind around. The gear-driven can opener takes less muscle and is more efficient. It costs under $6.

KITCHEN EQUIPMENT WITH GOOD NUTRITION IN MIND

Nonstick Pots and Pans
Fry pans were the first cookware marketed with nonstick finish. Now, almost every cookware and bakeware item is available with a nonstick finish. There are griddles, saucepans, casseroles, muffin pans, cookie sheets, Dutch ovens, egg poachers, cake pans, deep fryers, and waffle bakers. Using nonstick pans, you can cut in half or more the amount of oil usually used to saute.

Wok
A wok is an ancient form of cooking equipment originating with the Chinese. It is available in both electric and gas versions. It is relatively simple to operate and inexpensive. Its round bottom allows foods to be stir-fried with a minimum of oil. Preheat the wok, add a small amount of cooking oil, and lightly fry the food items for a very short period of time. Vegetables and thinly sliced meats are a favorite. Choose a wide (14 inches is good), deep wok so that you can keep foods moving while stir-frying.

Steamers
Cooking with steam enjoys tremendous popularity among the health-conscious. Although any product can be cooked with steam, vegetables have always been a favorite. In steam cookery the product does not come in contact with the cooking medium, only steam. Steam equipment can be either the pressure or nonpressure variety. The pressure cooker is quickly gaining the same popularity it had years ago. Its many virtues include the quick cooking of foods such as vegetables so they retain their color, flavor, and nutrients.

Many different types of pressurized and non-pressurized steamer equipment are available. The simplest and most inexpensive option is to buy a steamer basket (it costs less than $8) that fits into one of your covered pots. If you are interested in a set, a typical nonpressurized set may include an 8-quart stock pot, two steamer basket inserts (one with small holes for rice and one with larger holes for vegetables), and a cover with vents to release excess steam. The pressurized set will include a thick-walled pot and interlocking cover. Remember that the pressurized version will create very strong pressure of approximately 15 pounds per square inch (psi) and produce an internal temperature in excess of 250°F. In other words, if you should get burned by steam, it is really worse than being burned by boiling water!

Juice Extractor
With continuous emphasis on good health and cooking methods that promote low-fat and sufficient nutrient intake, the juicer is an excellent piece of equipment that has been an integral part of health food stores for a long time. An excellent juice extractor can be bought for under $100 that can make any kind of fruit or vegetable juice. It has a heavy-duty motor that extracts the juice from the fruit or vegetable and removes the pulp, which you must then clean out. The juicer can make fresh juices from various types of vegetables and fruits, either fresh, canned, or even frozen! Carrots, beets, and celery are popular vegetables, while strawberries, bananas, pears, apples, and raspberries are favorite fruits. Fruits that have an excessive water content such as melons are generally not used in the juicer. Although drinking juice is not as nutritious as eating the raw fruit or vegetable, fresh juice is tasty and certainly better for you than drinking soft drinks!

Hot-Air Popcorn Popper
A hot-air popcorn popper is an excellent method of providing low-calorie, high-fiber snacks. Hot air pops the popcorn in approximately five to ten minutes.

Fat Separator

The fat separator is a measuring cup with an unusual spout that allows you to pour out meat juices, stock, or soup without the fat, which remains in the cup. It is convenient when you need to degrease a sauce without waiting for the fat to become solid.

Two-Piece Nonstick Meat Loaf Pan

You can easily eliminate fat from meat loaf by using a two-piece set consisting of a ridged, perforated insert pan that permits fat to drain into a solid outer pan. Both pans are commonly coated with a nonstick finish such as Silverstone.

❖ ❖ ❖

CHAPTER EIGHT

MEAT AND POULTRY

MEAT

Meat is the flesh of domestic animals—beef and veal from cattle, pork and ham from hogs, and lamb from sheep. Meats are divided into two groups: red and white (based on color). Red meats include beef and lamb. White meats include veal and pork. Another group includes variety meats, which encompass liver, kidneys, heart, tongue, and sweetbreads (organs of the animal such as the intestines).

Purchasing

All meats are inspected by the U.S. Department of Agriculture for wholesomeness, in other words, that it is safe to eat. Some meats, but not all, are voluntarily graded. Beef, veal, and lamb are graded as prime, choice, or select. (Pork is not graded because there is little variation in quality.) The grade is determined by the age of the animal and the amount of marbling (fat) in the meat, and it indicates how tender, juicy, and flavorful the meat is. Prime, which is the top grade seen mostly in white tablecloth restaurants, has the most fat, while choice has less. Even though the difference in marbling between choice and select is small, select grades of meat are lower in fat. Most of the meats at the supermarket are choice. Select meats may be sold as a house brand or an economy meat.

If purchasing fresh meat, avoid any with a sour smell, slimy touch, or odd color such as brown or green—this indicates bacteria or mold. The color should be as follows.

- Beef: bright cherry red
- Pork: pale pink
- Lamb: pink
- Veal: pinkish white

Table 25 is a guide to how much to purchase.

Nutrition

Meat is a good source of many important nutrients, including protein, iron, copper, phosphorus, zinc, and B vitamins—thiamin, riboflavin, niacin, B6, and B12. Meat is, of course, also a significant source of fat, saturated fat, and cholesterol. Over the past number of years, the amount of fat (calories and cholesterol too) found in beef and pork has been trimmed—both because the animals are leaner and because the meats are being more carefully trimmed before you buy them.

These meats are indeed leaner and can be sensibly worked into your diet when lean cuts are chosen (see the following list) and they are well-trimmed; cooking methods are used that do not add fat (such as roasting or broiling); and serving sizes are kept sensible (3 ounces or less).

The lean cuts of meat include the following:

- Beef—Cuts from the round (eye of round, top round, bottom round, round tip); sirloin (top and bottom sirloin steak, top sirloin roast); extra lean ground beef (usually 15 to 18 percent fat).
- Pork—Cuts from the tenderloin, leg (fresh boneless ham)

❖ *Servings* Per Pound Chart—Veal* ❖

	Number of Servings
Rib	
Bone-in cuts (chops, roasts)	2½
Boneless roast	4
Short ribs	2
Shoulder	
Blade roast or steak	2½
Arm roast or steak	2½
Boneless shoulder roast	3½
Leg (Round)	
Boneless rump roast	3½
Leg cutlets	4
Boneless steak	4
Bone-in steak	3½
Foreshank and Breast	
Boneless breast	3
Bone-in breast	1½
Riblets	2
Cross cut shank	2
Loin	
Bone-in cuts (chops, roast)	2½
Boneless cuts	4
Sirloin	
Bone-in cuts	3
Boneless cuts	4
Other Cuts	
Veal for stew	4
Ground	4
Cubed steak	4
Cubes for kabobs	4

*A serving is about 3 ounces of cooked meat.

- Veal—All trimmed cuts except commercially ground and veal patties. (Some good choices include loin chop, rib chop, top round steak, or arm steak.)
- Lamb—Leg of lamb, loin chops

Some people think well-marbled meat tastes better than less well-marbled meat. However, the tasty cuts are not all high in fat. For example, well-trimmed cuts from the round (or rear leg) cuts of the animal are tender if prepared appropri-ately and they are lower in fat than well-marbled meat.

Storing

Fresh meat should be stored in the store's packaging for up to the number of days given in Table 26. For longer storage, either rewrap the meat or put another layer of wrap over the store's package. This is necessary because the plastic wrap used on meat lets some air into the package so if you freeze it as is, freezer burn will develop. Wrap tightly, getting out all the air, label with the name and date, and put into the freezer.

When thawing frozen meats, place the wrapped product in the refrigerator a day or two ahead and allow it to thaw completely or put it in the microwave oven set on a defrost or thaw cycle. Never thaw meat on the kitchen counter, as it could cause food poisoning.

Cooking Light and Healthy

To cook meat in a light and healthy manner, there are six simple steps to take.

1. Start with a lean meat.
2. Trim visible fat before cooking.
3. If using a dry heat cooking method, allow for the fat to pour off as the meat cooks.
4. If using a moist heat cooking method, chill the meat juices after cooking (or use a fat separator cup) to remove the fat.
5. If stir-frying, use a nonstick pan and a small amount of oil.
6. Trim off remaining visible fat before eating.

When cooking tender cuts of meat you will want to utilize the dry heat cooking methods. These include roasting, broiling, pan-broiling, grilling, stir-frying, and sauteing. When cooking less tender cuts of meat, you will want to choose a moist heat method such as braising. Table 27 shows which cooking methods work best with each cut of meat, and see also the general pointers, which summarize the steps involved in each method.

Some not-so-tender meats can be cooked with dry heat if they are marinated before cooking. Marinating can be used successfully to tenderize small cuts of meat such as flank steak (this is used

❖ *Table 25   Servings of Meat Per Pound* ❖

Knowing the approximate number of cooked servings to expect from a given piece of meat helps you judge quantities to buy. A serving is about 3 ounces of cooked, lean meat.

Servings-per-pound Chart—Beef

Roasts	Number of Servings	Pot Roasts	Number of Servings
Rib Eye Roast	3	Arm Pot Roast, Chuck	2
Rib Roast	2	Blade Roast, Chuck	2½
Rump Roast, Round	2	Bottom Round Roast	3
Rump Roast, Boneless, Round	3	Cross Rib Pot Roast, Chuck	2½
Tip Roast, Round	4	Heel of Round	2
Top Round	3	Shoulder Pot Roast, Boneless	2½
Eye of Round Roast	4		
		Braising Steaks	
Broiling Steaks		Arm Steak, Chuck	2½
Cubed Steak	4	Blade Steak, Chuck	2½
Flank Steak	4	Flank Steak	3
Porterhouse Steak, Loin	2½	Round Steak	3
Sirloin Steak	3	Tip Steak, Round	3
Rib Eye Steak	3		
Rib Steak	2	**Other Cuts**	
Rib Steak, Boneless	2½	Beef for Stew	4
T-Bone, Loin	2	Brisket	3
Tenderloin (Filet Mignon) Steak	3	Ground Beef	4
Top Loin Steak	2	Short Ribs	2
Top Loin Steak, Boneless	3	Beef Variety Meats (tongue, heart,	
Top Round	4	brains, sweetbread)	5
		Liver, Kidney	4

Servings-per-pound Chart—Pork

Roasts	Number of Servings	Other Cuts	Number of Servings
Leg (Fresh Ham), Bone-in	3	Back Ribs, Loin	1½
Leg (Fresh Ham), Boneless	4	Bacon (Regular), sliced	4
Smoked Ham, Bone-in	3	Canadian-Style Bacon, Loin	5
Smoked Ham, Boneless	4 to 5	Country-Style Back Ribs	1½
Smoked Ham, Canned	4 to 5	Country-Style Loin Ribs	2
Loin Blade, Bone-in	2	Cubes, Various	4
Top Loin (Rolled), Boneless		Hocks (Smoked or Fresh)	1½
(Smoked or Fresh)	3½	Pork Sausage	4
Center Loin	3	Spareribs	1¼
Smoked Loin	3	Tenderloin	4
Sirloin	2½		
Arm Picnic Shoulder (Bone-in)		**Variety Meats**	
(Smoked or Fresh)	2	Brains	5
Smoked Shoulder Roll	3	Heart	5
Blade Shoulder Boneless		Kidney	4
(Smoked or Fresh)	3	Liver	4
Chops and Steaks			
Blade Chops or Steaks	2½ to 3½		
Boneless Chops, Loin	4		
Loin Chops	2½		

❖ *Table 25 Continued* ❖

Servings-per-pound Chart—Pork	
Chops and Steaks	**Number of Servings**
Rib Chops	2½
Smoked (Rib or Loin) Chops	2½
Smoked Ham (Center Slice)	3½

Source: The Meat Board's Lessons on Meat (1990). National Live Stock and Meat Board. Reprinted with permission.

to make London broil) or round steak. Marinades contain an acid ingredient such as citrus juice, wine, or vinegar that penetrate the surface of the meat (only about ¼ inch) and tenderize it. Meat should always be marinated in the refrigerator, in a nonaluminum container (aluminum reacts with the acid in the marinade), and the meat should be turned frequently. Plan on about ½ cup marinade for every pound of meat. Do not marinate meat more than 24 hours (it will get overmarinated and mushy) and don't use the marinade as a sauce unless it is boiled first (to prevent food poisoning).

Testing for doneness in meat is crucial because the quality goes downhill rapidly when overcooked. Overdone meat is dry, tough, stringy, less flavorful, less juicy, and harder to carve.

Beef and lamb are the only meats that are served at various degrees of doneness. Pork and veal are always cooked to the stage of well done. Because some pork (it's only a very small percentage now) is contaminated with a parasite, it is

❖ *Table 26 Meat Storage Time* ❖

Food quality declines after the time shown on this chart.

	Storage Time			Storage Time	
	Days in the Refrigerator at 35° to 40°F (2° to 4°C)	Months in the Freezer at 0°F (−18°C) or Less		Days in the Refrigerator at 35° to 40°F (2° to 4°C)	Months in the Freezer at 0°F (−18°C) or Less
Fresh Meats			**Processed Meats**		
Roasts (beef and lamb)	3–5	6–12	Ham (whole)	7	1–2
			Ham (half)	5	1–2
Roasts (pork and veal)	3–5	4–8	Ham (slices)	3	1–2
			Luncheon meats	3–5*	Freezing not
Steaks (beef)	3–5	6–12	Sausage (dry, semi-	14–21	recommended
Chops (lamb)	3–5	6–9	dry)		
Chops (pork)	3–5	3–4	Sausage (smoked)	5–7	1
Ground and stew meats	1–2	2–3	Sausage (pork)	1–2	2–3
Variety meats	1–2	3–4	**Cooked Meats**		
			Cooked meat and meat dishes	3–4	2–3
Processed Meats					
Bacon	7	1	Gravy and meat broth	1–2	2–3
Frankfurters	7	½			

*After a vacuum-sealed package is opened.
Unopened vacuum-sealed packages can be stored in the refrigerator for up to 2 weeks.

❖ *Table 27 Recommended Cooking Methods* ❖

Retail Cut Name	Cooking Method	Retail Cut Name	Cooking Method
Beef		**Pork**	
Chuck Arm Pot Roast	Moist	Spareribs	Dry/Moist
Chuck Arm Steak	Moist	Fresh Ham, Whole, Boneless	Dry
Chuck 7-bone Pot Roast	Moist	Fresh Ham, Center Slice	Dry/Moist
Chuck Blade Roast/Steak	Dry/Moist	Smoked Ham	Dry
Chuck Shoulder Roast, Steak, Boneless	Moist	Smoked Pork Jowl	Moist
Chuck Top Blade Roast/Steak, Boneless	Moist	Cubed Steak	Dry/Moist
Chuck Under Blade Roast/Steak, Boneless	Dry/Moist	Ground Pork	Dry
Chuck Mock Tender	Moist	Sausage	Dry/Moist
Chuck Eye Roast, Boneless	Dry/Moist		
Shank, Cross Cuts	Moist	**Lamb**	
Brisket, Point/Flat Half, Boneless	Moist	Shoulder Chops	Dry/Moist
Flank Steak	Dry/Moist	Breast	Dry/Moist
Rib/Ribeye Roast/Steak	Dry	Shank	Moist
Loin, Top Loin Steak, Boneless	Dry	Rib Roast/Chops	Dry
Loin, T-bone Steak	Dry	Loin Roast/Chops	Dry
Loin, Top Sirloin Steak, Boneless	Dry	Leg Sirloin	Dry
Loin, Tenderloin Steak	Dry	Leg Center Slice	Dry
Round Steak	Dry/Moist	Leg Roast	Dry
Round, Heel of	Moist	Ground Lamb	Dry/Moist
Round, Top Roast/Steak	Dry	Shoulder Roast	Dry
Round, Bottom Roast	Dry/Moist		
Round, Bottom Steak	Dry/Moist	**Variety Meats**	
Round, Eye Roast/Steak	Dry/Moist	Brains	Dry/Moist
Round, Rump Roast, Boneless	Dry/Moist	Heart	Dry/Moist
Round, Bottom Roast/Steak	Dry/Moist	Kidney	Dry/Moist
Round, Tip Roast/Steak	Dry/Moist	Liver	Dry/Moist
Cube Steak	Dry/Moist	Sweetbreads	Dry/Moist
Beef for Stew	Moist	Tongue	Dry/Moist
Ground Beef	Dry/Moist		
		Veal	
Pork		Rump Roast	Dry
Shoulder Arm/Blade Roast/Steak	Dry/Moist	Cutlets	Dry
Smoked Shoulder Picnic	Dry/Moist	Ground Veal	Dry
Loin Roast/Chops	Dry/Moist	Blade Steaks, Arm Steaks, Round Steaks,	
Loin, Country Style Ribs	Dry/Moist	Cubed Steaks	Dry/Moist
Loin, Tenderloin Whole	Dry/Moist	Shoulder Roast	Dry/Moist
Smoked Loin Chops	Dry	Boneless and Bone-in Rib or Loin Chops	Dry/Moist
Smoked Canadian Style Bacon	Dry	Riblets, Boneless Breast, Cross Cut Shanks,	
Bacon	Dry	Veal Cubes	Moist

Source: *National Live Stock and Meat Board, reprinted with permission.*

recommended that you always cook pork well done, about 160°F. Doneness can be determined by a combination of several methods:

1. If cooking a roast, you can insert a thermometer and compare doneness according to a tem-

perature chart (see Table 28). Remember to keep the thermometer away from the bone, or it will register a higher than normal temperature.

2. When broiling, many chefs prefer to use the

❖ Table 28 Recommended Cooking ❖
Temperatures and Degrees of Doneness

Meat	Internal Temperature
Fresh Beef	
Rare*	140°F (60°C)
Medium rare	150°F (66°C)
Medium	160°F (71°C)
Well done	170°F (77°C)
Fresh Veal	170°F (77°C)
Fresh Lamb	
Medium rare	140°F (60°C)
Medium	155°F (68°C)
Well done	160°F (71°C)
Fresh Pork	160°F (71°C)
Cured Pork	
Ham, raw	165°F (74°C)
Ham, fully cooked	140°F (60°C)
Canadian bacon	160°F (71°C)

Degrees of Doneness

Rare:	140°F; red in center third, reddish pink to outer surface.
Medium rare:	150°F; reddish pink in center third, pink to light brown to outer surface.
Medium:	160°F; light pink in center, light brown to outer surface.
Well done:	170°F; light brown in center, darker brown to outer surface.

Note: Meat products continue to cook after removal from the heating appliance. It is not uncommon to encounter a 2° to 7°F post cooking temperature rise in the product. The extent of this rise depends on cooking conditions, such as rate of heating, length of standing time, and leaving the product covered or uncovered.
*Rare beef is popular, but you should know that cooking it to only 140°F means some food poisoning organisms may survive.

2. When broiling, many chefs prefer to use the touch-testing method. Rare meat is soft, medium meat is medium firm, and well-done meat is firm to the touch.
3. Another time-honored favorite method of checking the doneness of a broiled steak is cutting a small slit in the steak (now that's really cheating!) but is alright in terms of helping the novice developing the touch-test tech-

nique. Rare beef is pink on the edges and red in the center; medium beef has only a little pink in the center; well-done steak has no pink at all.

Roasting Roasting is a simple method of cooking but requires a relatively long cooking time. Red meats that are roasted usually refer to meat items (as opposed to baked goods) that are large in size, thawed if previously frozen, and cooked in an oven. The meat item may be seasoned, if desired. The meat should be placed on a rack in an open pan, fat side up without the addition of water or any other liquid. The meat should not come in contact with its drippings or else it will simmer. Next you place the meat thermometer in the thickest part of the meat, not touching the bone (or it will read a higher than normal temperature). A general oven temperature for roasting meat is 275°–350°F. Lower temperatures usually mean less shrinkage, extended cooking time, and ultimately a more juicy roast. Some commercial food service establishments use very large cuts of meat (such as a steamship round of beef) and roast at temperatures of 200°–250°F to avoid drying out and excessive doneness of the surface of the meat before the interior is cooked. Table 5 is a timetable for roasting, broiling, and braising.

The term "baking" is really the same as "roasting" when referring to meats. The use of either term depends strictly on the type of item being cooked. Typical items that are baked include some hams and most popularly the infamous "meat loaf" which may contain one or a combination of different ground meats—veal, pork, beef, turkey, etc. Although it is a simple item to make, it enjoys much popularity in the food service industry because of its low cost and many variations.

To carve the roasted meat, follow these directions.

1. Remove the meat from the oven and let it stand 15–30 minutes before carving. This will allow the juices to settle evenly throughout the meat and will provide you with very juicy pieces of meat.
2. When using a carving knife, be sure that it is very sharp. When you "hack away" at a roast

POINTERS FOR COOKING MEAT

General

1. Use dry heat cooking methods (roasting, broiling, grilling, stir-frying) for tender pieces and moist heat (braising) for not-so-tender (or tender) meats. Using dry heat on a not-so-tender piece of meat will result in dryness and toughness.

2. Use tongs, not a fork, to handle meat, so you don't lose any juices which keep the meat moist and tasty.

3. The larger the meat, the lower the heat. The thinner the meat the higher the heat. This is important for even cooking.

4. Always cut meat across the grain to make it more tender.

Roasting

5. Put meat fat side up on a rack in a roasting pan so the fat can baste the meat and the rack holds the roast out of the drippings.

6. Don't season before cooking because the seasoning won't penetrate. Also, salt interferes with the meat browning.

7. Use a moderate oven—275°–350°F is best. A moderate oven is important so the meat has the best flavor and taste, as well as yield. Cooking meat at higher temperatures significantly reduces the number of servings you will get out of it.

8. Turn the roasting pan around during cooking to make up for the uneven temperatures in the oven.

9. Use a thermometer to determine doneness, and remove the roast when it is 5–10 degrees below the desired reading because the meat continues to cook after being pulled from the oven.

10. Let the roast sit for at least 20–30 minutes before carving because the juices in the roast are still flowing and if cut too soon, the juices will flow from the meat.

Broiling and Grilling

11. These methods are not a great choice for pork or veal because these meats are served well done and broiling or grilling will dry them out too much.

12. Don't season meat before broiling or grilling because salt interferes with browning.

13. The more well done you want a piece of meat to be, or the thicker it is, the longer the cooking time and the further from the heat source. Otherwise, the outside of the meat will be cooked but the inside will not be done.

14. To make criss-cross grid marks when grilling meat, put meat diagonally on grill. When the side is half done, rotate the meat 90 degrees.

15. Turn meat on broiler when top is browned.

16. Turn meat on grill when the juices begin to flow on the top and the bottom has browned.

17. Touch-test meat frequently, using the following guidelines:
    - Rare—soft
    - Medium—medium firmness, some resistance when pressed
    - Well-done—firm, resists pressing with finger

Stir-frying

18. Cut up thin strips or diced portions of meat, poultry, fish, vegetables, or any combination.

19. Coat the cooking surface with a thin layer of oil or vegetable cooking spray.

20. Preheat equipment to high temperature.

21. Don't overload the pan because the food will not cook evenly or quickly.

22. Stir food rapidly during cooking.

23. When meat is almost done, add small pieces of vegetables such as broccoli, cauliflower, zucchini, sprouts, carrots, mushrooms, tomatoes, or green onions, as they cook quickly.

Braising

24. Before browning, make sure meat is dry. Coat small pieces of meat in flour and shake off excess. Do not season meat before cooking—instead season during the last 30 to 45 minutes of cooking.

25. Brown meat over high heat, then add liquid, reduce heat, and cover pot.

26. Cover the meat from one- to two-thirds with liquid unless it is a stew and then the meat is completely covered.

27. Cook meat until fork tender.

with a dull knife, you ruin its appearance and will end up with less meat. Either use a proper carving knife, straight or serrated edge, or use an electric knife.

3. If you want very thin slices, consider the use of a small, hand-operated slicer, or an electric slicer if available.

4. Always cut across the natural grain when carving—this helps tenderize the meat even more.

Broiling and Grilling Before broiling or grilling, you can season meats with your favorite seasoning (see Table 30), but it is suggested that you not salt the steaks—the juices will be drawn out from the meat and make the product drier. Place thicker cuts of meat and meat to be cooked well done farther from the heat. When using thinner cuts of meat (less than ½ inch) for broiling, you may place the meat on a rack while still frozen.

❖ *Table 29   Timetable for Roasting, Braising,* ❖
and Broiling Meats

Meat	Cooked at	Will Cook to	In About* (minutes/pound)
Roasting			
Beef or veal	300°–325°F	Rare	15–25
	300°–325°F	Medium	20–30
	300°–325°F	Well	25–35
Pork	300°–325°F	165°F—Well	30–40
Lamb	300°–325°F	Rare	20–30
	300°–325°F	Medium	25–35
	300°–325°F	Medium	30–40

Type/Cut			Time** (hours)
Braising			
Beef			
Large cut—pot roast			2½–3½
Small cut—round, rump, sirloin tip, brisket			1½–2½
Veal			
Boneless shoulder roast			2–2½
Boneless breast, rolled and tied			1½–2½
Arm/blade steak			¾–1
Round steak			½–¾
Loin/rib chops (½-inch thick)			8 to 10 minutes
Loin/rib chops (¾- to 1-inch thick)			20 to 25 minutes
Pork			
Shoulder chops			1–2
Lamb			
Shoulder chops			½–¾
Shoulder roast			1¾–2¾

❖ *Table 29 Continued* ❖

Kind and Cut of Meat	Approximate Thickness (inches)	Degree of Doneness	Approximate Total Cooking Time*** (minutes)
Broiling			
Beef steaks	1	Rare	10 to 15
Club, porterhouse, rib, sirloin,	1	Medium	15 to 20
T-bone, tenderloin	1	Well	20 to 30
	1½	Rare	15 to 20
	1½	Medium	20 to 25
	1½	Well	25 to 40
	2	Rare	25 to 35
	2	Medium	35 to 45
	2	Well	45 to 55
Hamburgers	¾	Rare	8
	¾	Medium	12
	¾	Well	14
Lamb chops	1	Medium	12
Loin, rib, shoulder	1	Well	14
	1½	Medium	18
	1½	Well	22
Cured ham slices	¾	Well	13 to 14
Cook-before-eating	1	Well	18 to 20

These times are only guidelines; there are many factors, such as the shape of the meat, that will affect the time. Have an oven thermometer ready to determine doneness.

**The actual time required will vary. Cook until meat is fork tender. Check larger cuts with a meat thermometer.*

***Meat at refrigerator temperature at start of broiling.*

You will find the meat holds its shape better than in a fresh state. Table 29 is a time guide to broiling meats.

Following are guidelines for outdoor grilling.

- Place grill in well-ventilated area.
- Use pyramid method to start charcoal fire 20 to 30 minutes before cooking.
- Meat cuts can be cooked using either direct or indirect heat. Tender cuts like steaks, chops, and ground patties are perfect for the faster cooking direct heat method. Medium tender cuts, large/thick cuts, and roasts are better suited for indirect heat.
- Use meat thermometer to determine doneness.
- Allow large cuts to "set" 15 minutes before carving.

- Use a marinade to add flavor and/or tenderize meat cuts.
- Total cooking time varies with the cut, temperature of meat (refrigerator or room temperature), temperature of the coals, outdoor temperature, and desired degree of doneness of the meat.
- Reports link outdoor grilling to a possible increased risk of cancer. Whether or not these risks are of concern to the majority of consumers, the National Cancer Institute has made these following suggestions; you may wish to follow any of these tips during outdoor grilling:
  - Choose leaner cuts of meat and trim meat of outside fat to reduce the fat that drips on the coals.

❖ Table 30 Sodium-free Seasonings for Meat ❖

Form of Meat	Spices	Recommended Amounts	Form of Meat	Spices	Recommended Amounts
Ground	Allspice	½ to 2 tsp per pound	Ground	Oregano, dried	2 tsp per pound
Stew meat	Bay leaf, dried	1 to 2 leaves	Chops, steaks	Paprika (for dredging)	½ tsp to ¼ cup flour
Ground	Basil, dried	1½ tsp per 1½ pounds			
Ground	Cinnamon	¼ to ⅓ tsp per pound	Ground	Parsley (flakes)	2 tbsp per 2 pounds
Ground	Chili powder, without salt	1 to 2 tbsp per pound	Steaks, chops (lamb)	Rosemary	¼ tsp per pound
Ground	Cayenne	½ to 1 tsp per 2 pounds	Steaks, chops	Tarragon	¼ to ½ tsp to basting
Ground	Coriander	½ tsp per pound	Chops, steaks	Thyme (for dredging)	¼ to ½ tsp to flour
Chops, steaks	Curry	1 to 2 tbsp per 2 pounds			
Ground	Cumin	¼ tsp per pound			
Roasts	Garlic, fresh	cut slits and/or bury pod in meat			
Chops, steaks	Garlic, fresh	rub surface			
Ground or chops	Garlic, powder	¼ tsp per ¼ cup basting			
Ground	Ginger, ground	⅛ tsp			
Ground	Mace	⅛ tsp per pound			
Ground	Marjoram	½ to 1 tsp per pound			
Ground or chops	Mint	¼ tsp per pound or mint jelly			
Ground	Mustard, dried	½ tsp per pound			
Ground	Pepper	½ tsp per pound			
Ground	Nutmeg	⅛ tsp per pound			

Avoid overuse of the following sodium-containing seasonings with meat:

anchovies	olives (green)
bacon	pickles (sweet and dill)
baking powder	relishes
baking soda	commercial salad dressings
barbecue sauce	sauerkraut
bouillon cubes	salt (plain or seasoned)
catsup	commercial soup or sauce
chili sauce	mixes
tomato sauce (regular)	teriyaki sauce
MSG (monosodium	commercial horseradish
glutamate)	Worcestershire sauce
mustard (prepared)	mayonnaise

- Precook meats containing more fat, like spareribs or ground beef, to remove some of the fat before grilling.
- Raise the level of the grill so meat is farther away from the coals.
- Grill meat in aluminum foil until the last few minutes of cooking.
- Clean grill after every use.

Pan-broiling Pan-broiling is done on top of the range in a fry pan and works best with beef as opposed to poultry, fish, and shellfish. This is a method that should only be used for very thin cuts of meat. The meat is placed in a preheated frying pan that does not contain oil or water and is left uncovered. As the meat is cooked slowly over medium heat, turn once and pour off the fat as it accumulates. This is a popular European technique due to the extreme shortage of oven and/or broiler space in traditionally small, older kitchens.

Stir-frying For stir-frying use a large, heavy skillet or, preferably, a wok. Either put a small amount of oil in the wok or use a vegetable cooking spray. The wok should be heated until very hot before you begin cooking. Because stir-frying is such a quick cooking process using high heat, it is a good idea to line up your ingredients by the wok before cooking. Here are some tips for preparing your ingredients.

- Partially freeze the meat so you can slice it very thin (this way it cooks quicker) against the grain into strips.
- Slice vegetables the same size and thickness as the meat so they cook evenly—diagonally slicing vegetables exposes more surface area so they cook quicker.

- Make sure none of the ingredients are watery—water will make the fat splatter.

Once you start cooking, be careful you don't overcook the meat. Also cook the firmest vegetables first and the more tender vegetables toward the end for even cooking. Only cook them until crisp-tender. Do not put too much into the wok at once or else they won't really get stir-fried and will wind up being soggy. Using a utensil keeps the food in motion.

Braising Braising is one of the most popular methods of moist heat cookery for meats. Both large pieces of meat, such as pot roast, are braised, as well as small pieces such as cubed or stew meat. The meat is coated with flour and lightly browned in hot oil to provide color for the meat and to seal in the juices.

A small amount of liquid, such as water, stock, wine, or fruit/vegetable juice, is added, and the meat is cooked until tender. If cooking cubed or stew meat, the meat is generally covered with liquid. If cooking a roast, liquid will generally cover from one-third to two-thirds of the roast. Table 5 is a time guide to braising meat. To remove the fat from the braising liquid at the end of cooking, use a fat separator cup (see Chapter 7) or refrigerate the liquid until the fat hardens and then lift off the fat.

Microwave Cooking With the growing popularity of the microwave oven, many meat dishes can be prepared in 20 minutes or less. Because microwaves vary from model to model, check your instruction booklet for actual cooking times and temperatures. As a general rule, most cuts should be microwaved at a lower power setting, such as medium or medium-low. Ground meat or reheated products may be cooked on higher power settings.

One of the keys to cooking meat in the microwave is the selection of the proper cut, in the appropriate size and shape. As a general rule, boneless cuts in uniform shapes and ground meats can be cooked successfully.

Here are some helpful microwave hints.

1. Roasts should not exceed 2 pounds and should have a uniform shape for best results.

2. Shape 1 pound of ground meat into 4½-inch-thick patties. Form a ¾-inch hole in the center of each, and top with seasoning mix for evenly cooked, well-browned burgers.

3. Arrange uniform meat, like patties or meatballs, in a circle, leaving a hole in the center of the circle.

4. Small portions cook faster than large portions and thin portions cook faster than thick portions.

5. Stir dishes with a high liquid content, like soup and stews, to redistribute the heat from the outside to the inside.

6. Cover meat with waxed paper to prevent the meat dish from drying out and to prevent splattering.

7. Use a rotating device to help facilitate uniform cooking, if possible.

POULTRY

Purchasing

All poultry and poultry products are inspected by the USDA to ensure that they are wholesome, unadulterated, and truthfully labeled. Inspection is mandatory and means the product is fit to eat. Of course, if you mishandle the product by, for instance, thawing it at room temperature, or if your supplier has mishandled the product, it may be unfit to eat.

There are different kinds of poultry, including chicken, turkey, duck, geese, guinea, and squab pigeon. Each kind of poultry is divided into classes that are based on age (Table 31). Age affects the tenderness of the bird and dictates the cooking method to use for maximum flavor and tenderness.

The following birds are mature and need moist-heat cooking such as simmering, steaming, braising, or pressure cooking to make them tender and develop their fuller flavor.

- Chicken: Mature chicken, hen, or fowl (sometimes called stewing chicken)
- Turkey: Mature turkey, old turkey
- Duck: Mature duck, old duck
- Goose: Mature goose, old goose
- Guinea: Mature guinea
- Pigeon: Pigeon

❖ Table 31 Poultry ❖

Kind/Class	Age	Weight (pounds)	Cooking Method*
Chicken			
Rock Cornish game hen	5–6 weeks	.75–2	Roast, broil, grill
Broiler	9–12 weeks	1.5–2.5	Roast, broil, grill
Fryer	9–12 weeks	2.5–3.5	Roast, broil, grill
Roaster	3–5 months	5–7	Roast, stew
Capon	4–5 months	6–9	Roast
Turkey			
Fryer-roaster	under 16 weeks	4–9	Roast
Young turkey	5–7 months	8–22	Roast
Duck			
Broiler or fryer duckling	under 8 weeks	2–4	Roast, broil
Roaster duckling	under 16 weeks	4–6	Roast
Other			
Young goose	under 6 months	6–10	Roast
Young guinea (related to pheasant)	about 6 months	.75–1.5	Roast
Squab pigeon	3–4 weeks	.75–1.0	Roast, broil, grill

*These are common cooking methods used with each different class of poultry. All of the above birds are young and tender and can be cooked using any cooking method.

Younger birds, which are most of what is available at the supermarket, are naturally tender and can be cooked using almost any style. Older birds are much less tender and must be cooked using moist heat, such as in stews.

In addition to purchasing whole birds, poultry parts are available and very popular; some examples are shown in the illustration. The following list explains some of the newer cuts of turkey breast that are available.

Fresh poultry should have unblemished skin without feathers or bruises. The skin should be smooth, soft, and moist without any indication of

Cuts of Turkey Breast	Description and Cooking Instructions*
Breast tenderloin	A separate muscle on the inside of each turkey breast half. The tenderloin lays against the bone and is easily removed. Broil or grill: 8–12 minutes per side (6 inches from heat) Bake at 400°F: 18–30 minutes
Breast cutlets	Cut from a boneless, skinless half turkey breast, against the natural meat grain, cutting down on a 45-degree angle, ⅛–¼ inch thick. Saute: 2–3 minutes per side Breaded, bake at 400°F: 6–8 minutes Unbreaded, bake at 350°F: 11–13 minutes
Breast slices	The same as cutlets, but cut ¼–⅜ inch thick. Saute: 3–4 minutes per side Breaded, bake at 400°F: 7–9 minutes Unbreaded, bake at 350°F: 13–15 minutes
Breast steaks	Cut from a boneless half turkey breast, ½–¾ inch thick. Broil or grill: 5–8 minutes per side

*Breast meat is done when the thickest part turns from pink to light in color. It is a very quick-cooking meat.

slime. The color of the skin, which ranges from white to deep yellow, is not a measure of nutrition value, flavor, tenderness, or fat content. The color is determined by the breed of bird and its diet.

Cut-up poultry

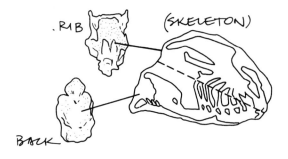

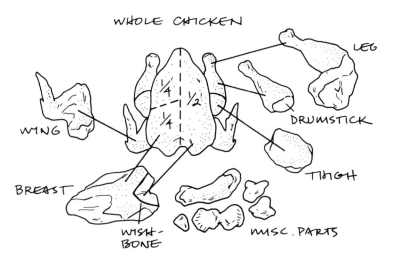

Chickens are generally fed corn and soybean meal, animal protein, and supplemental vitamins and minerals. Chickens with bright yellow skins also may have been fed feed containing marigold petals, alfalfa meal, or corn gluten meal, for example. Choose fresh poultry that is tightly wrapped in packaging free of tears, and check the label for any "sell by" or "best if used by" dates.

When buying frozen poultry, make sure the package is intact, rock hard, and stored below the frost line in the freezer. If you see much frozen moisture inside the package, the product has likely been thawed and refrozen. Discolored patches on the skin indicate freezer burn.

Due to concern about the amount of antibiotics given to chickens, what they are fed, and so on, some individuals choose to purchase organically grown chicken. This type of chicken is different than mass-produced chickens; it has much more flavor, but also tends to be tougher and more expensive. Organically grown chicken is commonly available at health food or natural food stores. Free-range chickens are also available—these are birds that have been raised outside of cramped cages, and generally have more flavor too.

Nutrition

In comparison to red meats, skinless white meat chicken and turkey are comparable in cholesterol but lower in total fat and saturated fat (Table 32). Chicken and turkey skin contains much of the bird's fat and should be removed before eating. If you compare the amount of fat in chicken to that found in turkey, you will no doubt be amazed. Chicken has about 50% more fat than turkey.

Chicken and turkey are rich in protein, niacin, and vitamin B6. They are also good sources of

❖ *Table 32   Nutritional Values* ❖
of Poultry Compared to Beef
(3.5 ounce cooked servings)

Name	Calories	Total Fat (grams)	Saturated Fat (grams)	Cholesterol (milligrams)
Chicken				
Dark and light meat, roasted, with skin	239	14	4	88
Dark meat, roasted, without skin	205	10	3	93
Light meat, roasted, no skin	173	5	1	85
Turkey				
Whole turkey, light and dark meat, without skin	150	3	1	98
Whole breast, meat and skin, roasted	189	7	2	75
Ground (burger)	193	11	3	58
Beef				
Lean hamburger, broiled, well-done	280	18	7	101
Rib roast, lean only, choice, roasted	243	14	6	80

Source: USDA Agriculture Handbooks

vitamin B12, riboflavin, iron, zinc, and magnesium. Chicken and turkey are always low in sodium.

Duck and goose are quite fatty, when compared to chicken and turkey, as they contain all dark meat.

Storing

When storing fresh poultry, remove it from the store's packaging and remove any giblets (neck, liver, gizzard, heart) because they spoil faster than the poultry itself. Rinse the poultry under cold water to remove the bacteria or other contaminants, pat dry with a paper towel, and store immediately wrapped loosely. Always wash your hands and work area thoroughly after handling raw

poultry. Store it in the coldest part of your refrigerator (where it won't drip onto any other food) and plan to use it within 1 to 2 days as it is quite perishable.

Fresh poultry can be frozen and stored in your freezer at 0°F or below for up to 6 months. Whole poultry and poultry parts should be repackaged in any type of moisture-resistant and airtight wrap such as freezer paper or heavy-duty aluminum foil to prevent freezer burn and the development of an off-flavor.

- If freezing a bird over 7 pounds, cut it into parts because it can't freeze fast enough in the home freezer and there will be a loss in quality.
- For poultry parts, wrap each one individually first in plastic wrap and then wrap them all together, as tightly as possible, in freezer paper or heavy-duty aluminum foil. This technique is especially helpful when the poultry parts are all different shapes.
- Always freeze poultry and stuffing separately because it would take too long for the stuffing to get frozen (and this may later cause food poisoning problems).

Date packages before storing and store so the freezing air will circulate around your packages and freeze them quickly. Poultry can remain frozen for 6 months (for parts) to 9 months (for whole birds).

Once cooked, poultry should not be held at room temperature, but should be put into the refrigerator right away, where it can be held for 3 to 4 days (stuffing and gravy for only 2 days). It is best to remove all the meat from the bones of a whole bird before you put it in the refrigerator. Wrap it loosely until completely cooled, then wrap tightly in plastic or foil.

Cooking Light and Healthy

To cook poultry in a light and healthy manner, do the following.

1. When roasting, broiling, or grilling, allow for the fat to drip away during cooking.
2. When braising, chill the meat juices after cooking (or use a fat separator cup) to remove the fat.

3. When stir-frying, use a nonstick pan and a small amount of oil.
4. Remove the skin before eating.

If you need to thaw the poultry before cooking, the safest and easiest way is to put it in the refrigerator ahead of time. Unless you are stewing or boiling poultry, you will need to thaw it. Thawing helps birds cook more evenly. Be sure to put the frozen product into some type of dish in case it drips. For thawing whole birds, use these times as a guide:

8–12 pounds	1–2 days
12–16 pounds	2–3 days
16–20 pounds	3–4 days
20–24 pounds	4–5 days

Thawing poultry parts requires 1 to 2 days in the refrigerator.

You can also thaw poultry in the microwave; follow manufacturer's instructions. Never thaw poultry at room temperature—some chicken is contaminated with a bacteria, Salmonella, that will grow like crazy at room temperature and possibly make you very sick.

Before cooking, some basic preparation must be done. The following rules should be followed to ensure delicious food that is safe to eat:

1. When handling raw poultry, be sure to select an area that is separate from the rest of the cooking area. For example, place a cutting board and knife at the far end of your counter.
2. Wash your hands thoroughly before, during, and after handling the poultry, without handling any other utensil, apron, or food. A really good technique is the use of plastic, disposable gloves.
3. Wash the poultry thoroughly under cold, running water. Run the water inside the cavity as well as on the outside to remove any blood that may be there.
4. After placing the bird into its cooking pan, thoroughly clean the work area with soap and water and dry off with a paper towel.

Before discussing the different ways to cook poultry, let's take a look at how to determine when poultry is done. Poultry should always be cooked

❖ **Table 33   Cooking Times for Poultry** ❖
Roasting at 325°F

Type of Poultry	Weight (pounds)	Approximate Cooking Time (hours)
Cornish game hen*	1¼–1½	1
Whole chicken,* unstuffed	2	1–1¼
Whole chicken,* unstuffed	3	1¼–1½
Whole chicken,* unstuffed	4	1½–2
Whole chicken,* unstuffed	5	1¾–2¼
Chicken parts, unstuffed (with bones)	1	¾–1
Boneless chicken	1	20–40 minutes
Whole turkey, unstuffed	6–8	2¼–3¼
Whole turkey, unstuffed	8–12	3¼–4
Whole turkey, unstuffed	12–16	4–4½
Whole turkey, unstuffed	16–20	4½–5
Whole turkey, unstuffed	20–24	5–5½
Whole turkey, stuffed	6–8	3–3½
Whole turkey, stuffed	8–12	3½–4½
Whole turkey, stuffed	12–16	4½–5½
Whole turkey, stuffed	16–20	5½–6½
Whole turkey, stuffed	20–24	6½–7

*These items are first put into a 425°F oven for 15 minutes to sear the surface of the bird and retain its natural juices. Then, the oven is lowered to 325°F for the rest of the cooking.

to the stage of well done and be juicy, not dry. Follow some simple rules:

1. Follow a cooking time guide (Table 33).
2. In order to be sure it is cooked well done, insert a meat thermometer in the thickest part of the thigh (not touching the bone), which should have an internal temperature of at least 180°F. The breast should cook to 170°F, and stuffing to 165°F. Do not overcook, as it will dry out.
3. The internal juices should be clear and not red.
4. The skin should be golden brown and the joints should be easily removable.
5. If you have stuffed the bird, be sure that the internal temperature of the stuffing is a minimum of 165°F. When birds are stuffed prior to cooking, it is best to cook at a lower temper-

ature and extend the cooking time to avoid overcooking the bird.

Age affects the tenderness of the bird and dictates the cooking method to use for maximum flavor and tenderness. Younger birds are naturally tender and can be cooked using any cooking method. Older birds are tough and therefore require moist-heat cooking methods (braising, simmering, poaching) to tenderize the meat.

Roasting   All young poultry may be roasted because their meat is tender. Although poultry is usually oven-roasted, it may also be spit-roasted or barbecued. Poultry roasts nicely because the skin (and the fat in it) keeps the bird moist during cooking.

A common practice in cooking large birds is to initially truss the bird, which means to tie the legs and wings together to make a compact unit. Trussing helps the bird cook evenly (otherwise the extended legs and wings will cook quicker than the breast) and have a more attractive appearance. The following are guidelines for trussing a bird:

1. Stand the bird on its end, breast toward you, and grab the neck bone. Wrap the center of a clean string (about 4 to 5 times the length of the bird) around the neck bone. The string is now in back of the chicken.
2. Lay the chicken on its back, and bring the string toward the tail end of the bird. Bring string forward, and cross over the ankles, pulling string tight.
3. Bring string up toward wing joint and flip the bird over.
4. Cross the string over the wings, pull tight, and tie securely. Cut off excess string.
5. Tuck wings under string to secure.

If you are planning on stuffing poultry, only stuff just before cooking. It may seem like a good idea to save time by stuffing your turkey in advance, but that's inviting trouble, because harmful bacteria can multiply in the stuffing and cause food poisoning. The cavity of the bird should be stuffed lightly, because stuffing expands as it cooks. Allow three-fourths of a cup of stuffing

for each pound of ready-to-cook poultry. Extra stuffing may be baked separately.

To keep the stuffing in a whole bird, you need to close the neck and body cavities. Fold the neck skin over the back and fasten with a skewer, trussing pins, or toothpicks. Twist the wingtips under the back of the turkey to rest against the neck skin. To close the body cavity, use skewers, or tuck ends of legs under a band of skin at the tail, or into metal "hock-locks," if provided, or tie legs together with clean string.

To roast, place the bird backside down (so the breast develops a crisp, golden color) on a rack in a roasting pan. You may want to rub the skin with oil to prevent cracking and blistering, although it isn't absolutely necessary. Start roasting at a high temperature—425°–450°F—to sear the surface of the bird and retain its natural juices. Then, the oven can be lowered to 325°–350°F for the rest of the cooking.

Whole birds and larger roasts should be allowed to stand 10–20 minutes before carving to avoid losing the juices when you slice the meat. The accompanying illustration shows how to carve a turkey.

Broiling and Grilling   Halves of tender young birds and fryer parts are best for broiling or grilling to ensure that the product is thoroughly cooked. Poultry is broiled or grilled slowly when compared to fish to prevent drying while ensuring doneness in the center.

Whether broiling or grilling, always season before cooking, and preheat the broiler or grill to moderately hot. Use tongs for turning to avoid piercing the poultry and losing valuable juices.

When broiling, place the chicken on a nonstick broiling pan and place about 3 inches from the heat. Cook until the outside is browned and the inside is cooked, but still moist and juicy, about 8 to 15 minutes per side. The actual cooking time will depend on the size of the poultry and intensity of the heat.

When grilling, place bone-in chicken pieces skin side down on a covered grill. Cook for 20 minutes, then turn and cook until the juices run clear, about 15 minutes more. Boned pieces will cook in about 8 to 12 minutes.

How to carve a turkey

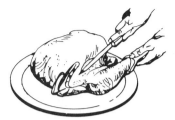

1. Separating the leg.

To remove the drumstick and thigh, hold the drumstick firmly with the fingers and pull it away from the body. At the same time, cut through the skin between the leg and the rest of the body. With the skin cut, the entire leg will pull away freely from the body.

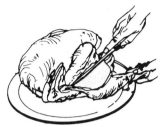

2. Removing the leg.

Pull the leg away from the body. If the joint connecting the leg to the backbone doesn't snap free, use a knife to sever it. Completely cut the dark meat away from the body by following the body contour with a knife.

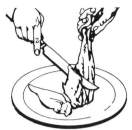

3. Slicing the dark meat.

Place the leg on a separate plate and cut through the connecting joint. The drumstick and thigh may now be individually sliced. Holding the drumstick with a napkin and tilting it at a convenient angle, slice toward the plate.

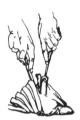

4. Slicing the thigh.

Hold the thigh firmly on the plate with a meat fork. Make even slices, parallel to the bone. Arrange the slices of dark meat on a plate. Repeat this process for the other leg.

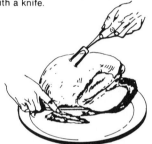

5. Preparing the breast.

Place the knife parallel and as close to the wing as possible. Using the meat fork to anchor the turkey, make a deep cut into the breast meat. Cut right to the bone. This is your base cut. All breast slices will stop at this vertical cut.

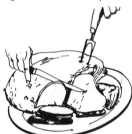

6. Carving the breast.

After you have made the base cut, begin slicing the breast meat. Start halfway up the side, carving downward and ending at the base cut. Start each new slice slightly higher up on the breast. Make your slices thin and even. Since poultry dries out quickly, slice only as needed.

Braising   Braising is actually a two-step process in which cut-up poultry, such as chicken, is sauteed or browned quickly, then liquid is added and the pot is covered. Cooking may be done on top of the stove or in a slow oven. Cooking time will vary from 40 minutes to 1½ hours. The poultry is done when it is fork tender and firm to the touch. A favorite braised chicken dish is chicken cacciatore, which means "hunter's style." The chicken is lightly browned and has seasonings, tomatoes, and other vegetables added to it and is simmered until the chicken is cooked.

Poaching   Poaching is cooking in a gently simmering liquid such as water, chicken stock, or white wine. Poaching is usually used to cook older birds, as it tenderizes them. Poaching is also used to cook whole birds for salad or cooked-chicken dishes.

To poach, bring the liquid to a boil and put in the poultry. Make sure the liquid covers the poultry completely. Reduce heat to a simmer; the liquid should barely bubble. The chicken is done when it is fork tender, the flesh changes color, and feels firm (but not hard). Poaching takes about 35 minutes per pound for whole birds, or about 12 minutes for chicken breasts. Be sure not to overcook (this is a common problem with poaching) as the poultry will be dry (even though it was cooked with a liquid).

GROUND BEEF, GROUND CHICKEN, AND GROUND TURKEY: A COMPARISON

❖ ❖ ❖

Ground meat has always enjoyed much popularity—it's inexpensive and very versatile in cooking. Recently ground beef has had some competition—ground chicken and ground turkey, the new kids on the block. Now don't expect to use these new products in the all-American entree, hamburgers, and enjoy the same juiciness and tenderness. Burgers made with ground turkey or ground chicken are quite different from those made with ground beef. A turkey burger is tight-textured and on the dry side. While ground chicken is certainly moister and more flavorful than ground turkey, it may still not be acceptable to your palate. To ease this problem, there's a simple solution: combine some ground poultry with beef. An acceptable ratio for taste as well as content is two parts poultry and one part lean ground beef, but you may want to first try a 50-50 combination. (Doing the same for meat loaf also produces a flavorful product that has less fat and saturated fat.) Ground chicken and turkey work really well in recipes that are sauced or spiced, like chili, lasagna, stuffed cabbage, sloppy joes, spaghetti sauce, and enchiladas.

For making burgers, you may want to add one egg white to each pound of ground turkey to add moisture. Follow these cooking guidelines.

- Broil: Broil on a nonstick pan 4 inches from the heat for 4 to 5 minutes on each side. Burger is thoroughly cooked when it springs back to the touch.
- Grill: Place burgers on hottest area of nonstick grill (or spray grill with vegetable oil) for 1 to 2 minutes on each side to brown. Then move burgers to outside of grill and continue to cook 3 to 4 minutes on each side until burger springs back when touched.
- Bake: Bake in 350°F oven for 15–20 minutes.

Be careful when purchasing ground chicken or turkey labeled "breast meat." Otherwise, the product will include ground up poultry parts and skin (and five times more fat).

If you want to stick to ground beef, it is available in different forms with varying fat contents. Although there may be variation from store to store, ground chuck is usually higher in fat than ground round, and ground sirloin is leaner than ground round. Some supermarkets label their ground beef regular (often 75 percent lean or fat-free), lean (often 80 percent lean), and extra lean (often 85 percent lean). Because these terms are defined differently depending on where you shop, it is best to ask your supermarket meat manager about the exact fat content in the ground meats, or select a sirloin steak and ask the butcher to trim it well and grind.

Another type of ground beef you may find at the supermarket is even lower in fat than ground sirloin and is 93 percent fat-free. This new low-fat ground beef, currently being used in some fast-food hamburgers, is made from very lean beef mixed with water and a binder to keep it moist. The binder may be carageenan (a carbohydrate derived from red seaweed), oat bran, or soy protein (derived from soybeans). These plant-derived ingredients help maintain the moisture in the cooked products.

Here is how it compares to other ground meats.

Product (3 ounces cooked)	Calories	Fat
Low-fat ground beef	149	7 grams
Extra lean ground beef	161	12
Lean ground beef	238	15
Ground turkey	183	10

If using low-fat ground beef at home, be aware that it cooks more quickly because of the lower fat content. It also tastes differently than regular ground beef: less meaty and less juicy. For this reason, it is probably best in combination dishes such as meat sauce and meat loaf. Here are some cooking tips when using low-fat ground beef.

- Do not overmix as overmixing creates a firm, compact texture.

- When making meat loaf or meatballs, do not use additional liquids (except sparingly) as the product may come out soft.
- When making hamburgers, do not squash them—it will take out the moisture and make them dry.

TURKEY DELI MEATS

❖ ❖ ❖

The variety of turkey deli meats never ends, as you see from this list. Why is there such interest in these products? It stems from the fact that, in most (but not all) cases, they contain less fat and saturated fat than their meat counterparts. However, you still need to read the label and check on the amount of fat per serving. Try to choose one with 4 grams of fat per ounce or less.

Turkey ham tastes like its pork look-alike, but generally with less than 5 percent fat. Since ham is defined as thigh meat, cured and smoked turkey thigh meat becomes turkey ham, and is available in reduced salt versions, too. Turkey ham comes in chunks, diced, or ground, or pre-sliced for instant use for breakfast or sandwiches.

Turkey franks are often lower in fat and calories but have the traditional all-American flavor. In some cases when the skin is ground in, such franks may be as fatty as their beef and pork counterparts. Try to select a frank with less than 6 grams of fat/frank.

Turkey bologna is made from lean turkey, and is seasoned, smoked, and cooked.

Turkey pastrami is lean and full of traditional pepper and garlic flavor. This dark turkey deli favorite is perfect for sandwiches, luncheon plates, or in an omelet.

Turkey sausages, such as Kielbasa, Polish and Italian sausage, are made from dark turkey meat that is cured, seasoned, smoked, and cooked.

Canadian bacon has its turkey counterpart. Some processors call it Canadian-style turkey ham.

RECIPES

CHICKEN-BEEF BURGERS

1 green onion
1 lb ground chicken
8 oz lean ground beef
½ cup soft whole wheat bread crumbs
3 tbsp barbecue sauce
3–4 grinds of black pepper
1 tsp Worcestershire sauce
⅛ tsp salt

1. Preheat grill.
2. With scissors, snip green onion finely into medium bowl. Add chicken, beef, bread crumbs, barbecue sauce, pepper, Worcestershire sauce, and salt, and mix well. Shape into patties, about ¾-inch thick.
3. Cook on preheated grill to desired doneness, about 5 minutes on each side for medium.

Serves 6

Nutrition Analysis:

Calories 182
Carbohydrate . . . . .3 grams
Fiber . . . . .0 grams
Fat . . . . .11 grams
Cholesterol . . . . .51 milligrams
Sodium . . . . .180 milligrams

BROILED MARINATED BEEF TOP LOIN

1 lb beef top loin, well trimmed
½ cup dry white wine
¼ cup low-sodium soy sauce
2 cloves garlic, minced

2 tbsp freshly squeezed lime juice
2 tbsp brown sugar
¼ cup sliced scallions
½ tsp freshly ground pepper

1. Stir together the wine, soy sauce, garlic, lime juice, brown sugar, scallions, and pepper. Place the beef in a dish. Pour the marinade over it. Cover and refrigerate for 24 hours, turning the meat 2 or 3 times while it marinates.
2. Preheat the broiler.
3. Drain the beef and then broil it, approximately 10 minutes on each side for medium rare.

Serves 4

Nutrition Analysis:
```
Calories . . . . . . . . . . . . . .215
Carbohydrate. . . . . . . . . .10 grams
Fiber . . . . . . . . . . . . . . . .0 grams
Fat. . . . . . . . . . . . . . . . . .7 grams
Cholesterol. . . . . . . . . . .64 milligrams
Sodium. . . . . . . . . . . . . .652 milligrams
```

BEEF STROGANOFF

¾ lb beef top round steak, boneless, trimmed
¼ lb fresh mushrooms, sliced
½ cup beef broth, condensed (low-sodium)
1 tbsp tomato juice
1 tsp Worcestershire sauce
⅛ tsp pepper
2 tbsp flour
1 cup low-fat yogurt or light sour cream
2 cups noodles, cooked, unsalted

1. Slice beef across the grain into strips ⅛-inch wide and 3 inches long.
2. Wash and slice mushrooms.
3. Cook beef strips and mushrooms in nonstick frying pan (use vegetable cooking spray) until brown.
4. Add broth, tomato juice, and seasonings. Cover and simmer 45 minutes.
5. Mix flour and low-fat yogurt until smooth. Stir into beef mixture. Cook, stirring constantly until thickened.
6. Serve over noodles.

Serves 4

Nutrition Analysis:
```
Calories . . . . . . . . . . . . . .281
Carbohydrate. . . . . . . . . .28 grams
Fiber . . . . . . . . . . . . . . . .2 grams
Fat. . . . . . . . . . . . . . . . . .8 grams
Cholesterol. . . . . . . . . . .78 milligrams
Sodium. . . . . . . . . . . . . .206 milligrams
```

BEEF AND VEGETABLE STIR-FRY

¾ lb beef round steak, boneless
1 tsp oil
½ cup carrots, sliced
½ cup celery, sliced
½ cup onions, sliced
1 tbsp soy sauce
⅛ tsp garlic powder
Dash pepper
2 cups zucchini squash, cut into thin strips
1 tbsp cornstarch
¼ cup water

1. Trim all the fat from steak. Slice steak across the grain into thin strips about ⅛-inch wide and 3 inches long. (Partially frozen meat is easier to slice.)
2. Heat oil in frypan. Add beef strips and stir-fry over high heat, turning pieces constantly, until beef is no longer red, about 3 to 5 minutes. Reduce heat.
3. Add carrots, celery, onion, and seasonings. Cover and cook until carrots are slightly tender, 3 to 4 minutes.
4. Add squash; cook until vegetables are tender-crisp, 3 to 4 minutes.
5. Mix cornstarch and water until smooth. Add slowly to beef mixture, stirring constantly.
6. Cook until thickened and vegetables are coated with a thin glaze.

Serves 4

Nutrition Analysis:
Calories 168
Carbohydrate. . . . . .8 grams
Fiber . . . . .2 grams
Fat. . . . . .5 grams
Cholesterol. . . . . .54 milligrams
Sodium. . . . . .210 milligrams

BEEF AND VEGETABLE FAJITAS

1 lb flank steak
1 large onion, sliced
1 sweet red pepper, sliced into strips
1 garlic clove, finely chopped
¼ cup lime juice
1 tbsp olive oil
1 tbsp balsamic vinegar
2 tbsp fresh coriander, chopped
¼ tsp ground cumin
⅛ tsp salt
8 flour tortillas

1. Place steak, onion, and red pepper in shallow dish. Combine garlic, lime juice, oil, vinegar, coriander, cumin, and salt; pour over steak and vegetables. Toss, cover, and refrigerate 2 hours.

2. Preheat broiler. Broil steak 8 to 10 minutes, one side; turn. Add vegetables; broil 10 more minutes or until meat is done. Cut meat at 45-degree angle in thin slices. Mound steak and veggies in tortillas; fold and serve.

Serves 4

Nutrition Analysis:
Calories 419
Carbohydrate. . . . . .43 grams
Fiber . . . . .2 grams
Fat. . . . . .12 grams
Cholesterol. . . . . .72 milligrams
Sodium. . . . . .119 milligrams

VEGETABLE PORK STIR-FRY

¾ lb pork tenderloin, cut in strips
1 tbsp vegetable oil
1½ cups sliced fresh mushrooms
1 large green pepper, cut in strips
1 zucchini, thinly sliced
2 ribs celery, diagonally sliced
1 cup thinly sliced carrots
1 clove garlic, minced
1 cup low-sodium chicken broth
2 tbsp light soy sauce
1½ tbsp cornstarch
3 cups hot cooked rice

1. Brown pork strips in oil in large skillet over high heat.

2. Push meat to side of skillet; add vegetables. Stir-fry vegetables approximately 3 minutes.
3. Combine broth, soy sauce, and cornstarch; add to skillet and cook until clear and thickened. Serve over rice.

Serves 6

Nutrition Analysis:
Calories 262
Carbohydrate. . . . . .36 grams
Fiber . . . . .3 grams
Fat. . . . . .5 grams
Cholesterol. . . . . .40 milligrams
Sodium. . . . . .302 milligrams

BRAISED VEAL STEAK WITH VEGETABLES

2 tsp vegetable oil
¾ lb veal shoulder arm steak, cut ¾- to 1-inch thick
¼ tsp salt
⅛ tsp coarse grind black pepper

1 small onion, thinly sliced
¼ cup water
3 medium unpeeled red potatoes, halved
½ lb snow peas, strings removed

1. Heat 1 teaspoon of the oil in 12-inch nonstick skillet. Add veal shoulder arm steak and brown, turning once. Remove veal from skillet. Sprinkle with salt and pepper, reserve.
2. Cook onion in skillet in remaining oil over medium heat until crisp-tender, about 3 minutes. Return veal to skillet. Add water. Cover and simmer over low heat 25 minutes. Arrange potatoes in skillet. Cover and continue cooking veal and potatoes until tender, 25 to 40 minutes. Add snow peas and continue cooking, covered, until peas are crisp-tender, about 5 minutes.
3. Arrange veal, potatoes, and snow peas on plate.

Using a fat separator cup, pour the fat off the pan liquid. Cook the defatted pan liquid over high heat until slightly thickened and spoon over veal steak.

Serves 3

Nutrition Analysis:

Calories 388
Carbohydrate. . . . . .42 grams
Fiber . . . . .4 grams
Fat. . . . . .8 grams
Cholesterol. . . . . .132 milligrams
Sodium. . . . . .258 milligrams

CHICKEN AND ZUCCHINI

3 chicken breast halves, boneless, without skin
2 tsp oil
1 clove garlic, cut in fourths
1 tbsp soy sauce, low-sodium
⅓ cup celery, thinly sliced
2-ounce can mushroom slices, drained
1 cup zucchini squash, cut in thin strips
2 tsp cornstarch
3 tbsp water

1. Slice chicken into thin strips, about ⅛-inch wide. (It is easier to slice chicken thinly if it is partially frozen.)
2. Heat oil in nonstick frypan. Add chicken and garlic.
3. Cook, stirring constantly, until chicken turns white, about 5 minutes. Remove garlic pieces.

4. Stir in soy sauce.
5. Add celery, mushrooms, and squash.
6. Cook, covered, until vegetables are tender crisp, about 4 minutes.
7. Mix cornstarch with water until smooth. Add slowly to chicken mixture, stirring constantly.
8. Continue cooking until ingredients are coated with a thin glaze, about 1 minute.

Serves 4

Nutrition Analysis:

Calories 183
Carbohydrate. . . . . .4 grams
Fiber . . . . .1 gram
Fat. . . . . .8 grams
Cholesterol. . . . . .62 milligrams
Sodium. . . . . .275 milligrams

LEMON BAKED CHICKEN

3 tbsp lemon juice
1½ tbsp. oil
1 tbsp onion, very finely chopped
¼ tsp salt
⅛ tsp paprika
4 chicken breast halves, boneless, without skin

1. Mix all ingredients except chicken.
2. Place chicken pieces in shallow baking pan.
3. Pour lemon mixture over chicken pieces.
4. Bake at 400°F (hot oven) until chicken is tender,

about 1 hour. Baste chicken several times during baking with liquid in pan.

Serves 4

Nutrition Analysis:

Calories 242
Carbohydrate. . . . . .1 gram
Fiber . . . . .0 grams
Fat. . . . . .10 grams
Cholesterol. . . . . .83 milligrams
Sodium. . . . . .202 milligrams

CHICKEN CURRY

¼ cup onion, chopped
2 cups tart apple, unpared, chopped
1 tbsp oil
2 tbsp flour
½ tsp salt
⅛ tsp ground ginger
1 tsp curry powder
1 cup skim milk
1½ cups chicken, cooked, diced
¼ cup raisins
2 cups brown rice, cooked, unsalted

1. Cook onion and apple in oil until tender.
2. Stir in flour, salt, ginger, and curry powder.
3. Add milk slowly, stirring constantly; cook until thickened.
4. Add chicken and raisins. Heat to serving temperature.
5. Serve over rice.

Serves 4

Variation: Fish Curry In place of chicken, use 1 lb fresh or frozen haddock fillets, without skin; omit raisins. Thaw frozen fish in refrigerator overnight. Cook fish in 1 cup boiling water for 2 minutes. Drain. Break into bite-size pieces. Proceed as in basic recipe.

Nutrition Analysis:

Calories 406
Carbohydrate. . . . . .45 grams
Fiber . . . . .2 grams
Fat. . . . . .11 grams
Cholesterol. . . . . .73 milligrams
Sodium. . . . . .360 milligrams

BAKED TURKEY TENDERLOINS IN BARBECUE SAUCE

2 turkey breast tenderloins (8-oz each) cut in half
2 tbsp water
¼ cup cider vinegar
¼ cup catsup
½ tsp dry mustard
½ tsp Worcestershire sauce
3 tbsp minced onion
1 clove garlic, minced or pressed
salt and pepper to taste
1 drop Tabasco sauce

1. Preheat oven to 350°F.
2. Arrange turkey pieces in a baking dish. Combine remaining ingredients and mix well. Spoon over turkey.

3. Bake, uncovered, in 350°F oven 15–20 minutes or until turkey turns from pink to light in color in deepest part. Baste once or twice.

Serves 4

Nutrition Analysis:

Calories 144
Carbohydrate. . . . . .6 grams
Fiber . . . . .0 grams
Fat. . . . . .1 gram
Cholesterol. . . . . .76 milligrams
Sodium. . . . . .210 milligrams

TURKEY TENDERLOIN BUNDLES

½ cup carrots, julienned (¼-inch)
1 turkey breast tenderloin (approx. ½ lb)
⅛ tsp garlic powder
⅛ tsp dried rosemary leaves
⅛ tsp salt

dash pepper
2 green onions, sliced into eighths
2 rings sweet red pepper
1 tbsp white wine

1. Preheat oven to 400°F.
2. Place carrots in center of 12 × 16-inch foil rectangle. Top with tenderloin and sprinkle with garlic powder, rosemary, salt and pepper. Arrange onions and pepper over tenderloin. Fold edges of foil up to form a bowl shape. Pour wine over tenderloin.
3. Bring two opposite foil sides together above food; fold edges over and down to lock fold. Fold short ends up and over.
4. Place foil bundle on a small cookie sheet; bake 20–25 minutes or until meat reaches 170°F.

(Check for doneness by opening foil bundle carefully and inserting meat thermometer in thickest part of meat.)

Serves 2

Nutrition Analysis:
Calories 135
Carbohydrate. . . . . .4 grams
Fiber . . . . .1 gram
Fat. . . . . .1 gram
Cholesterol. . . . . .71 milligrams
Sodium . . . . .182 milligrams

FREEZ'N BAKE TURKEY CUTLETS OR SLICES

1 egg white
1 tbsp water
½ cup seasoned bread crumbs
1 pound turkey breast cutlets or slices, ⅛- to ⅜-
   inch thick

1. In shallow bowl beat egg white and water together. Set aside.
2. Spread bread crumbs over shallow plate.
3. Dip turkey into egg mixture, then into crumbs.
4. Arrange breaded turkey slices on a cookie sheet. Freeze 30 to 45 minutes. Transfer frozen turkey slices to self-closing freezer bag and return to freezer until ready to bake.
5. When ready to prepare, preheat oven to 400°F.

6. Spray cookie sheet with nonstick cooking oil. Arrange frozen cutlets or slices on sheet; bake approximately 9 minutes for ⅛-inch slices and 13 minutes for ⅜-inch slices or until turkey slices are no longer pink in center.

Serves 4

Nutrition Analysis:
Calories 135
Carbohydrate. . . . . .3 grams
Fiber . . . . .0 grams
Fat. . . . . .1 gram
Cholesterol. . . . . .71 milligrams
Sodium . . . . .87 milligrams

TURKEY SLOPPY JOES

2 tsp cooking oil
1 lb ground turkey breast
1 cup onion, thinly sliced
½ cup green pepper, chopped
1 cup reduced-calorie, reduced-sodium
   catsup
¼ cup sweet pickle relish
1½ tsp chili powder
1 tsp Worcestershire sauce
½ tsp seasoned salt
½ tsp garlic powder
¼ tsp celery seed
8 hamburger buns, toasted

1. In a large skillet, over medium heat, saute ground turkey, onion, and green pepper 5 minutes or until turkey is no longer pink. Add catsup, relish, chili powder, Worcestershire sauce, seasoned salt, garlic powder, and celery seed. Bring to a boil. Reduce heat to low; cover and simmer 30 minutes.*
2. To serve, spoon turkey mixture over bottom halves of buns. Place top halves of buns over turkey mixture.
   *Mixture may be prepared to this point, cooled and stored in a covered bowl in the refrigerator overnight. Reheat mixture when ready to serve.

Serves 8

Nutrition Analysis:

Calories 221
Carbohydrate. . . . . .29 grams
Fiber . . . . .1 gram
Fat. . . . . .3 grams
Cholesterol. . . . . .21 milligrams
Sodium . . . . .649 milligrams

❖ ❖ ❖

CHAPTER NINE

SEAFOOD

Seafood includes both finfish (usually just called "fish"), such as flounder and tuna, and shellfish, such as shrimp and scallops. There are two types of shellfish: mollusks (which are the true shellfish with hard shells) and crustaceans (which have segmented shells and jointed legs). Examples of mollusks include abalone, clams, oysters, and scallops. Examples of crustaceans include crabs, crayfish, lobsters, and shrimp (see Table 34). Octopus and squid, even though they lack shells, are also considered shellfish.

Recently the safety of fish products has come into question. There have been concerns of chemical contamination, bacteria, viruses, parasites,

and toxins. This topic is discussed in detail in Chapter 6 including precautions you should take to ensure seafood safety in your home.

Regarding nutrition (see Table 35), fresh and frozen seafood are excellent sources of protein and are also:

- relatively low in calories, fat, and saturated fat when compared to meat
- a good source of omega-3 fatty acids
- low to moderate in cholesterol content
- low in sodium
- a good source of certain vitamins (such as vitamins E and K and niacin) and minerals (such as iodine and potassium)

❖ *Table 34 Shellfish* ❖

Crabs	Shrimp	Crawfish	Lobsters	Univalves	Bivalves		Cephalopods
Alaska King Crab	Blue Shrimp	Fresh Water	American	**Abalone**	**Clams**	**Oysters**	Octopus
Blue Crab	Brown Shrimp	Crayfish	Lobster		Butter Clam	Eastern/	
Dungeness Crab	California Bay	Sea Crawfish	Rock Lobster	**Conch**	Geoduck Clam	Atlantic	Squid
Jonah Crab	Shrimp	Western	Slipper Lobster		Hard or Quahog	Oyster	
Red Crab	Northern Shrimp	Crayfish	Spiny Lobster	**Snails**	Clam	Gulf Oyster	
Soft Shell Crab	Pink Shrimp			Cockles	Littleneck Clam	Olympia Oyster	
Snow Crab	Rock Shrimp			Sea Snails	Pismo Clam	Pacific Oyster	
	White Shrimp				Razor Clam	South American	
					Soft Clam/Steamer	Oyster	
					Surf or Skimmer		
					Clam	**Scallops**	
						Bay Scallop	
					Mussels	Calico Scallop	
					Blue Mussel	Sea Scallop	
					California Mussel		

❖ Table 35   Seafood Nutrition Chart (based on 3½-ounce portions) ❖

Species	Calories	Fat (grams)	Saturated Fat (grams)*	Cholesterol (milligrams)
Finfish				
Carp, cooked, dry heat	162	7	1	84
Cod, Atlantic, cooked, dry heat	105	1	—	55
Grouper, cooked, dry heat	118	1	—	47
Haddock, cooked, dry heat	112	1	—	74
Halibut, cooked, dry heat	140	3	1	41
Herring, Atlantic, cooked, dry heat	203	12	3	77
Mackerel, Atlantic, cooked, dry heat	262	18	4	75
Perch, cooked, dry heat	117	1	—	115
Pike, Northern, cooked, dry heat	113	1	—	50
Pollock, Walleye, cooked, dry heat	113	1	—	96
Pompano, cooked, dry heat	211	12	5	64
Salmon, Coho, cooked, moist heat	185	8	1	49
Salmon, Sockeye, canned, drained solids with bone	153	7	2	44
Sea bass, cooked, dry heat	124	3	1	53
Smelt, Rainbow, cooked, dry heat	124	3	1	90
Snapper, cooked, dry heat	128	2	—	47
Swordfish, cooked, dry heat	155	5	1	50
Trout, Rainbow, cooked, dry heat	151	4	1	73
Tuna, Bluefish, fresh, cooked, dry heat	184	6	2	49
Whiting, cooked, dry heat	115	2	—	84
Shellfish				
Clam, cooked, moist heat	148	2	—	67
Crab, Alaska King, cooked, moist heat	97	2	—	53
Crayfish, cooked, moist heat	114	1	—	178
Lobster, Northern, cooked, moist heat	98	1	—	72
Oyster, Eastern, cooked, moist heat	137	5	1	109
Scallops, raw	88	1	—	33
Shrimp, cooked, moist heat	99	1	—	195

A dash (—) means less than 1 gram of saturated fat.
Source: *United States Department of Agriculture.*

Certain fish are fattier than others (Table 36). Although they contain more fat, it is still less than the fat contained in equivalent servings of most meats. More important, the type of fat found in these fish is rich in health-promoting fatty acids (key components of fats) known as omega-3's. Omega 3's are polyunsaturated fatty acids found almost exclusively in fish and shellfish. They have various health benefits, as follows.

- Reduce the chance of developing heart disease and may reduce damage from heart disease
- Usually lower blood triglyceride (fat) levels
- May improve heart functioning

- Can modestly lower blood pressure, resulting in less chance of heart attack and stroke
- May improve symptoms of arthritis and psoriasis

Shellfish, as well as fatty fish, are higher in omega 3's than lean fish, although lean fish still contain some.

Shellfish, as a family, got an unfair reputation in the past for being high in cholesterol. This was the result of outdated scientific methods that detected cholesterol-like substances as well as real cholesterol in shellfish, so cholesterol readings for many shellfish were mistakenly high. Certain

❖ *Table 36   Fat Content of Fish* ❖

Low-Fat Fish (fat content less than 2.5 percent)	Medium-Fat Fish (fat content 2.5–5 percent)	High-Fat Fish (fat content over 5 percent)
Cod	Bluefish	Albacore tuna
Croaker	Swordfish	Bluefin tuna
Flounder	Yellowfin tuna	Herring
Grouper		Mackerel
Haddock		Sablefish
Pacific halibut		Salmon
Pollock		Sardines
Red snapper		Shad
Rockfish		Trout
Sea bass		Whitefish
Shark		
Sole		
Whiting		

shellfish—shrimp and crayfish—are higher in cholesterol than other seafood, but a 3½-ounce portion of either still has less cholesterol than one egg. Shellfish is also very low in saturated fat, so the net effect of eating shellfish is that it's no worse than eating chicken without the skin. Prominent heart experts no longer see any reason to place limitations on specific shellfish for their patients with high blood cholesterol—that is, if portion sizes are not excessive and they have a moderate intake of saturated fats.

Canned seafoods have much higher levels of sodium. By rinsing canned seafood, you can remove some of the sodium. Many canned seafood products are packed in oil or water. The water-packed is a better choice to reduce total fat.

FISH

Purchasing

When purchasing fish, there are several things you need to consider.

1. What kind to buy.
2. What form it should be in—whole, drawn, dressed, fillets, steaks, stick, portions.
3. If you want it to be fresh, frozen, or processed (such as canned).
4. How to choose high-quality fresh and frozen fish.

When considering what type of fish to purchase, you may want to consider flavor and texture. Table 37 is a guide to flavor and texture of fish. Table 38 gives additional information on many of the popular types of fish.

Both fresh and frozen fish are marketed in quite a few different forms and it is advantageous to know them, as shown in the accompanying diagrams. Many kinds of seafood are also available canned, such as tuna, salmon, and sardines. They come packed in water or oil. The following guidelines will help you determine how much you need to purchase.

- Whole or round fish: 1½ lb whole fish yields three 4-oz portions
- Drawn fish: 1 lb yields two 4-oz portions
- Dressed fish: 1 lb yields two and one-half 4-oz portions
- Steaks: 1 lb yields three to four 4-oz portions
- Fillets, stick, and portions: 1 lb yields three to four 4-oz portions

When buying fresh fish, first look over the way it is displayed. Although you don't have access behind the supermarket seafood counter, ask your seafood salesperson to confirm that it is held at 32°F and is cold to the touch. Fish should not be lying in water or juices, and seafood that does not have any skin or shell to protect it should not be in direct contact with the ice. Also, only buy fish that doesn't smell fishy—a fishy odor indicates large levels of bacteria. A slightly seaweedy or cucumber-like odor is okay.

Fresh fillets and steaks should have firm, elastic flesh and retain true color; pearly white for flounder, sole, and haddock; reddish for tuna (except albacore, which ranges from light beige to rosy beige); grayish for bluefish, and pink to red and orange-red for trout and salmon. They should have a fresh-cut appearance with no drying or browning or curling up around the edges. If cut fish is left too long in a display case, the flesh begins to separate and may get slimy.

Whole fish, whatever the variety, has certain characteristics that indicate freshness. Fresh fish should never have a sour or ammonia odor. Here is what to look for when buying whole fish.

Market Forms of Fish

Whole or Round

This, as the term suggests, means the fish is whole, just as it comes from the water. Nothing has been removed.

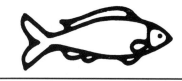

WHOLE

Drawn

The fish has been gutted (the insides removed) and the fins and scales have usually been removed as well.

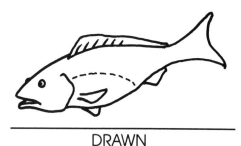

DRAWN

Dressed

The fish has been gutted and scaled, the fins removed, and usually the head and tail cut off as well.

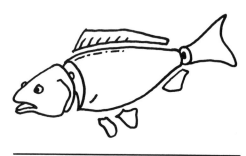

DRESSED/PAN-DRESSED

Steaks

These are cross-section slices, from ¾ to 1½ inches thick, of larger dressed fish. Steaks usually have a piece of the backbone in the center.

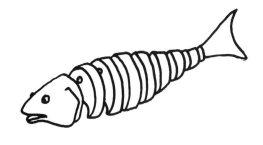

STEAKED

Chunks

These are cross-section pieces cut thicker than steaks. They may have a piece of the backbone.

Fillets

Fillets are the sides of the fish cut away from the backbone. They are often boneless and skinless, though the skin of fatty fish is usually left attached to the fillets. That way it holds together better during cooking. Sometimes small bones called pins are present. They can be easily removed. Fillets are the most popular market form in America.

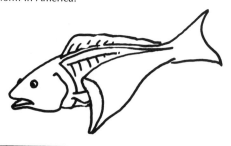

FILLETED

Butterfly Fillet

Not a common market form but occasionally found, these are the two fillets of a fish held together by the uncut flesh and skin of the belly.

Sticks and Portions

Sometimes blocks of fish are cut into sticks and portions. These are available breaded or not breaded, precooked or uncooked, usually in the frozen seafood section.

❖ *Table 37   Flavor Guide to Fish* ❖

Mild Flavor	Moderate Flavor	Full Flavor
Delicate Texture	**Delicate Texture**	**Delicate Texture**
Cod	Black Cod	Bluefish
Crabmeat	Buffalo	Mussels
Flounder	Butterfish	Oysters
Haddock	Lake Perch	
Pollock	Lingcod	**Moderate Texture**
Scallops	Whitefish	Canned Salmon
Skate	Whiting	Canned Sardines
Sole		Mackerel
	Moderate Texture	Smoked Fish
Moderate Texture	Canned Tuna	
Crawfish	Conch	**Firm Texture**
Lobster	Mullet	Clams
Rockfish	Ocean Perch	Marlin
Sheepshead	Shad	Salmon
Shrimp	Smelt	Swordfish
Walleye Pike	Surimi Products	Tuna
	Trout	
Firm Texture		
Grouper	**Firm Texture**	
Halibut	Amberjack	
Monkfish	Catfish	
Ocean Catfish	Drum	
Sea Bass	Mahimahi	
Snapper	Octopus	
Squid	Pompano	
Tautog	Shark	
Tilefish	Sturgeon	

- Bright, clear, full (sometimes protruding) eyes. As a fish ages, the eyes become cloudy and sunken.
- Bright red or pink gills; gray, brown, or green gills are a sign of age.
- Moist, shiny skin with scales that adhere tightly and with distinct colors and markings.
- Firm, elastic flesh that springs back when pressed gently with the finger. With time, the flesh becomes soft and separates from the bones.

When buying frozen fish, check to be sure the package was stacked below the frost line of the freezer case. Look for packages that still have their original shape with the wrapping intact and no visible ice or blood. Fish that has been thawed and refrozen may have a sour smell, a brown color at the edges of the fillet, a dried out appearance, or excessive frost or ice in the packaging. Be sure the fish is solidly frozen with no discoloration, freezer burn, or bad odor.

Storing

Fresh fish should be stored at 30°–32°F—about 10 degrees cooler than most refrigerators—so put seafood in the coldest spot in your refrigerator. (Don't worry—it doesn't freeze until the temperature gets below 28°F.)

When storing fresh fish, make sure they are wrapped well in moisture-proof paper or an airtight plastic bag or container. Rewrap purchased fish if it was not properly wrapped in the store. Fresh fish should be used 1 to 2 days from purchase, preferably within one day. Fattier fish is more fragile than lean fish, so definitely plan to cook fattier fish, such as tuna and mackerel, within a day.

Cooked fish should be sealed tightly, promptly refrigerated, and eaten within 3 or 4 days.

Fish cannot be frozen as long as red meat and poultry because it is high in polyunsaturated fats, which are more prone to oxidation than saturated fats. Changes in texture also occur after a period of time. Therefore, it is particularly important to label all frozen fish clearly with the date and use it within a day after it's thawed.

If you want to freeze fresh fish that you have purchased, make sure it is still of high quality and wrap it tightly in plastic bags or wrap designed for freezing. Make sure all the air is pressed out before sealing. Lean fish can be frozen for 4 to 6 months, fattier fish for 2 to 3 months.

Fish should be frozen as quickly as possible; avoid slow freezing. To do so, about 2 hours before freezing, set the freezer thermostat to its coldest setting and rearrange the contents so the seafood packages can be placed in direct contact with the walls and floor of the freezer. Here are some other freezing tips.

- Do not overload the freezer; as a general rule, freeze no more than 2 to 3 pounds of seafood per cubic foot of freezer space in a 24-hour period.

❖ Table 38 Guide to Fish ❖

Name/Varieties	Characteristics	Availability*	Market Forms
Bluefish	Fatty flavorful fish, flesh turns from blue to grey when cooked, loose, flaky texture	Year-round	Whole, drawn, filleted
Cod	Lean, mild-flavored, moist fish with white, firm flake; most commonly used fish in the U.S.; scrod is a small, young cod	Year-round	Drawn, dressed, steaked, filleted, frozen, breaded raw or cooked sticks and portions
Flounder (summer or fluke, winter, sand dab)	Lean fish with a white flesh, fine flakes, and mild, delicate flavor when cooked	Primarily July–December	Drawn, dressed, filleted, frozen, breaded raw or cooked fillets and portions
Grouper (Red grouper)	Lean white fish similar in texture and flavor to red snapper	Year-round	Whole, steaked, filleted
Haddock	Lean fish with white, firm flake, delicate flavor, member of the cod family	Year-round	Drawn, dressed, filleted, frozen, breaded raw cooked fillets, sticks, and portions
Halibut	Lean, white, mild-flavored fish	Primarily April–October	Whole, drawn, dressed, steaked, filleted
Mackerel (Spanish mackerel, King mackerel)	Fat, firm flesh with rich flavor and slightly dark color	Almost year-round	Whole, drawn, dressed, steaked, filleted
Perch (Ocean perch— redfish, freshwater perch—yellow)	Lean, mild-flavored white flesh with firm texture and fine flakes	Year-round	Whole, drawn, dressed, filleted, frozen, breaded raw or cooked fillets and portions
Pompano	Fatty fish with rich, well-flavored flesh, expensive	Year-round	Whole, filleted
Salmon (Atlantic, chinook, sockeye or red, cohoe or silver, chum, humpback or pink)	Pink-to-red flesh; fatty, strong-flavored fish with meaty texture	August–November	Dressed, steaked, filleted, frozen, canned, smoked
Shad	Fatty fish with rich sweet flavor, very bony	February–May	Whole, drawn, filleted, canned, smoked
Shark (Mako, blue)	Like swordfish, except soft and a little moister, less expensive	Year-round	Steaked
Snapper (Mangrove, silk, yellowtail)	Lean fish; firm, delicate, white flesh with large flakes; red skinned	Year-round	Whole, filleted
Sole (Dover, lemon or English, petrale)	Lean fish with white flesh, mild sweet flavor, member of the flounder family	Primarily July–December	Whole, filleted, breaded sticks and portions, stuffed
Swordfish	Fatty fish with firm dense texture; delicate flavor; expensive	Year-round	Steaks
Trout (lake, river, brook, rainbow)	Fatty fish with rich, fine-textured flavor; flesh may be white or pinkish-red	Year-round	Whole, drawn, filleted, steaked

❖ *Table 38 Continued* ❖

Name/Varieties	Characteristics	Availability*	Market Forms
Turbot (blue halibut, gray halibut, Newfoundland turbot, Greenland halibut)	Lean fish with snowy white, moist, finely textured flesh	July–November	Dressed, filleted
Whitefish	Fatty fish with flaky, white flesh and slightly sweet flavor	Year-round	Whole, drawn, dressed, filleted, frozen, smoked

Availability refers to buying fresh fish. Many types of fish are available year-round frozen or canned.

- Once the packages are frozen, place them where the temperature is most stable, generally away from the door, allowing space for air circulation.

Thaw frozen fish in the refrigerator for ½ to 1½ days depending on size.

Cooking Light and Healthy

Fish can be prepared in countless delicious ways. Because it is naturally tender, it lends itself to every kind of cooking method. Any cooking method (except frying of course) makes fish a light and healthy dish as long as minimal amounts of oil or margarine, if any, are used. Following are some general pointers for successful seafood preparation.

- **Cook fresh fish soon after purchase, the same day if possible.**
- **Cook frozen fish that has been thawed within a day.** Fillets, steaks, and portions up to 8 ounces can be cooked directly from the frozen state to prevent excessive drip loss during cooking and for convenience (just double the length of the cooking time). However, if you plan to bread the fish first, partially thaw the fish (you can microwave it for a few seconds) so it can be breaded successfully. Never thaw frozen breaded or battered fish sticks or portions before cooking, because the breading will become soggy.
- **Don't overcook fish.** It is tender as it comes from the water. Very little cooking is needed to develop flavor or soften connective tissue.

Cook only until the product becomes firm and opaque but is still moist and juicy. When fish cooks, it lightens in color and turns opaque white or light gray. To test for doneness, slide a knife tip into the thickest part of the fish and check the color. If it is still dark and translucent, it needs more cooking. If it is solid white, the fish is done. Don't cook fish until it flakes or separates. By this time, it has shrunk, toughened, and dried out.

- **Do not overseason fish.** Fish and shellfish generally have a delicate flavor that is easily overwhelmed. A seafood and its sauce should complement each other.
- Fish adapt well to almost all cooking methods, but because of a tendency to dry out during cooking using dry heat (baking, grilling, and broiling), **lean or low-fat fish are better when cooked using moist heat.** Dry heat methods are fine if lean fish is basted with a sauce before baking, broiling, or grilling or brushed lightly with a minimal amount of oil. Use the ideas suggested here for marinades, sauces, condiments, and herbs and spices that can be used to keep fish moist during cooking and flavor fish as well.

To cook fish, use the 10-minute guideline for determining doneness when baking, grilling, broiling, poaching, or sauteing fish. Here is how it works.

1. Measure the fish at its thickest point. If the fish is stuffed or rolled, measure it after stuffing or rolling.

2. Cook fish about 10 minutes per inch, turning it halfway through the cooking time. For example, a 1-inch fish steak should be cooked about 5 minutes on each side. Pieces less than ½ inch thick do not have to be turned over.

3. Add 5 minutes to the total cooking time for fish cooked in foil.

4. Double the cooking time for frozen fish that has not been defrosted.

5. Shorten the cooking time when poaching or frying because both water and oil make fish cook faster.

6. Use time only as a **guideline** for determining doneness—always check the fish for doneness a few minutes before the end of the estimated cooking time.

Table 39 lists approximate cooking times for fish and shellfish.

Now let's take a look at different cooking methods.

Baking Baking is a particularly easy way to prepare fish. Whole fish, whole stuffed fish, fillets, stuffed fillets, steaks, and chunks of fish may all be baked. Use pieces of fish of similar size for even cooking. To bake, preheat the oven to 425°F. Rinse the fish under cold water and pat dry with paper towels. If baking a whole fish, pat the inside dry. Lightly oil a shallow baking dish (or use vegetable oil spray or a nonstick pan) and place fish in it, skin side down if baking fillets.

To prevent the fish from drying out (this applies particularly to leaner fish), you can do a number of things besides adding oil.

- Wrap the fish in aluminum foil or parchment paper.
- Cover the fish with chopped vegetables which will help flavor the fish while at the same time keeping it moist (such as a combination of onions, celery, and carrots; or mushrooms and onions; or onions, tomatoes, and red and green peppers).
- Use a bread crumb topping or other coating—first dip the fish in 1 egg white combined with ¼ cup skim milk or dip in ½ cup buttermilk.
- Brush on a minimal amount of low-fat Italian salad dressing or a thin layer of vegetable oil.

❖ **Table 39   Approximate Cooking Times** ❖
for Fish and Shellfish

Finfish (minutes per inch thickness)

Amberjack 10	Sheepshead 10
Black Cod 10	Skate 8
Bluefish 9	Smelt 8
Buffalo 10	Snapper 12
Butterfish 10	Sole 8
Catfish 10	Sturgeon 9
Cod 10	Swordfish 8
Croaker 10	Tautog 12
Drum 10	Tilefish 12
Flounder 10	Trout 9
Grouper 12	Tuna 6
Haddock 10	Walleye Pike 8
Halibut 8	Whitefish 10
Lake Perch 8	Whiting 10
Lingcod 10	
Mackerel 9	**Shellfish (minutes)**
Mahimahi 10	Bay Scallops 1½
Marlin 8	Clams 5–7 until open
Monkfish 12	Crab (live) 5–8
Mullet 9	Crawfish 2–3
Ocean Catfish 10	Lobster 12 for first pound, 6 for
Ocean Perch 10	each additional pound
Pollock 10	Mussels 3–4 until open
Pompano 9	Octopus 1–1½ hours
Porgy 12	Oysters 2–3 until edges curl
Rockfish 10	Sea Scallops (large) 5
Salmon 9	Shrimp (medium) 3
Sea Bass 12	Shrimp (large) 4
Shad 10	Squid Rings 1–1½
Shark 9	

To enjoy the taste of "fried" fish without excessive fat, bake fish fillets, dredging them in seasoned flour, dipping them in an egg white beaten with a little water, and coating them with bread crumbs. Place fish in a shallow, lightly oiled (or nonstick) baking pan and dot with margarine or oil. Bake 6 to 12 minutes per inch of thickness until fish is just opaque throughout.

To bake prepared breaded frozen fish products, follow the directions on the package.

Broiling Steaks, whole fish, split whole fish, and fillets can all be broiled. To broil fish, preheat broiler pan. Rinse fish under cold water and pat dry with paper towels. Season it on all sides if desired with pepper, herbs, and lemon juice.

GUIDE TO MARINADES, SAUCES, CONDIMENTS, HERBS, AND SPICES FOR SEAFOOD

❖ ❖ ❖

MARINADES

Combine ingredients such as wine, vinegar, lemon, or any citrus juice along with a mild-flavored cooking oil and your choice of other flavoring agents to create tangy marinades for seafood. A basic oil-based marinade uses 1 cup vegetable oil, ½ cup lemon juice or vinegar, ½ teaspoon each of salt and pepper, 1 clove minced garlic, 3 tablespoons fresh chopped or 2 tablespoons dried herbs such as tarragon, basil, parsley, thyme, or oregano, alone or in combination.

For less fat and more convenience, use bottled salad dressing (low-fat products work fine) like Italian, vinaigrette, or Dijon flavor. For a fresh summery taste, you can marinate fillets of fish with a higher fat content in lime juice (3 tablespoons juice per pound of fish) for 1 hour.

To make a marinade, thoroughly blend all ingredients. If marinating whole fish, make 3 to 4 slits into the flesh down to the bone on each side so the marinade penetrates. Marinate 1 to 4 hours in the refrigerator, turning fish or shellfish about every hour. The longer the fish marinates, the more flavor will be absorbed. But don't marinate fish overnight like beef or poultry—it will turn mushy. Always drain the marinade from the fish before cooking and discard it (it could contain harmful bacteria or other substances). Use reserved fresh marinade during cooking for basting. Baste at least once during cooking.

WHITE WINE MARINADE

½ cup light olive oil
¼ cup dry white wine
1 clove garlic, finely minced
½ tbsp tarragon leaves
½ tbsp Dijon-type mustard
Salt and pepper to taste

TOMATO-ORANGE MARINADE

6 oz no-salt V-8 juice
¼ cup frozen orange juice concentrate
¼ cup minced onions
1 small clove garlic, minced

SAUCES AND CONDIMENTS

Soy sauce (try low-sodium) and teriyaki sauce, which contain no fat, can be used in marinades or brushed on fish and shellfish before grilling, broiling, baking, steaming, or microwaving. Tomato sauces and jarred salsas are also low-fat and can be poured over fish before baking or heated and added after poaching and sauteing. Cocktail sauce and tartar sauces (make your own with reduced-calorie mayonnaise and relish) are traditional condiments for fish and seafood. Or you can make your own sauce by combining fresh tomatoes with herbs as seen here.

TERIYAKI SAUCE

½ cup low-sodium soy sauce
2 tbsp dry sherry
½ tbsp sugar
1 clove garlic, finely minced
½ tbsp finely grated fresh gingerroot or ½ tsp
    dried ground ginger

TOMATO BASIL SAUCE

2 large ripe tomatoes, diced
3 tbsp fresh basil, chopped
2 tbsp olive oil
1 tbsp balsamic or other vinegar
Juice of 1 lemon (about 3 tablespoons)
1 small clove of garlic, minced

LEMON SAUCE

3 tbsp lemon juice
1 tbsp Dijon mustard
1 tbsp margarine, melted
¼ tsp freshly ground pepper

HERBS AND SPICES

Basil, bay leaf, dill, oregano, paprika, pepper, seasoned peppers, tarragon, thyme, rosemary, sage, marjoram, chervil, chives, fennel, ginger, and garlic nicely complement the flavor of seafood.

Lightly oil the broiler pan or use a nonstick pan or vegetable oil spray. If broiling a small whole fish, slash the skin on both sides and turn it over halfway through broiling. Arrange fish fillets, skin side down in a single layer. Place fish, 1 inch thick or less, 3 to 4 inches from the heat source; place thicker pieces 5 to 6 inches away. Fillets under 1 inch thick do not need to be turned over. Baste with a marinade, such as low-fat salad dressing, during cooking.

To broil frozen fish, double the cooking time and turn the fish over halfway through broiling.

Grilling Grilling is particularly well suited to thick cuts of fish, such as whole fish, steaks, and kabobs, but fillets may also be grilled. Nonstick grills are ideal for cooking fish without having to oil the grill. It can also be helpful to use a hinged grilling basket or aluminum foil that has been punctured to allow air flow, particularly with more delicately textured fish. Prior to placing on the heat, spray the basket with vegetable cooking spray (unless the basket is nonstick). When not using a basket or the foil method, pre-oil the unheated grill rack. Always use super clean grill racks and baskets.

Rinse the fish under cold water and pat dry with paper towels. For fish that is 1 inch thick or less, place the grill 2 to 4 inches above the coals or heat source; for thicker pieces, 5 to 6 inches away. Cook fish and shellfish over a medium-hot fire. Cook on one side for half the cooking time, basting frequently. Turn over and continue grilling and basting until done. Marinades and sauces, such as low-fat Italian salad dressing, add flavor and keep the fish moist when grilled.

The exact cooking time will depend on the thickness of the fish, the type of fire (wood, char-coal, gas, electric), the distance of the fish from the heat source, and whether you use a covered or an open grill. Watch carefully and do what professionals do—peek inside to check for doneness. Grill until the fish is just opaque throughout. As a rule, shellfish cooks faster than finfish.

Sauteing Sauteing is ideal for thinner fish fillets. (Shucked oysters, shrimp, scallops, and squid also lend themselves quite well to this cooking method.) To saute, first rinse the fish under cold water and pat dry with paper towels. If desired, lightly flour the fish to help seal in the juices. Using a heavy skillet, heat up 1 tablespoon vegetable oil and add fish to the pan, being careful not to crowd because the fish will become soggy.

Cook about 6 to 12 minutes per inch thickness until fish is just opaque throughout. Turn fish over halfway through cooking. For thicker fish, reduce heat to medium. Drain fish on paper towels and season.

Stir-frying Stir-frying small pieces of fish (or shellfish) together with an assortment of colorful vegetables is a quick, easy way to make a healthy, tasty entree. Shrimp and scallops are very easy to cook this way; if using fish, be sure it is a firm-fleshed fish like halibut, tuna, shark, or grouper. Cooked crab meat or surimi (imitation) seafood may be added at the end and cooked just long enough to warm through. Stir-frying is a very fast technique, so have everything ready to go before heating the oil.

Using a wok or large skillet, lightly coat the bottom and sides with vegetable oil. Add raw seafood (cooked seafood should be added at the end to warm it) and stir-fry, tossing gently to coat on all sides, until about three quarters done, anywhere from 2 to 4 minutes. Shrimp will turn pink, scallops and fish opaque or white. Remove to a warm platter and continue by stir-frying the vegetables and making a light sauce if desired. Return the seafood to the wok or skillet and cook 1 to 2 minutes longer. Serve at once.

Poaching   Poaching is cooking in a gently simmering liquid such as lightly seasoned lemon water, fish or vegetable stock, or dry white wine. Poaching works well for fish in any form.

To prepare a whole, dressed fish for poaching, rinse it under cold water. Bring the liquid to a boil in a fish poacher or in a large skillet or saute pan and add the fish or shellfish. Reduce to a simmer; the water should barely bubble. Gently cook 6 to 12 minutes per inch thickness of fish until it is just opaque throughout. It is not necessary to turn fish when poaching. Check before the time is up—poaching usually cooks seafood a little quicker. Remove when the fish turns from translucent to opaque or white and is firm but still moist. Reserve the liquid to make a sauce for the fish.

A fish poacher with a long-handled rack to hold the fish is very handy for poaching whole fish, especially a large one. If you have a large fish to poach but no fish poacher, you can improvise by wrapping the fish in cheesecloth and draping the ends over the sides of a large pot or covered roasting pan. Be sure to keep the ends away from the burner. When the fish is done, lift it out of the broth using the loose ends of cheesecloth as handles.

Steaming   Whole fish, chunks, steaks, and thick or rolled-up fillets are all suitable for steaming. (Shellfish is also excellent steamed.) Steaming, like poaching, is ideal for those who want to avoid adding extra fat. To steam fish, fill a steamer or large saucepan fitted with a steaming rack and a tight cover with about 1 inch of plain or seasoned water, such as fish stock. Just make certain that it's a mild liquid, one that will not overpower the flavor of the fish. The water should not rise above the rack.

Bring liquid to a boil. Reduce to a simmer. Wash the fish, place on the rack, and place the rack in the pot. Cover tightly. Steam until done—steam cooks quickly so check frequently for opaque flesh. Be careful to open the lid away from you to let the steam out of the pot.

Microwave cooking   Almost all kinds of fish can be prepared in the microwave oven. Watch closely when you try a new seafood recipe for the first time using the microwave. If a range of times is given, start with the shortest one. You can always put the dish back in the oven and cook it a little longer, but you cannot turn the clock back if it has cooked too long. Write the correct time down on the recipe for future reference. Split-second timing is the secret to cooking seafood in the microwave.

Fish cooked in the microwave is done when the flesh has just begun to change from translucent to opaque or white and when it is firm but still moist. Fish will continue to cook after it has been removed from the microwave, so take the dish out before it looks done—when the outer edges are opaque with the center still slightly translucent. Allow the fish to stand, covered, for a few minutes before serving to let the heat distribute evenly and the fish to finish cooking. Here are some additional tips for cooking in the microwave.

Cooking Finfish in the Microwave Oven
- Defrost frozen fish before cooking.
- Use a shallow microwave-proof dish to hold the fish.
- Make several diagonal slashes through the skin of whole fish to prevent it from bursting.
- Arrange fillets in a dish with the thicker parts pointing outward and the thinner parts toward the center of the dish. Rolled fillets cook more evenly by microwave than flat fillets.
- Cover the dish and vent by turning back a corner.
- Allow 3½ to 6 minutes per pound of boneless fish cooked on high (100 percent power) as a guide. Rotate the dish halfway through the cooking time.
- Cook side dishes first and keep them covered while cooking the fish. They will retain heat longer than fish.

- Brush fish with stock or juice before microwaving.

Cooking Shellfish in the Microwave
- Arrange a single layer of shellfish in a shallow dish and cover with plastic wrap turned back at one corner for venting.
- Allow 2 to 3 minutes per pound of thawed shucked shellfish cooked on high (100 percent power). Stir and rotate halfway through the cooking time. Allow to stand for one-third of the cooking time after removing from the oven. (For example, if you cook ½ pound of shucked shellfish for 1 minute and 30 seconds, allow it to stand for 30 seconds before serving.) Be careful not to overcook.

- Place clams, mussels, or oysters in the shell in a single layer in a shallow dish. Cover with plastic wrap, venting at one corner. Cook for 2 to 3 minutes on high (100 percent power). Check and remove pieces as they open. Continue until all have opened. 1 pound will take 12 to 15 minutes.

SHELLFISH

The illustration shows the many types of shellfish available. This section will give useful information on the following forms of shellfish: clams, crabs, lobsters, oysters, scallops, and shrimp.

The flavor of shellfish ranges from mild to full. Scallops, lobster, crawfish, and squid have a mild

Types of shellfish

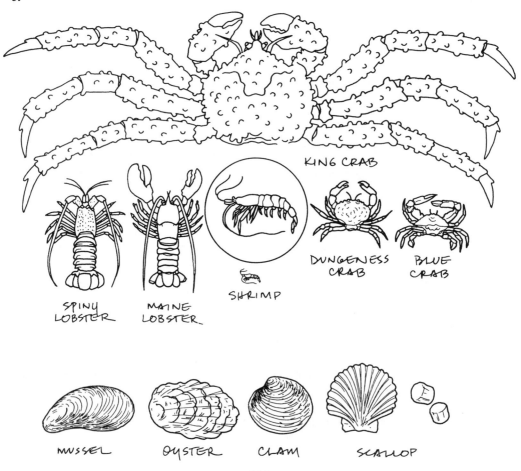

KING CRAB

SPINY LOBSTER

MAINE LOBSTER

SHRIMP

DUNGENESS CRAB

BLUE CRAB

MUSSEL

OYSTER

CLAM

SCALLOP

flavor. Octopus has a moderate flavor, and mussels, oysters, and clams have a full flavor.

Clams

Purchasing Clams are a smooth-shelled species and are found on both the East and West coasts. Hard-shell and soft-shell clams are the two major kinds of clams on the East coast. Hard-shell clams, or quahogs, have different names depending on their size.

- **Littlenecks** are the smallest and tenderest.
- **Cherrystones** are medium sized and the most common.
- **Chowders** are the largest and because they are tough, they are cut up for use in chowder or for frying.

Soft-shell clams, also called steamers or longnecks, have a long tube that extends from between the shells. They are often used in fritters and in New England clam chowder.

Clams are sold live in the shell, shucked (fresh or frozen), canned (whole or chopped), and frozen breaded (raw or cooked). When buying live clams, make sure they have:

- Tightly closed shells (if the shells open slightly, tap with a knife and they should close; discard if they don't close)
- Moist shells that are not cracked, chipped, or broken
- Mild odor

Don't buy live clams that have broken shells or a bad odor. Shucked clams should have plump meat, a mild odor, and a pale to deep orange color. Clams are available year-round. Plan on 12 littlenecks, 4 cherrystones, or 12 soft-shell steamers for one serving (about 4 ounces). For shucked clams, plan on ¼ pound per serving.

Storing Live clams carry around their own seawater environment inside their shells. They should be stored at refrigerator temperatures in a shallow pan covered with a wet cloth. Keep damp but not wet. They can be kept up to 2 or 3 days. Shucked clams should be stored in their own juices in a container with a tight lid in the coldest section of your refrigerator. They should be used

in 1 to 2 days. Cooked clams can keep 3 to 4 days in the refrigerator when covered.

To freeze clams, first shuck them over a bowl to save the liquid from inside the shell (this will be used to store them in). Wash the shucked clams in cold water or brine (1 teaspoon salt to 1 cup water) to remove any sand; place in small freezer containers (3 cup size or less) and cover with liquid. Add clean brine if needed to cover the meats, but leave ½ inch headroom to allow for expansion during freezing. Cover, label, and freeze. Once frozen, check that the meats are covered; if not, add more brine solution. They can be stored in the freezer for up to 3 months.

Handling and Cooking Purging freshly caught clams of sand is an important preliminary step. To purge clams, place them in a large container and cover with ⅓ cup of vinegar to ½ gallon water. Leave for 20 to 30 minutes and change the water. Next, scrub the shells under cold running water. The illustrations show you how to shuck a clam, as explained here:

1. Place a clam in the palm of your hand with the hinge between the thumb and index finger. Take a clam knife or dull paring knife and line it up along the base.
2. Curl the fingers of the hand holding the clam around the back of the knife and apply slow steady pressure until the knife slides in. Twist the knife to open the shell wide enough to cut the muscle on top.
3. Break off the top shell and keep the clam level to avoid losing the juice. Cut the clam away from the bottom shell by scraping with the knife point.

If you find it very difficult to shuck clams, try warming them very briefly—just until they open wide enough to insert the knife. This can be done in the microwave or conventional oven or by steaming or boiling. It is also helpful to freeze the shellfish or to wash it and place it in the freezer for 15 to 30 minutes before shucking.

Only cook clams that are alive, as evidenced by their closed shell. Clams can be cooked by steaming, poaching, baking on the half shell, or simmering in soups and chowders. Clams are cooked when the shell opens. Remove them one by one as they open and continue cooking until all are done. Shucked clams become plump and opaque when cooked. Do not overcook, as overdone clams are tough.

Crabs

Purchasing   There are various kinds of crabs available to the consumer.

1. Alaskan King crab: Largest of the crabs, range in size from 6 to 24 pounds, cooked immediately after harvest, usually purchased as clusters (3 legs and 1 claw attached to a shoulder), legs, or claws
2. Alaskan snow crab: Smaller than King crab and less expensive, cooked immediately after harvest, usually purchased as clusters
3. Blue crab: From the East coast, a small crab ranging from 4 ounces to 1 pound (averages 5 ounces), used often for frozen crabmeat.
4. Soft-shell crab: Molting blue crabs that have shed their hard shells, when deep fried or sauteed they may be eaten shell and all
5. Dungeness crab: From the West coast, ranges from 1½ to 4 pounds in size, very sweet meat
6. Stone crab: Popular in the Southeast, only the claws are eaten, comes from the Gulf of Mexico

Crabs are available live (they taste best this way) and cooked frozen meat or cooked frozen in the shell. When bought live, make sure there is some leg movement. Frozen crab is available year-round. Fresh is available during warm months in the producing areas. For one serving (about 4 ounces), plan on an 8-ounce King or snow crab, 4 whole blue crabs, 8 blue claws, a 12-ounce whole Dungeness crab, 2 whole soft-shell crabs, or 8 ounces of stone crab claws.

Storing   Live crabs should be kept in the refrigerator for only one to two days in moist packaging (seaweed or damp paper strips).

Cooked crabmeat can be placed in freezer bags and wrapped tightly. The meat will be better protected if frozen in a prepared dish, such as a casserole. Maximum storage time is 1 to 2 months.

Handling and Cooking   Crabs should be alive before cooking. To clean a soft-shell crab, do the following **before** they are cooked.

1. Place the crab top side up on the work surface. With a pair of kitchen scissors, cut off the head about ¼ inch behind the eyes. Be sure the yellowish sand bag (stomach) is removed and discarded. Rinse well under cold running water and pat dry.
2. Turn the crab on its back and cut off the tail flap, or apron, which is triangular in females, T-shaped in males. First, pry the apron up with your fingers, then pull it down and away. Discard the apron and the intestinal tract, which is attached to it.
3. Peel back the pointed shell and scrape away the gills on each side. Rinse the crab with cold water and pat dry.

Don't clean soft-shell crabs until you are ready to cook them. The crab may then be dredged in flour for sauteing or breaded or battered for deep-frying. Sauteed or deep-fried soft-shell crabs take about 3 minutes each.

Hard-shell crabs do not need to be prepared before cooking. They are usually simmered for 10 to 15 minutes in salted water and then cooled rapidly in ice water. They can also be steamed. To pick the meat out of a Dungeness or other hard-shell crab, do the following (a nutcracker comes in handy to break claws and legs).

1. Grasp a front claw and twist it, breaking it off where it meets the body. Repeat with other claw and legs. Crack each piece and remove the meat.
2. Break off the pointed shell on the underside.
3. Pry off broad top shell. Discard the gills, spongy parts, and stomach (behind eyes) under shell.
4. Place knife blade down center of crab's body; tap the knife with a mallet to cut in half. Repeat to cut each half into chunks, placing knife blade between leg joints. Pry out meat.

Frozen crabmeat is already cooked—just heat through before serving.

How to shuck a clam

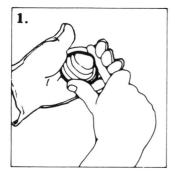 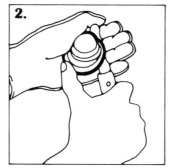 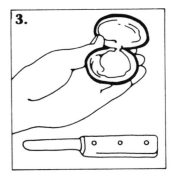

Lobsters

Purchasing   The most popular lobster is the northern lobster. It has a large tail, four pair of legs, and two large front claws. Its shell is dark green, or blue-green, and it turns red when cooked. Lobsters can be purchased live or frozen (whole or the tail only). Cooked meat (either fresh or frozen) is also available. Lobster is normally sold live by the pound: a jumbo lobster is over 2.5 pounds, a large lobster is 1.5 to 2.5 pounds, a quarter lobster is 1.25 to 1.5 pounds, and a chicken lobster is under 1 pound.

The spiny or rock lobster is not a true lobster, but a type of crayfish. The only usable meat of the spiny lobster is found in the tail, and it is less sweet than lobster.

When buying live lobster, make sure there is some leg movement and that the lobster's tail curls under when picked up. Lobsters are available year-round. Plan on a 1- to 1¼-pound lobster per serving (4 ounces meat) or one 6-ounce tail.

Storing   Store lobsters in the refrigerator in ventilated containers. Keep moist with seaweed, lettuce leaves, or damp paper towels or cloth. Never store in an air-tight container as they will suffocate and die. Live lobsters and cooked lobster meat should be used in 1 to 2 days.

Cooked lobster meat can be placed in freezer bags and wrapped tightly. The meat will be better protected if frozen in a prepared dish, such as a casserole. Maximum storage time is 1 to 2 months.

Handling and Cooking   Live lobster (make sure there is movement of the legs and claws) are often cooked live by throwing them into boiling water (this kills them instantly) and simmering for 12 minutes for the first pound, 6 for each additional pound. When boiling lobsters, the shells turn red quickly, but that is no indication of doneness. Don't boil lobster—it toughens the meat. Lobsters can also be split and cut up in preparation for broiling.

To split a lobster for baking or broiling, do the following.

1. To kill the lobster instantly, place it on a cutting board on its back and insert the tip of a large knife between the eyes.
2. Continue cutting back to the end of the tail. Work the knife down to the back shell to split the lobster.
3. With your hands, crack the back of the shell by spreading the lobster open.
4. With a paring knife, remove the intestinal tract, which resembles a long thin vein running the length of the lobster. Remove the sandy sac (stomach) beneath the eyes.
5. With a sharp blow of the back of the knife, crack the claws to expose the meat.

Whole or cut-up lobster can also be cooked by baking, sauteing, or simmering in sauce or soup.

Oysters

Purchasing   Oysters have a rough shell with scalloped edges. They vary in size, texture, and flavor according to where they are harvested.

- Eastern oysters are taken from the waters of the Atlantic
- Olympia oysters are very small oysters taken from Puget Sound
- Pacific oysters are found along Oregon and Washington coasts
- Japanese oysters are giant oysters found in the Pacific

Oysters can be purchased live in the shell, shucked (fresh or frozen), breaded (raw or frozen), and canned. When buying live oysters, make sure they have:

- Tightly closed shells (if the shells open slightly, tap with a knife and they should close; discard if they don't close)
- Moist shells that are not cracked, chipped, or broken
- Mild odor

Shucked oysters should be plump, with a mild odor, and creamy white in color, but they vary naturally to include green, red, brown, and pink colorations. They should be in a clear liquid. Oysters are available year-round, but are best in fall and winter. Plan on 4 large oysters (in the shell) per serving (4 ounces) and ¼ pound shucked oysters per serving.

Storing Live oysters should be stored at refrigerator temperatures in a shallow pan covered with a wet cloth. Keep damp but not wet. They can be kept up to 3 or 4 days. Shucked oysters should be stored in their own juices in a container with a tight lid in the coldest section of your refrigerator. They should be used in 2 to 3 days.

To freeze shucked oysters, follow the directions for clams.

Handling and Cooking At least one hour before shucking, scrub the oysters under cold running water. Discard any oysters that don't have tightly closed shells or shells that close once jiggled. Put them flat on a tray and place them in the refrigerator. This helps them relax. The illustration shows the steps for shucking; to shuck, do the following.

1. Shucking an oyster is a question of leverage, not force. To open, place it flat side up, and with a cloth or towel, press it firmly against

How to shuck an oyster

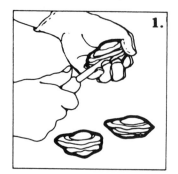

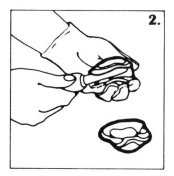

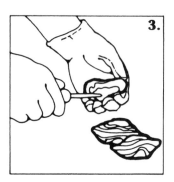

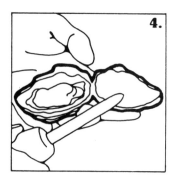

the work surface. Do not hold it in your hand and try to open it in the air as you would a clam. Place the tip of the oyster knife between the shell near the hinge.

2. Twist the knife up while pushing it in until you hear a snap (that means the hinge is broken).

3. Twist to open the shell wide enough to slide the knife inside the top shell to cut the muscle that closes the shell. Avoid cutting the flesh of the oyster (or it will lose its plumpness).

4. Lift the top shell off. Keep the oyster level at all times to save the juice. Cut the lower end of the muscle from the bottom shell to loosen the meat. Remove any pieces of shell that may be in the meat.

Cooking methods for oysters include poaching, baking on the half-shell, in soups and stews. Oysters in the shell are cooked when the shell opens. Shucked oysters are done when they become plump and opaque and the edges start to curl.

Scallops

Purchasing The scallop is actually the muscle that opens and closes the shell. This sweet-flavored, creamy white muscle is the only part of the scallop eaten by Americans, but Europeans eat the entire scallop. There are several different kinds of scallops.

- Bay scallops are caught off the Eastern coast of the United States, the Gulf of Mexico, and the North Sea. They are smaller and often considered more delicate than other varieties.
- Calico scallops are primarily found in the South Atlantic and are usually available breaded only.
- Sea scallops are caught off the coasts of the New England and Middle Atlantic states. They are larger and are often cut into smaller pieces.

Scallops are always sold shucked. To be fresh, they should display the following characteristics.

- Mild, sweet odor
- Moist-looking but not displayed in liquid or in direct contact with ice
- Varying color—the smaller bay and calico scallops are usually creamy white, with occasional light tan or pink coloration; the larger sea scallops are also usually creamy white, though they might show light orange or pink color, which is natural

Scallops are available year-round. Plan on ¼ pound per 4-ounce serving.

Storing Scallops can be stored for 1 to 2 days covered in the refrigerator. A fishy smell or brownish color indicates spoilage. To freeze scallops, poach them first and pack them in their own juices. Maximum storage is 3 months.

Handling and Cooking The only preparation for scallops is to wash them quickly in cold water and pull off the small, tough tendon that is on the side of each scallop. Scallops can be cooked in almost any way that fish can, such as baking, broiling, sauteing, and poaching. Scallops turn milky white or opaque and firm when done. Sea scallops take 3 to 5 minutes to cook through; the smaller bay scallops take 2 to 3 minutes.

Shrimp

Purchasing Shrimp is a small crustacean that looks somewhat like a small lobster without claws. The edible portion of the shrimp is the tail section. These tails are graded according to the number per pound in unpeeled form. This unit is known as count and is important because the cost and use are based on this. Generally the larger the shrimp, the higher the price. There are many varieties of shrimp, such as brown, pink, and white, but after cooking, all shrimp are the same color. The term **prawn** is sometimes used to mean large shrimp. The term **green shrimp** refers to raw shrimp in the shell.

Shrimp can be purchased in several forms.

- Green shrimp—raw in the shell
- Peeled and deveined—raw with the shell and vein removed
- Peeled, deveined, and cooked

These three forms are usually sold frozen (unless it is locally produced) because shrimp is highly perishable. Shrimp is also available frozen and breaded (raw or cooked), canned, and butterflied (split in the shell). Following are characteristics of fresh raw and cooked shrimp.

How to peel and devein shrimp

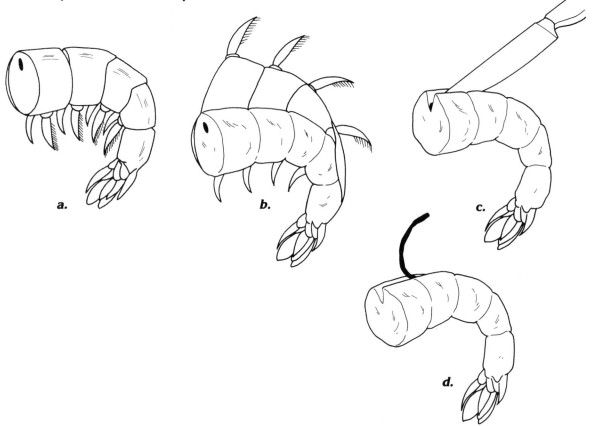

a.   b.   c.

d.

Raw shrimp

- Firm meat
- Translucent shells with grayish green, pinkish tan, or light pink tint and a minimum of black spots or edges
- Moist but not displayed in liquid

Cooked shrimp in the shell

- Firm white meat with pink or reddish shells
- Moist but not in direct contact with ice

Shrimp are available year-round. Plan on ⅓ pound of headless, unpeeled shrimp per serving (4 ounces), and ¼ pound of peeled and deveined shrimp or cooked meat per serving.

Storing Fresh shrimp should be stored in the refrigerator and used within 1 to 2 days. Frozen shrimp should be kept at or below 0°F, and their maximum storage time is 4 to 6 months.

Handling and Cooking Shrimp to be served hot must be peeled and deveined before cooking. If shrimp is to be served cold, it is usually peeled and deveined after cooking to maintain flavor.

To peel and devein shrimp, do the following, as shown in the illustration.

1. Break off the head and discard (a). Starting at the head end, grasp the legs on one side and peel the shell around and off the body (b). Several segments may be done at once. The tail section may be left on for appearance.
2. Make a shallow cut down the outer curve of the shrimp with a paring knife (c) and remove the vein found just below the surface (d).

Shrimp can be cooked by baking, broiling, simmering, sauteing, and deep-frying. Raw shrimp turn pink and firm when cooked. Cooking time depends on the size; it takes from 3 to 5 minutes

TUNA FISH

❖ ❖ ❖

The largest seafood industry in the United States—tuna—was developed back in 1903 when sardines were in short supply. Today there are four main species of tuna marketed here.

1. Albacore—the only white meat tuna, has a mild flavor and creamy white color
2. Yellowfin—the most popular tuna for canned chunk light tuna
3. Bluefin—this tuna is also canned as chunk light tuna
4. Skipjack—smallest of the four tunas, canned as chunk light tuna

When buying canned tuna fish, there are various pack styles.

- Solid white tuna—when the label states "solid white," only large pieces of albacore tuna are used (this is the more expensive product)
- Chunk light—this pack style uses smaller pieces of tuna that have a darker color and fuller flavor than albacore
- Oil pack—the tuna is packed in a mixture of soybean oil and vegetable broth seasoned with salt
- Water pack—the tuna is packed in water and therefore has fewer calories (about 60 fewer calories for every 3 ounces of tuna fish)

Besides canned tuna, fresh raw tuna is available. If you've never had it, you don't know what you're missing. Fresh raw tuna does not look at all like its canned counterpart; indeed, it ranges in color from light to dark red, depending on the species. Much of fresh tuna is cut into boneless steaks and fillets, steaks probably being more popular. Because fresh tuna has a firm texture, it holds together well during cooking and can be easily grilled (a 1-inch steak cooks in only 10 minutes), broiled, baked, stir-fried, or poached as follows.

Cooking Method	Guidelines	Time (minutes/lb)	Temperature
Grill	Baste during cooking. Turn once.	6–12	High
Bake	Use a nonstick pan. Brush with oil/lemon juice mixture or low-fat Italian salad dressing.	8–10	425°F
Broil	Use a nonstick pan. Brush with oil/lemon juice mixture or low-fat Italian salad dressing. Broil 4 inches or less from heat. Turn once.	8–12	High
Stir-fry	Cut tuna in ½-inch strips. Stir-fry fish first, remove, then stir-fry vegetables and add fish back to cook for one minute.	6–10	High
Poach	Poach in stock with wine vinegar and herbs.	10–12	Simmer

to boil, steam, or saute 1 pound of medium size shrimp in the shell. If overcooked, the meat will be tough and rubbery.

Boiling is a quick, convenient way to cook shrimp. You don't have to boil shrimp in plain old water. Instead, to 2 cups of water or stock, add 3 tablespoons of red wine vinegar or lemon or lime juice, and a tablespoon of pickling spice. In place of the pickling spice, try bay leaves, thyme, garlic powder, paprika, or ground white or black pepper. These different combinations will impart some additional flavor to the dish.

WHAT IS SURIMI?

❖ ❖ ❖

A new fish product that has become available to consumers is surimi seafood. The word "surimi" is derived from the Japanese term for restructured food. It is currently made from Alaska pollock, a mild white-fleshed fish, because of its gelling qualities, light color, and good texture.

Surimi is prepared under strict controls at sea or on shore. The fillet portion of fresh-caught fish is minced, washed, and strained to yield a concentrated fish paste. Small quantities of salt, sugar, and/or sorbitol are added to stabilize the protein. The paste is frozen for transportation to further processing plants where it becomes raw material for unique food products.

Surimi is processed into consumer food products, such as imitation crabmeat, by blending it with binders such as starch or egg white. Real shellfish, a shellfish extract, or artificial shellfish flavoring is added to make it taste like shellfish. Then it is fabricated into the shape, texture, and color of shellfish. Manufacturers have developed a flake style for salads as well. Surimi products are marketed under a number of names, such as imitation crabmeat and imitation lobster tail.

RECIPES

ITALIAN FISH ROLL-UPS

1 lb flounder or cod fillets, fresh or frozen, without skin
9-oz package frozen French-style green beans
2 tbsp onion, chopped
½ cup boiling water
8-oz can tomato sauce (low-sodium may be used)
¼ tsp oregano leaves
¼ tsp basil leaves
⅛ tsp garlic powder
1 tbsp grated Parmesan cheese

1. Thaw frozen fish in refrigerator overnight. Divide fish into 4 servings.
2. Add beans and onion to boiling water. Cover and boil gently until beans are tender crisp, about 7 minutes. Drain.
3. Place ¼ of the bean-onion mixture in middle of each fish portion.
4. Start with narrow end of fillet and roll. Place in baking pan with end of fillets underneath.
5. Mix tomato sauce, oregano, basil, and garlic powder. Pour over fish roll-ups.
6. Sprinkle with cheese.
7. Bake at 350°F (moderate oven) just until fish flakes easily when tested with a fork, about 35–45 minutes.

Serves 4

Nutrition Analysis:

Calories 169
Carbohydrate. . . . . .9 grams
Fiber . . . . .2 grams
Fat. . . . . .2 grams
Cholesterol. . . . . .73 milligrams
Sodium. . . . . .520 milligrams

BAKED FISH FILLETS

1 lb fresh or frozen ocean perch, cod, or flounder fillets
2 tsp margarine, melted
1 tbsp lemon juice

½ tsp salt
¼ tsp paprika
1 tsp parsley, chopped

1. Thaw frozen fish in refrigerator overnight.
2. Spray a shallow baking pan with vegetable spray. Place fillets in a single layer, skin side down, in pan.
3. Mix margarine, lemon juice, salt, and paprika. Spoon over fillets.
4. Bake at 350°F (moderate oven) until fish flakes easily when tested with a fork, about 10–20 minutes.
5. Garnish each serving with parsley.

Serves 4

Nutrition Analysis:

Calories 130
Carbohydrate. . . . . .0 grams
Fiber . . . . .0 grams
Fat. . . . . .3 grams
Cholesterol. . . . . .58 milligrams
Sodium. . . . . .372 milligrams

SHARK KABOBS

1 8-oz can juice-packed pineapple chunks
¼ cup sherry
1 tbsp low-sodium soy sauce
2 tsp brown sugar
½ tsp ground ginger
½ tsp dry mustard
1 clove garlic, minced
1 lb shark steaks, cut into 1-in. cubes
1 green pepper, cut into 1-in. squares

1. Drain pineapple, reserving juice. For marinade, combine pineapple juice and remaining ingredients. Reserve 1 tbsp for cooking. Place shark cubes, pineapple, and green pepper in a shallow dish; add marinade. Cover and refrigerate for at least 1 hour.
2. Drain marinade. Thread fish, pineapple, and green pepper alternately on 4 skewers.
3. Place skewers on shallow baking pan and broil about 4 to 6 inches from heat source for 4 to 5 minutes. Turn skewers, brush with reserved marinade. Broil 4 to 5 minutes longer or until fish is opaque or white and firm.

Serves 4

Nutrition Analysis:

Calories 185
Carbohydrate. . . . . .15 grams
Fiber . . . . .1 gram
Fat. . . . . .4 grams
Cholesterol. . . . . .43 milligrams
Sodium. . . . . .220 milligrams

ITALIAN-STYLE MICROWAVED HALIBUT STEAKS

1 lb halibut steaks, approximately 1-inch thick
¼ cup low-calorie Italian dressing
1 tbsp lemon juice
¼ tsp pepper
¼ tsp paprika

1. Place steaks in a microwave dish. Combine remaining ingredients and pour over fish. Cover dish and refrigerate 30 minutes, turning once.
2. Turn back one corner of cover for venting. Cook 4 to 5 minutes on HIGH (100%), rotating dish ¼ turn after 2 minutes. Let stand 2 to 3 minutes before serving. Fish is done when it is opaque or white and firm.

Serves 4

Nutrition Analysis:

Calories 141
Carbohydrate. . . . . .1 gram
Fiber . . . . .0 grams
Fat. . . . . .4 grams
Cholesterol. . . . . .37 milligrams
Sodium. . . . . .179 milligrams

BASIL-BAKED COD FILLETS

½ lb cod, haddock, lingcod, or orange roughy fillet
1 tsp olive oil
1 tsp lemon juice
¼ tsp dried basil, crushed
⅛ tsp black pepper
dash salt
2 plum tomatoes, cored and cut crosswise into thin
  slices
2 tsp grated Parmesan cheese

1. Pat fish dry and cut into two serving pieces.
   Combine oil and lemon juice in a baking dish.
   Add fish and turn to coat both sides. Sprinkle
   with basil, pepper, and salt. Overlap tomatoes in
   even layer on fish and sprinkle with Parmesan
   cheese.
2. Cover with foil and bake at 400°F, about 10–15
   minutes or until fish is opaque or white and
   firm.

Serves 2

Nutrition Analysis:

    Calories 152
    Carbohydrate. . . . . .7 grams
    Fiber . . . . .1 gram
    Fat. . . . . .4 grams
    Cholesterol. . . . . .48 milligrams
    Sodium. . . . . .118 milligrams

FISH BAKED WITH SUMMER SQUASH, ONION, AND HERBS

2 tsp vegetable oil
1 lb orange roughy, cod or other firm, white fish
  fillets
2 medium onions, thinly sliced
2 medium zucchini, thinly sliced
2 medium yellow squash, thinly sliced
⅓ cup freshly squeezed lemon juice
¼ tsp salt
½ tsp freshly ground pepper
3 tbsp freshly chopped herbs—any combination of
  thyme, tarragon, chives, parsley, dill
lemon wedges to garnish

1. Preheat the oven to 400°F. Coat bottom of a 9
   × 12-inch ovenproof baking dish with the oil.
   Spread half the sliced onion, zucchini, and
   yellow squash over the bottom of the dish. Lay
   the fish fillets on top of the vegetables. Cover
   the fish with the remaining onions and squash.
   Sprinkle the lemon juice over the dish and then
   the salt and pepper. Cover tightly with
   aluminum foil.
2. Bake the fish for about 45 minutes, until the fish
   is firm and opaque and the vegetables are
   tender. Just before serving sprinkle the herbs
   over the top. Serve with lemon wedges.

Serves 4

Nutrition Analysis:

    Calories 154
    Carbohydrate. . . . . .15 grams
    Fiber . . . . .2 grams
    Fat. . . . . .3 grams
    Cholesterol. . . . . .37 milligrams
    Sodium. . . . . .185 milligrams

BROILED SESAME FISH

1 lb cod fillets, fresh or frozen
1 tsp margarine, melted
1 tbsp lemon juice
1 tsp dried tarragon leaves

⅛ tsp salt
dash pepper
1 tbsp sesame seeds
1 tbsp parsley, chopped

1. Thaw frozen fish in refrigerator overnight or defrost briefly in a microwave oven. Cut fish into four portions.
2. Place fish on a broiler pan lined with aluminum foil. Brush margarine over fish.
3. Mix lemon juice, tarragon leaves, salt, and pepper. Pour over fish.
4. Sprinkle sesame seeds evenly over fish.
5. Broil until fish flakes easily when tested with fork—about 12 minutes.
6. Garnish each serving with parsley.

Serves 4

Nutrition Analysis:

Calories 103
Carbohydrate. . . . . .0 grams
Fiber . . . . .0 grams
Fat. . . . . .2 grams
Cholesterol. . . . . .49 milligrams
Sodium. . . . . .137 milligrams

No-Mayo Tuna Salad

2 cans (6½ ounces each) tuna fish, water-packed, well-drained
1 tart apple (Granny Smith), unpeeled and diced
½ cup diced celery
¼ cup balsamic vinegar

1. In bowl, combine tuna, apple, and celery. Add enough balsamic vinegar to bind.

Serves 4 (sandwiches)

Nutrition Analysis:

Calories 149
Carbohydrate. . . . . .9 grams
Fiber . . . . .1 gram
Fat. . . . . .1 gram
Cholesterol. . . . . .15 milligrams
Sodium. . . . . .319 milligrams

❖ ❖ ❖

CHAPTER TEN

DAIRY AND EGGS

Dairy products and eggs are among the most versatile foods that are part of many recipes. You cannot overlook the fact that in addition to the many advantages of nutrition, dairy products and eggs are generally inexpensive, and many lower-in-fat versions are available.

MILK

Although milk is consumed as a beverage, it is classified as a food. Cold milk not only serves as a delightful beverage, but is also used in cooking and baking. Milk provides substantial amounts of calcium and is a very inexpensive source of protein in the diet. It serves as a primary ingredient in various drinks including cocoa, milkshakes, and eggnogs, a real holiday favorite.

It seems that the age of the long-necked glass milk bottle that required shaking prior to consumption was not so long ago. In the early stages of milk processing, the consumer received milk that was "pasteurized" (heated to kill harmful germs) but not "homogenized." When milk was not homogenized and allowed to stand, the lighter fat would float to the top and the thinner milk would settle below. In other words, the top contained "cream" and the bottom clear liquid was "skim milk." Upon shaking prior to use, the consumer created a "temporary emulsion" (a combination of fat and liquid) and the milk would become smooth and blended. Since fat and liquid do not combine permanently under normal circumstances, the milk would start to separate within a few minutes after shaking. Today's milk

products are homogenized to create a permanent bond between the milk and cream. In addition, the cardboard containers help to better preserve some nutrients.

Purchasing

Milk is available in many forms. The following is a breakdown of different milks and their uses:

Whole milk Whole milk is characterized by a smooth, rich flavor. It contains a fat content of at least 3.5 percent and has enjoyed popularity as both a beverage and food for many decades.

Low-fat milk Low-fat milk is very popular. There are two major types of low-fat milk at the supermarket: 1 percent or 2 percent. The product's name declares the percentage of milk fat.

Skim milk Skim milk must have a fat content of less than 0.5 percent. It has a "cloudy" appearance and lacks the richness in taste of either whole or low-fat milk. If you are accustomed to drinking either whole or low-fat milk, skim milk will have a watery flavor. As you drink skim milk over a period of time, the flavor becomes pleasant and you will adjust to it.

Chocolate milk Chocolate milk is made by adding sweeteners and chocolate to milk. The milk may be whole, low-fat, or skim.

Cultured buttermilk Buttermilk is made most often by adding a bacterial culture to fresh, pasteurized skim milk. The bacteria convert the sugar in milk, lactose, into lactic acid, thereby giving buttermilk a thick consistency and tart and buttery taste. Buttermilk is enjoyed as a beverage and is used in baking when sour milk is needed. It is also used in making salad dressings and some cold soups.

Eggnog Eggnog is a mixture of dairy ingredients (cream, milk, partially skimmed milk or skim milk), eggs, and sweeteners. It may be flavored with rum extract, nutmeg, vanilla, or other flavorings. Commercial eggnog is pasteurized so there shouldn't be any concern about the safety of the egg yolks in this product.

Lactase-treated milk Milk that has been treated with the enzyme lactase is particularly helpful for individuals who have lactose intolerance. Lactose intolerance or lactase deficiency, is a disease caused by a lack of the enzyme lactase, which is needed by the intestine to split lactose into its two components for absorption. After drinking milk or eating a dairy product with lactose, the lactose-intolerant individual experiences symptoms that include abdominal cramps, bloating, and diarrhea. Lactase-treated milk is ready to drink or be used in recipes as it has only 30 percent of the lactose found in regular milk. Eight fluid ounces of LactAid brand milk contains only 3 grams of lactose, compared with 12 grams in regular milk, and is nutritionally identical to regular milk.

Certified milk Also called raw milk, certified milk is not pasteurized. It can only be sold by certain dairies.

Canned whole milk or UHT milk Did you notice in the supermarket one day that there were little paper cartons, looking just like juice, that were indeed milk, and it wasn't even under refrigeration? Well, milk has gotten high-tech. Using a process called ultra-high temperatures, whole milk can be packaged in sterilized, sealed containers and stored at room temperature. It is identical in composition to fresh, whole milk and tastes close to it as well. It can be kept unrefrigerated for up to 3 months or up to the date stamped on it. Chill it before serving and refrigerate after opening.

Evaporated milk and evaporated skim milk These products are made by heating milk to stabilize the milk protein, then removing about 60 percent of the water. Both products are sold in cans. Evaporated milk has 7.5 percent milk fat; evaporated skim milk has no more than 0.5 percent milk fat. They are used mostly in cooking and baking. One-half cup of either product can be reconstituted with one-half cup of water to make 1 cup of milk.

Sweetened condensed milk and skimmed milk These products also have about 60 percent of their water removed. What makes them different is that they are heavily sweetened, usually with sugar. Sweetened condensed milk has 8 percent milk fat; sweetened condensed skimmed milk has no more than 0.5 percent milk fat. They are used mostly in cooking and baking.

Nonfat dry milk (powdered milk) This product is made by removing the water from pasteurized skim milk. It is popular because it is generally cheaper to use than buying liquid milk, it is convenient, and has a good shelf life. It can be easily reconstituted with water—3 tablespoons to 8 ounces of water. Although it doesn't have the taste of fluid milk, it is acceptable to use in baking and cooking.

When purchasing fresh milk, make sure the label states that the milk is pasteurized, homogenized, and fortified with vitamins A and D. Also check the pull date, which indicates when the product should be withdrawn from retail sale. This date allows for several days storage time in your refrigerator. Also, buy milk in cartons or tinted glass bottles, not clear glass bottles or plastic. Certain nutrients in milk, such as riboflavin, are destroyed by light. Last, only buy milk that has been refrigerated properly and is not on the edge of the milk case getting warm.

Nutrition
Milk is a good source of:

- High-quality protein
- Carbohydrate
- Riboflavin
- Vitamins A and D (if fortified)

- Calcium and other minerals such as phosphorus, magnesium, and zinc

Table 40 compares the nutritional content of whole, 2 percent, 1 percent, and skim milk. By switching from whole milk to skim, you save about 60 calories and reduce the amount of fat to almost zero.

Buttermilk has about the same nutritional composition as the milk from which it was made—in most cases, skim milk. Evaporated milk, when mixed with an equal part of water, has about the same nutritional value as an equal amount of fresh milk. Condensed milk is much higher in calories than fresh fluid milk due in large part to the high fat content (of the regular version only) and the added sugar. Nonfat milk, when mixed with water, has about the same nutritional value as an equal amount of skim milk.

Storing

Fresh milk is very perishable and should be stored in the refrigerator for up to 4 days after the pull date (whole milk stays fresher longer than either skim or low-fat milks). If the milk goes bad (it will smell terrible and look curdled) before this time, it is probably because the dairy, the store, or possibly you, mishandled the milk and let it warm up one or more times. Always close the container the milk is in (so the milk doesn't ab-

sorb other odors in the refrigerator) and don't let the container sit on the kitchen table during meals. If you do pour milk into a pitcher to sit out at room temperature for more than 15 minutes, do not pour it back into the milk container. Keep it separate as it is no longer as fresh. Also, use milk in the order of purchase.

Foods made with milk, such as pudding and custard, should be covered tightly in the refrigerator and used within 3 to 4 days.

Evaporated, condensed, and nonfat dry milk can all be stored unopened at room temperature for at least one year or, if available, use the dating code marked on the container. Once opened, evaporated and condensed milk should be poured into another container, refrigerated, and used within 5 days. Once reconstituted, nonfat dry milk should be refrigerated and used within 5 days.

Cooking Light and Healthy

Milk products are a very important part of many recipes. The addition of milk products can create a creamy consistency to many sauces, help dissolve dry ingredients in baked products, or simply add good nutrition and flavor to a food. Substituting low-fat or skim milk for whole milk works well in most cooking and baking recipes to reduce the fat content. Evaporated skim milk can be used in place of half-and-half in some recipes such as soups.

When cooking with milk, remember a very important rule—use a moderate heat and heat the milk slowly (but not too long) to avoid "curdling"—a grainy appearance with a lumpy texture. From a scientific point of view, milk "curdles" when the casein (the name of the protein in milk) separates out of the milk. When adding food products to hot milk products, remember to add slowly either with a spoon or using a wire whisk if preparing a sauce to avoid lumps. Be especially careful when adding foods high in acid—milk has a tendency to curdle very quickly if not beaten quickly.

Another problem with milk is the creation of a top layer of "skin"—a film that forms on top of the milk during cooking. It can be prevented by keeping the pot of milk covered. A final problem with milk is scorching—when milk sticks to the

❖ Table 40 Calories and Fat in Milk ❖ and Cream

Product	Serving Size	Calories	Fat (grams)
Skim milk	1 cup	86	0.5
1% milk	1 cup	102	3
2% milk	1 cup	121	5
Whole milk	1 cup	150	8
Half-and-half	1 tablespoon	20	2
Light cream (coffee cream)	1 tablespoon	29	3
Light whipping cream, fluid	1 tablespoon	44	5
Heavy whipping cream, fluid	1 tablespoon	52	6
Sour cream	1 tablespoon	26	3

bottom of the pot during cooking and eventually starts to burn, making the food you are cooking taste terrible. Because milk is very sensitive to direct heat, heat it slowly; in some cases you will need to heat milk in a double boiler.

CHEESE

Cheeses are a versatile food and can be used in many different applications. Cheeses have a variety of flavors ranging from mild to very sharp and can be an important ingredient in a recipe as well as a great snack.

Purchasing

Cheese is made from various types of milks—cow's and goat's being the most popular. In many parts of the world cheese is produced from various other sources of milk: sheep, reindeer, yak, buffalo, camel mares, and donkeys. Cheese is produced when bacteria or rennet (or both) are added to milk and the milk then curdles. The liquid, known as the whey, is separated from the solid, known as the curd, which is the cheese. It is thought that cheese was discovered by accident thousands of years ago in the ancient Far East.

Cheese can be divided into different categories depending on texture or whether it has been ripened (also called cured). The texture of cheese varies from soft, semisoft, firm, to hard. Ripened cheeses are those that have been fermented with bacteria or molds. By contrast, unripened cheeses are fresh and untreated. Unripened cheeses are generally more perishable than the ripened cheese. The processing time is very short since no time is needed for ripening. When the cheese is manufactured, it is packaged and sold with a relatively short expiration date versus the ripened cheeses. Popular types of unripened cheeses include ricotta cheese and cottage cheese.

The ripened cheeses need many months to age and develop into a marketable cheese. Examples are provolone and Parmesan cheese. For those of you who love blue cheese (and are willing to pay extra as a salad dressing when dining out), the blue vein in the cheese is a "mold" that has been carefully controlled and adds the characteristic flavor to the blue cheese. This cheese also needs months of aging to create a ripening effect.

When a cheese or combination of cheeses is manufactured into another type of cheese, this is referred to as a "processed cheese." Whereas natural cheeses are made directly from milk or whey, processed cheeses are a modified form of natural cheeses that have been ground or shredded from a variety of natural cheeses. Processed cheeses, which contain more sodium than natural cheeses, take many forms:

- Pasteurized process cheese—a combination of cheddar and other cheeses with emulsifiers to make it smooth (for this reason, these cheeses melt better); includes American cheese
- Pasteurized process cheese foods and spreads—made like process cheese except for the addition of optional ingredients such as cream, milk, buttermilk, nonfat dry solids, or whey; it contains more moisture and less fat than process cheese
- Cold pack cheese—made by mixing ripened cheeses without heat

Table 41 is a guide to many of the different types of cheeses available.

When purchasing cheese, check for mold—even when it is in airtight packaging. Mold commonly appears as white, blue, or green fuzzy spots. Also check for dryness—the cheese will have darker edges if this is the case. Many processed cheeses are dated with sell by or use by dates, so check for one. Make sure the cheese has been kept cold. Only four types of cheese do not require refrigeration—cold pack cheese, cold pack cheese food, pasteurized process cheese food, and pasteurized process cheese spread—until opened.

Nutrition

On the positive side, cheese is an excellent source of nutrients such as protein and calcium. However, because most cheeses are prepared from whole milk or cream, they are also high in saturated fat and cholesterol. Ounce for ounce, meat, poultry, and most cheeses have about the same amount of cholesterol. But cheeses generally have much more saturated fat.

Determining which cheeses are high and low in saturated fat and cholesterol can be confusing

❖ Table 41 A Guide to Cheeses ❖

Cheese	Characteristics	Uses
Unripened		
Cottage	Mild, slightly acid flavor; soft, open texture with tender curds of varying size; white to creamy white	Appetizers, salads, cheesecakes, dips
Cream	Delicate, slightly acid flavor; soft, smooth texture; white	Appetizers, salads, sandwiches, desserts, and snacks
Neufchatel	Mild, acid flavor; soft, smooth texture similar to cream cheese but lower in fat; white	Salads, sandwiches, desserts, snacks, dips
Ricotta	Mild, sweet, nutlike flavor; soft, moist texture with loose curds (fresh Ricotta) or dry and suitable for grating; white	Salads, main dishes such as lasagna and ravioli, and desserts, mostly in cooked dishes
Soft, Ripened		
Bel paese	Mild, sweet flavor; light, creamy-yellow interior; slate-gray surface; soft to medium-firm, creamy texture	Appetizers, sandwiches, desserts, and snacks
Brie	Mild to pungent flavor; soft, smooth texture; creamy-yellow interior; edible thin brown and white crust	Appetizers, sandwiches, desserts, snacks, salads
Camembert	Distinctive mild to pungent flavor; soft, smooth texture— almost fluid when fully ripened; creamy-yellow interior; edible thin white or gray-white crust	Appetizers, desserts, and snacks
Limburger	Highly pungent, very strong flavor and aroma; soft, smooth texture that usually contains small irregular openings; creamy-white interior; reddish-yellow surface	Appetizers, desserts, snacks, sandwiches
Semisoft, Ripened		
Blue	Tangy, piquant flavor; semisoft, pasty, sometimes crumbly texture; white interior marbled or streaked with blue veins of mold; resembles Roquefort	Appetizers, salads and salad dressings, desserts, and snacks
Brick	Mild, pungent, sweet flavor; semisoft to medium-firm, elastic texture; creamy white-to-yellow interior; brownish exterior	Appetizers, sandwiches, desserts, and snacks
Gorgonzola	Tangy, rich, spicy flavor; semisoft, pasty, sometimes crumbly texture; creamy-white interior, mottled or streaked with blue-green veins of mold; clay-colored surface	Appetizers, salads, desserts, and snacks
Mozzarella (also called Scamorza)	Delicate, mild flavor; slightly firm, plastic texture; creamy white	Main dishes such as pizza or lasagna, sandwiches, snacks, and salads
Muenster	Mild to mellow flavor; semisoft texture with numerous small openings; creamy-white interior; yellowish-tan or white surface	Appetizers, sandwiches, desserts, and snacks
Port du Salut	Mellow to robust flavor similar to Gouda; semisoft, smooth elastic texture; creamy white or yellow	Appetizers, desserts, and snacks
Roquefort	Sharp, peppery, piquant flavor; semisoft, pasty, sometimes crumbly texture; white interior streaked with blue-green veins of mold	Appetizers, salads and salad dressings, desserts, and snacks
Sap sago	Sharp, pungent, cloverlike flavor; very hard texture suitable for grating; light green or sage green	Grated for seasoning
Stilton	Piquant flavor, milder than Gorgonzola or Roquefort; open, flaky texture; creamy-white interior streaked with blue-green veins of mold; wrinkled, melon-like rind	Appetizers, salads, desserts, snacks, in cooked foods

❖ Table 41 Continued ❖

Cheese	Characteristics	Uses
Hard, Ripened		
Cheddar (often called American)	Mild to very sharp flavor; smooth texture, firm to crumbly; light cream to orange	Appetizers, main dishes, sauces, soups, sandwiches, salads, desserts, and snacks
Colby	Mild to mellow flavor, similar to Cheddar; softer body and more open texture than Cheddar; light cream to orange	Sandwiches, snacks, cooked foods
Edam	Mellow, nutlike, sometimes salty flavor; rather firm, rubbery texture; creamy-yellow or medium yellow-orange interior; surface coated with red wax; usually shaped like a flattened ball	Appetizers, salads, sandwiches, sauces, desserts, and snacks
Gouda	Mellow, nutlike, often slightly acid flavor; semisoft to firm, smooth texture, often containing small holes; creamy-yellow or medium yellow-orange interior; usually has red wax coating; usually shaped like a flattened ball	Appetizers, salads, sandwiches, sauces, desserts, and snacks
Gruyere	Nutlike, salty flavor, similar to Swiss, but sharper; firm, smooth texture with small holes or eyes; light yellow	Appetizers, desserts, snacks, fondue and other cooked dishes
Monterey (Jack)	Semisoft; smooth, open texture, mild flavor; Cheddar-like; hard when aged	Appetizers, sandwiches, salads
Parmesan	Sharp, distinctive flavor; very hard, granular texture; yellowish white	Grated on cooked (Italian) dishes, salads, as seasoning
Provolone	Mellow to sharp flavor, smoky and salty; firm, smooth texture; cuts without crumbling; light creamy yellow; light-brown or golden-yellow surface	Appetizers, main dishes, sandwiches, desserts, and snacks
Romano	Very sharp, piquant flavor; very hard, granular texture; yellowish-white interior; greenish-black surface	Seasoning and general table use; when cured a year, it is suitable for grating
Swiss (also called Emmentaler)	Mild, sweet, nutlike flavor; firm, smooth, elastic body with large round eyes; light yellow	Sandwiches, salads, snacks, fondue and other cooked dishes

because there are so many different kinds on the market: part-skim, low-fat, processed, and so on. Not all reduced fat or part-skim cheeses are always low in fat; they are only lower in fat than similar natural cheeses. For instance, one reduced-fat cheddar gets 56 percent of its calories from fat—considerably less than the 71 percent of regular cheddar, but not super lean either. The trick is to read the label. For less fat, saturated fat, cholesterol, and calories, choose a cheese made from skim milk or low-fat milk with 4 grams of fat or less per ounce. Table 42 is a guide to fat in cheeses.

Besides cheeses that contain less fat, there are cheeses coming on the market with no fat. Examples include nonfat cream cheese and nonfat American processed cheese. In addition, some companies are beginning to use the fat substitute Simplesse in low-fat cheeses.

If watching your sodium intake, be aware that cheese is fairly high in sodium. Natural cheeses, such as cheddar, have less sodium than processed cheeses, such as American. Also, low-fat cheeses quite often have more sodium than their regular counterparts. Read labels carefully.

Storing
Because of their fat content, many cheeses readily absorb refrigerator odors, resulting in a poor-tasting product. Therefore, store all cheeses tightly in plastic wrap or foil (except blue cheese—wrap loosely). Cheeses also need to be wrapped tightly to prevent them from drying out. Hard and firm

❖ *Table 42 Guide to Fat in Cheeses*[†] ❖

Lowfat 0–3 g fat/oz	Medium Fat 4–5 g fat/oz	High Fat 6–8 g fat/oz	Very High Fat 9–10 g fat/oz
Natural Cheeses			
*Cottage Cheese (¼ c) Dry curd	*Mozzarella *Part skim*	Bleu Cheese	Cheddar
Cottage Cheese (¼ c) Lowfat 1%	*Ricotta (¼ c) *Part skim*	*Brick	Colby
Cottage Cheese (¼ c) Lowfat 2%	String Cheese *Part skim*	Brie Camembert	*Cream Cheese (1 oz = 2 Tbsp)
Cottage Cheese (¼ c) Creamed 4%		Edam Feta	Fontina *Gruyere
Sap Sago		Gjetost Gouda	Longhorn *Monterey Jack
		*Light Cream Cheese (1 oz = 2 Tbsp)	Muenster Roquefort
Look for special lowfat brands of mozzarella, ricotta, cheddar, and monterey jack.	*Look for reduced fat brands of cheddar, colby, monterey jack, muenster, and swiss.*	Limburger Mozzarella, *whole milk* Parmesan (1 oz = 3 Tbsp) *Port du Salut Provolone *Ricotta (¼ c), *whole milk* Romano (1 oz = 3 Tbsp) *Swiss Tilsit, *whole milk*	
Modified Cheeses			
Pasteurized process, imitation, and substitute cheeses with 3 g fat/oz or less.	Pasteurized process, imitation, and substitute cheeses with 4–5 g fat/oz.	Pasteurized Process Swiss Cheese Pasteurized Process Swiss Cheese food Pasteurized Process American Cheese Pasteurized Process American Cheese food American Cheese Food Cold Pack Imitation and substitute cheeses with 6–8 g fat/oz.	*Some pasteurized process cheeses are found in this category—check the labels.*

[†]*Check the labels for fat and sodium content. 1 serving = 1 oz. unless otherwise stated.*
*These cheeses contain 160 mg or less of sodium per 1 oz.
Source: *Reprinted by permission of the American Heart Association, Alameda County Chapter, 11200 Golf Links Road, Oakland, CA 94605.*

cheeses keep from a week to several months in the refrigerator, while semisoft and soft cheeses are much more perishable and can keep only one to two weeks. For unripened cheeses, such as cottage cheese and cream cheese, check the "sell by" or "use by" date. These products should last at least several days beyond the sell by date.

In general, the firmer cheeses hold up longer than the soft cheeses, such as ricotta and Brie.

Cooking Light and Healthy
There are several ways to use cheese in light and healthy cooking.

- Use less cheese than the recipe calls for.

- Substitute low-fat cheeses for regular ones.
- Use a mixture of half regular cheese and half low-fat cheese.
- Use a regular cheese, but use a strong-flavored one and use less of it than called for in the recipe.

Recipes for Low-Fat Macaroni and Cheese, Cheesy Macaroni and Vegetables, and Mushroom and Spinach Lasagna appear on pages 181–182.

When cooking with cheese, observe some simple guidelines.

1. Use low heat. It is best to use as low a heat as possible, because cheese has a tendency to toughen when subjected to high heat due to its high protein content. Avoid "boiling" at all costs.
2. Use short cooking times. Most recipes will require the addition of cheese at the end of the recipe to avoid overcooking. Remember to stir often to enhance the blend of flavors and establish a good, smooth consistency.
3. Grate the cheese. The best way to add a cheese to a recipe is to grate it. Grating will break the cheese into small, thin pieces that will melt and blend quickly and evenly into the end product.

CREAM

Cream is used in many ways in the kitchen, such as in sauces, soups, hot and cold beverages, baked goods, and when whipped, as a topping for desserts and hot beverages.

Purchasing
There are several types of cream. Most have been pasteurized. In some cases you may find ultrapasteurized cream at the supermarket. In comparison to pasteurized cream, ultrapasteurized cream has a much longer shelf life but does not whip as well.

Heavy whipping cream or heavy cream Heavy cream is a very thick, semifluid liquid that is at least 36 percent fat (by weight). It is often used as a topping after a short period of whipping and can be used in sauces. Remember not to overbeat heavy cream or it will turn into butter!

Light whipping cream or whipping cream Light whipping cream contains 30–35 percent milk fat. Whipping cream labeled as ultrapasteurized does not whip as well as regular whipping cream, but does have a longer shelf life.

Light cream Light cream is also called table cream or coffee cream. It has a fat content of 18–30 percent (usually it's 18 percent). It too has a strong, rich flavor and is often used as an ingredient in both sauces and baked products. It can't be successfully whipped.

Half-and-half Half-and-half (half milk, half cream) normally has a fat content of 10–12 percent. Its consistency is heavy and the flavor is still rich. Like light cream, it can't be successfully whipped.

Sour cream Sour cream is made from pasteurized cream (with 18 percent milk fat content) to which bacteria are added. The bacteria convert the milk sugar lactose into lactic acid, thereby giving the product its thick consistency and tangy taste.

Prepared whipped cream Whipped cream is available in aerosol cans. It also contains sweeteners and stabilizers.

Whichever style you buy, be sure the container is clean, tightly sealed, and cold. Check for a date code on it as well.

Nutrition
Although cream does contain some nutrients, it mostly supplies fat (see Table 40).

Storing
Cream is very perishable and should be kept refrigerated in its closed carton. Do not leave cream out on the kitchen table while you are having your morning coffee—keep it cold! Observe the "use by" date on the carton. If "sell by" dates are used, allow 3 to 4 days beyond the date. For sour cream, allow about 10 days past the "sell by" date. If sour cream gets moldy, even if it is just a few dots, throw it out. Cream that has been ultrapasteurized can be kept refrigerated (unopened) for up to 6 weeks. Once opened, it can keep 1 week.

Cooking Light and Healthy

In recipes, you can substitute lower-in-fat products for cream, such as:

Instead of:	Use:
1 cup heavy cream	1 cup evaporated skim milk
1 cup light cream	1 cup low-fat yogurt
1 cup sour cream	1 cup reduced fat sour cream, part or all plain low-fat or nonfat yogurt

When cooking with sour cream and yogurt, don't let it boil or it may curdle due to the high heat. To prevent separation, you can mix in 1 tablespoon flour per ½ cup sour cream or 1 cup of yogurt before cooking.

There are a number of substitutions for real whipped cream. At the very least, you can whip light whipping cream rather than heavy whipping cream. They won't always be acceptable and some may work better for you on certain foods than others. In any case, try them out and jot down those that work well.

- Whip ½ cup light whipping cream and fold into ½ cup plain or vanilla nonfat yogurt.
- Use low-fat plain vanilla yogurt.
- Blend low-fat cottage cheese and vanilla, mix in sugar if desired.
- Whip well-chilled evaporated skim milk and fold in vanilla and cinnamon.

If you decide you must have **real** whipped cream (in moderation anything is fine), use light whipping cream. Make sure the cream is cold, as cold cream whips better than warm cream. For best results, place the cream, bowl, and beaters into the freezer for about 10 minutes before whipping. Use a bowl that is deep enough for the beaters to fit and small enough for the beaters to maintain contact with the cream. Beat rapidly, scraping the bowl frequently for 2 to 3 minutes, until you get stiff peaks. Don't overbeat—the product will be granular and turns into butter. That is all it usually takes. If adding sugar to the cream, do so after whipping because it makes the cream harder to whip and less stable. Also, use confectioner's rather than granulated sugar for a smoother product. One cup whipping cream yields two cups whipped. It is best to use whipped cream right away, but it can be put into the refrigerator, covered, for a few hours.

ICE CREAM AND ICE MILK

Ice cream is the food produced by freezing, while stirring, a pasteurized mix composed primarily of milk, egg yolks, sweeteners, and flavorings. Ice cream is one of the most popular treats.

Purchasing

In order to be labeled as ice cream, a product must have at least 10 percent fat by weight. Premium ice creams have much more than the minimum required: about 16 percent fat. By comparison, ice milk, which is prepared from the same ingredients as ice cream, has 2–7 percent fat. Ice milk usually has more sugar added.

Ice cream varies, in taste as well as cost, in three ways.

- The amount of fat. The more fat an ice cream contains, the richer it tastes and the more expensive it is.
- The kind of flavoring. Ice cream contains natural flavorings, artificial flavorings, or a combination of both. Natural flavorings make a better quality ice cream that is then more expensive. If only natural flavorings are used, the product is called vanilla ice cream; if both natural and artificial flavorings are used, it is called vanilla flavored ice cream; if only artificial flavorings are used, it is called artificially flavored ice cream.
- The amount of air in the ice cream. All ice cream has air in it—less than half of the product can be air if it is to be labeled as ice cream. Air cells act as a cushion that keep the ingredients from forming into a solid, icy mass. The cranking of an ice cream freezer whips air into the mixture. Premium ice creams have less air in them than lesser brands. That's why premium ice cream always weighs more than equivalent volumes of cheaper brands. Since the amount of air is not stated on the label, you

NONDAIRY DESSERT TOPPINGS

❖ ❖ ❖

Nondairy dessert toppings, such as Dream Whip®, look like whipped cream and have a similar taste, but are made primarily of vegetable oils. Are they healthier? Not really, despite their claims of being "light" and "less fat." Many provide 1 gram of fat per tablespoon, just like whipped cream. What's worse, though, is that many nondairy toppings use highly saturated vegetable oils called tropical oils, which include coconut, palm, and palm kernel oils, so the product contains **more** saturated fat than whipped cream.

Nondairy dessert toppings are available either frozen or in aerosol cans. Check for any dating code to make sure it is fresh. Frozen toppings can be kept in the freezer for one year. Once thawed, it can stay in the refrigerator for 7 days and can even be refrozen for a few more months.

might want to use a scale at the supermarket to compare similar volumes, such as one pint containers.

Make sure any ice cream or ice milk you buy is well below the frost line of the freezer or, preferably, in a freezer with a door. Make sure the container is rock solid and clean. If it feels sticky or looks frosty, it has probably thawed and refrozen.

Nutrition

Ice cream and ice milk are a source of calcium, riboflavin, and protein. Ice cream is also a significant source of fat, as seen in Table 43. There are some brands of ice cream available that are made with fat substitutes. More of these products will be coming on the market in the years to come. Ice milk also has less fat.

Storing

Ice cream and ice milk are best kept in a plastic container with tightly fitting lid in the freezer. This helps prevent it from drying out and absorbing flavors from other food. If kept in the original carton, place plastic wrap over the top of the ice cream before putting the lid on. This gives some added protection from the development of ice crystals. Ice cream and ice milk last about 2 months in the freezer. For best quality, it is best to use within 2 weeks.

YOGURT

Yogurt is an ancient food, but it remained relatively obscure in the United States until about 20 years ago. Americans ate an average of 4.1 pounds of yogurt per person in 1990, four times as much as in 1970, according to the U.S. Department of Agriculture. Europeans eat even more yogurt than we do, as much as 17 pounds per person annually, according to the National Yogurt Association.

Why is yogurt more appealing than ever before? It carries a reputation for being a healthy food, and indeed it is quite nutritious, particularly in its low-fat and nonfat forms. In addition to the claim of promoting long life, yogurt has been touted by some researchers as a cure for digestive ills, high cholesterol levels, and even cancerous tumors in animals. The focus for these health claims is primarily on the bacteria added during yogurt production. The bacteria, Lactobacillus bulgaricus and Streptococcus thermophilus, ferment, or culture, ordinary milk into a tart, creamy gel. But does yogurt really do all these things?

❖ **Table 43   Calories and Fat in** ❖
Ice Cream, Ice Milk, and Frozen Yogurt

Dessert	Serving Size	Calories	Fat (grams)
Premium Vanilla ice cream (16% fat)	1 cup	349	24
Vanilla ice cream (10% fat)	1 cup	269	14
Vanilla ice milk	1 cup	184	6
Vanilla soft-serve ice milk	1 cup	223	5
Frozen yogurt, vanilla	1 cup	240	varies

Scientific studies have not convincingly supported many claims about yogurt's healing properties.

However, yogurt is definitely beneficial to individuals who cannot digest lactose, a kind of sugar found in milk products. Many people in the world, including some 40 million Americans, are lactose intolerant. The condition is very common except among people of European ancestry. For the lactose intolerant, dairy products containing significant amounts of lactose cause diarrhea, abdominal cramps, and nausea. Yogurt is easier to digest because enzymes from the yogurt bacteria break down some of the lactose during the fermentation process. There's also preliminary evidence that once the yogurt's eaten, the bacteria may continue to help break down lactose in the intestinal tract. Yogurt may also help manage diarrhea caused by antibiotic therapy by reestablishing the "good" bacteria killed along with the bad during treatment.

Purchasing

Yogurt has been made basically the same way for centuries. First, cow's milk (in many countries, it's goat's or sheep's milk) is pasteurized to kill unwanted bacteria. Then it's cooled to about 113°F, and the yogurt bacteria are added. The mixture is kept lukewarm for a number of hours, then chilled, allowing time for the bacteria to grow until the mixture becomes a tart, acidic gel.

To make their products last longer on store shelves, manufacturers may heat-treat their yogurts after fermentation. While this doesn't affect the calcium content of the yogurt, it does kill the live cultures, the very ingredient many people expect in a yogurt. If the manufacturer heat-treats the yogurt after fermentation, the label must say "heat-treated after culturing." If the yogurt contains living bacteria, the label may say "active yogurt cultures," "living yogurt cultures," or "contains active cultures." Don't be confused by a label that says "made with active cultures." All yogurts are made this way, but only the brands that are not heat-treated after fermentation retain their living cultures.

There are three main types of yogurt to choose from:

1. Unflavored, plain yogurt
2. Flavored, containing no fruit (such as vanilla, lemon, or coffee)
3. Flavored and containing fruit, may be of two styles:
   - Sundae-style—fruit is at the bottom of the container with plain or flavored yogurt on top; this product is normally stirred before eating
   - Blended-style (also called Swiss-style)—fruit blended throughout plain or flavored yogurt

Whichever style you buy, be sure the container is clean, tightly sealed, and cold.

In addition to fresh yogurt, there is **frozen yogurt**. Frozen yogurt is available either soft-serve or hard. Like fresh yogurt, it must have the two types of bacteria added during processing. Other than that, frozen yogurts may bear little resemblance to their fresh counterparts. For one thing, frozen yogurts are often very sweet. Tart frozen yogurt introduced in the 1970s didn't catch on with consumers looking for an ice cream substitute. Today's frozen yogurts taste more like desserts because they are not fermented as long as non-frozen yogurt. Therefore, they're less acidic than non-frozen yogurt and taste sweeter.

Frozen yogurts also may not have the same amount of living bacteria as their non-frozen counterparts, if they're alive at all. Some manufacturers make frozen yogurt by fermenting milk the traditional way, then freezing the mixture. Others make a kind of ice milk mixture and add the bacteria later. As a result, the number of live culture organisms in frozen yogurt varies greatly between brands.

Nutrition

Yogurt is a good source of:

- Protein
- Calcium, phosphorus, and potassium
- Riboflavin and vitamin B12

Yogurt contains the same fats that are found in the milk product it was made from. Whole milk yogurts contain at least 3.5 grams fat per half-cup, low-fat contains between 0.5 and 2 grams fat, and nonfat yogurts contain less than 0.5 grams fat.

❖ Calories and Fat in Yogurt ❖ (1-cup portion)

Type of Yogurt	Calories	Fat (grams)
Whole milk, plain	139	7
Low-fat, plain	144	4
Low-fat, vanilla or coffee flavored	194	3
Low-fat, fruit flavored	225	3
Nonfat, plain	127	0

The calorie content of fresh yogurt varies dramatically due to two major factors: the fat content and whether sweeteners are added. Many yogurts with fruit also have a lot of sugar or other sweetener added to help preserve the fruit. For fewer calories and sugar, you are better off buying plain yogurt and adding your own fruit, fresh or canned, or fruit spread. For less fat, choose a nonfat or low-fat yogurt.

Like fresh yogurt, frozen yogurt varies in the amount of fat it contains. On the high end are yogurts with as much fat as ice cream—about 14 grams/cup. On the low end are nonfat yogurts. With or without active cultures, frozen yogurt can be a healthier option than ice cream (that is, of course, without the chocolate chip topping). Try to choose a frozen yogurt with no more than 4 grams fat/cup.

Storing
Store yogurt in the refrigerator up to the "use by" date or 7 to 10 days past the "sell by" date. If you open the container and find some liquid sitting on top of the yogurt, don't worry; it's still safe to eat. Just drain off the liquid or stir it into the yogurt. Mold and gas bubbles signal spoilage.

Cooking Light and Healthy
Plain yogurt, either nonfat or low-fat, can be substituted for many ingredients higher in fat in salad, salad dressings, soups, sauces, and desserts. Here are some examples.

- Substitute plain yogurt for mayonnaise. In situations where the taste of mayonnaise is desired, use half reduced calorie mayonnaise and half yogurt. This works well for dishes such as potato salad, cole slaw, tuna salad, cold pasta salads, and appetizers.
- Substitute plain yogurt for sour cream in dips and salad dressing recipes.
- In baking, substitute plain yogurt for sour cream in recipes for pancakes, waffles, loaf breads, and muffins.
- In baking, substitute 1 cup plain yogurt for 1 cup light cream.
- In cooking, substitute 1 cup plain yogurt for 1 cup sour cream.
- On baked potatoes, use plain yogurt instead of sour cream. Mix with fresh herbs.
- Mix plain yogurt with ricotta cheese (made from skim milk) and use as a spread on toast, bagels, and crackers.
- For whipped cream, whip ⅓ cup heavy cream and fold in ⅔ cup plain yogurt.

Where you want a creamy texture, drain the yogurt first to remove some of the liquid. Because of yogurt's acidity, you may want to decrease the amount of other acidic ingredients in your recipe, such as lemon juice.

When cooking with yogurt, use only low heat. High temperatures may cause separation, evaporation of liquid, and a curdled appearance. To help keep yogurt from separating during cooking, blend one tablespoon of cornstarch (unless the recipe calls for flour to be mixed with it) with a few tablespoons of yogurt, then stir mixture into remaining yogurt to be used and proceed according to recipe. Yogurt might also become thin if it is overmixed, so do not overstir.

Yogurt can also be used to make tasty desserts. Make a yogurt parfait by alternating layers of yogurt and fruit or layers of a variety of yogurts. Make a pie by blending yogurt, fresh or frozen fruit, and 1 cup whipped cream. Pour into pie shell and freeze.

Some healthy toppings for frozen yogurt include the following.

- Pureed fruit sauce or fruit spread
- Crushed oatmeal cookies
- Wheat germ
- Chopped dried fruit
- Fresh fruits

EGGS

Eggs are truly a unique food product—they provide versatility and can be used for any meal. Eggs are available at all times of the year at consistently low prices. Eggs not only are traditional breakfast foods, but are used in many breads, pies, cakes, custards, beverages, entrees, to name a few.

Purchasing

Eggs are sold according to their grade and size. Standards for both grade and size are established by the USDA. Grade refers to the quality of the egg and the shell when it is packed. Grades are AA, A, and B. The grade of an egg has nothing to do with whether it is nutritious or wholesome. Instead, grade is based on freshness as well as the interior quality of the egg white and yolk. Lower grade eggs have a thinner white and flatter yolk than higher grade eggs. U.S. Grade A is the most common grade available and has a 30-day shelf life. Grade AA is not often seen because it has a 10-day expiration date.

Eggs come in various sizes: jumbo, extra large, large, medium, small, and peewee. Eggs are sized by weight, so in a given box, some eggs may be below size and others above. One dozen of each size eggs must meet the minimum weight per dozen set for that size, as listed.

Most recipes are based on the use of large eggs. To substitute another size, use Table 44.

Always buy eggs from refrigerated cases. Check the carton to make sure it contains only clean, uncracked eggs and check the date on it; it is normally the last date of sale. Unfortunately, sell by dates are not required in all states.

There is no difference between brown- and white-shelled eggs. Shell color is determined by the breed of the hen and it does not affect the grade, nutritive value, flavor, or cooking performance of the egg. Brown eggs are often more expensive because they come from larger hens that require more food.

Egg substitutes are available that are low in cholesterol, but not always low in fat. They are often made from egg whites and vegetable oil.

Nutrition

Eggs are very nutritious and full of high-quality protein as well as varying amounts of many vitamins and minerals. The current concern with overconsumption of eggs stems from the fact that they are very high in cholesterol—213 milligrams per egg (compare that to the 300 milligrams suggested maximum we eat daily). One egg also contributes 5 grams of fat, of which 1.5 grams are saturated fat.

Storing

Store eggs in the carton they came in because the carton will help keep out odors the eggs might absorb; it also helps prevent the loss of carbon dioxide and moisture from the eggs which causes them to age quicker (this is especially true in frost-free refrigerators). Also, keep eggs refrigerated as they maintain freshness better this way.

Size	Minimum Net Weight (ounces per dozen)
Jumbo	30
Extra large	27
Large	24
Medium	21
Small	18
Peewee	15

❖ **Table 44   Substituting Egg Sizes** ❖

If the Recipe Calls for Large Eggs:	Substitute			
	Jumbo	Extra Large	Medium	Small
1	1	1	1	1
2	2	2	2	3
3	2	3	3	4
4	3	4	5	5
5	4	4	6	7

Eggs should be stored with the large end up to keep the yolk centered.

As an egg ages, the yolk flattens and the thick section of the white becomes watery and thins out. Stale eggs also usually have a "rotten egg" odor that smells like sulfur.

You can store raw egg whites in a tightly covered container in the refrigerator for 4 to 5 days. Yolks, if covered with water, can be refrigerated for 2 to 3 days. Hard-cooked eggs should be refrigerated in their shells and can be held for up to one week.

Egg substitutes can last 1 year in the freezer and, once thawed, 7 days in the refrigerator.

Cooking Light and Healthy

Before discussing cooking, it is important to discuss a problem with contaminated eggs that has received much media attention. A few years ago you could tell a potentially contaminated egg by its broken or dirty shell. Now a perfectly fine-looking egg may contain the disease-causing bacteria, Salmonella enteritidis. Salmonella is passed into the egg before the shell is formed by an infected hen, so it's impossible to know by appearance if an egg is contaminated. Perhaps 1 in 200 eggs is affected by salmonella. The following is a list of precautions to prevent foodborne illness when using eggs and poultry. If you cook eggs so they are done and eat them right away, there shouldn't be any problems.

Purchasing

1. Check the expiration date on the carton.
2. Make sure the carton is clean and each egg is not cracked.
3. Make sure the eggs have been under refrigeration.

Storage

4. Refrigerate at 45°F or below.
5. Store eggs properly:
   • Hard-cooked—refrigerate for up to 1 week
   • Fresh—refrigerate for up to 3–5 weeks as indicated by the date code
6. Store newer eggs behind older eggs.
7. Refrigerate hard-boiled eggs—that means Easter eggs too (they can stay out of refrigeration for coloring and hunting, but that's it)!

Preparation/Cooking

8. Don't use cracked eggs—throw out!
9. Cook both yolk and white until firm. Avoid soft- or medium-cooked eggs, soft omelets, runny scrambled eggs, and coddled eggs.
10. Do not use raw eggs in recipes that don't require further cooking, such as mayonnaise, Caesar salad, mousses, homemade eggnog, and hollandaise sauce.
11. Do not reuse a container after it has had raw egg mixture in it until it is washed thoroughly.
12. Use an egg separator, instead of the egg shells themselves, to separate the white from the yolk.
13. If a recipe calls for eggs at room temperature, take the eggs out of the refrigerator about 30 minutes before you need them.
14. Eat all egg dishes right away; otherwise refrigerate them promptly.

If you find blood spots in a cracked egg, don't be alarmed. It does not indicate a fertile egg, as some people might have you believe, or bacterial problems. Simply remove the blood spot with the tip of a knife or egg shell, and it is perfectly safe to eat the egg.

There are several ways to decrease the number of whole eggs you use in cooking and baking.

1. To make scrambled eggs and omelets, use one whole egg and add extra egg whites to make larger servings.
2. In baking, replace one whole egg with 2 egg whites, and two whole eggs with one whole egg and two or three egg whites.
3. Make French toast with bananas and skim milk (see recipe on page 185) rather than eggs and regular milk.
4. Use ½ cup egg substitute to equal one whole egg.

Eggs can be cooked in many ways: baked, cooked in the shell, poached, fried, and scrambled. The use of nonstick pans and vegetable cooking sprays has enjoyed much popularity. You can reduce the caloric content substantially by avoiding butter or margarine and at the same time enjoy a good product. When making fried eggs, scrambled eggs, and omelets, the use of nonstick pans and vegetable cooking sprays are important to keep down the amount of fat.

When cooking eggs, always use low to medium temperatures to prevent overcooking. Overcooked eggs are tough and rubbery.

Cooking eggs in the oven is not as popular as it once was. This form of cookery generally requires a liquid that keeps the eggs from drying out. The best known form of oven cookery for eggs is the "Shirred Egg" dish. Shirred eggs require the use of a special baking dish that will not crack when subjected to the intense heat of the 350°F oven. The dish is first coated with vegetable spray. Then the whole egg is taken out of the shell and placed into the cup, milk is added, and then the egg is baked until the white is firm and the yolk is hard and glossy (about 10–12 minutes).

A simple method of cooking eggs is by leaving them in their shells. Cooking eggs to various degrees of hardness can be accomplished by either placing the eggs directly into boiling water and reduce to simmering, or by first placing them into cold water and bringing to a simmer. The following is a simple guide:

| Soft-Cooked Eggs | 3–5 minutes |
| Hard-Cooked Eggs | 15–20 minutes |

Hard-cooked eggs should be chilled down immediately with ice cold water in order to prevent the "green ring" (it's harmless) that appears on the yolk. It is best to peel the eggs while still warm, especially if the eggs are very fresh. Fresh eggs are more difficult to peel.

To make **poached eggs**, simply break the egg onto a plate, and gently slide it into a pot of simmering water. Some chefs prefer to add a teaspoon of vinegar to help the white become solid. This method is not recommended because it has a tendency to make the white too tough. As the egg instantly cooks, its white will congeal into a rounded mass within a few minutes. The egg can be removed with a large slotted spoon or with a flat vegetable skimmer. The egg can be served on top of toast. Many stores sell devices that are specially designed to cook poached eggs and give them a nice, rounded shape—a good investment if you consume them on a regular basis.

Fried eggs can easily be made either "sunny side up" (you know, staring at you!) or turned over and cooked to the desired degree of doneness. Regardless of the type of dish prepared, remember to use strictly fresh eggs which will insure maximum flavor and best appearance. Although many theories exist on how to hold "fried eggs," we have never found one that equaled the quality of one "made to order."

When cooking breakfast for many people, **scrambled eggs** is probably the easiest method of cooking eggs. The egg mixture seasoned lightly with pepper and perhaps some milk can be prepared ahead of time and kept refrigerated. Scrambled eggs are made simply by pouring the egg mixture into a hot nonstick pan and stirring with a fork or other utensil in a circular motion. Although scrambled eggs do hold better than other forms of breakfast egg dishes and are sometimes held on a brunch buffet table, preparing them as close to serving time as possible is still best in terms of product quality.

Omelets are merely a variation of scrambled eggs. The difference is that when the egg mixture is added to the pan, stir the mixture only a few strokes and let the mixture cook. Variations on the plain French omelet (recipe on page 184) are endless—western style may include diced turkey ham, peppers, and onions; Spanish style may include a tomato sauce with peppers and onions; low-fat cheeses may be added; jellies, potatoes, and so on may also be added. An omelet can be your personal creation. As the bottom starts to brown, tip the pan and flip one half of the omelet over the other.

An interesting style of omelet is called a foamy omelet (recipe on page 184), and it may even be served for dessert. To prepare as a dessert, follow the recipe; when the bottom is cooked, add fresh apples in the center, fold one half over the other, and finish baking in the oven for a few minutes. For service sprinkle with powdered sugar and serve—a real treat.

Custards are discussed in Chapter 16. Although the main ingredients in custards are eggs and milk, it is possible to use fewer eggs and skim milk and still have a nice product. See the recipe for vanilla custard on page 274.

RECIPES

LOW-FAT MACARONI AND CHEESE

½ pound elbow macaroni
1 cup Low-Fat White Sauce (recipe on page 298)
1 tsp brown mustard
dash of cayenne pepper
½ lb low-fat sharp cheddar cheese, shredded
⅓ cup skim milk
2 tbsp freshly grated Parmesan cheese
1 tbsp freshly grated Romano cheese
1 oz yellow cheddar cheese, grated

1. Cook macaroni until tender, about 8 to 10 minutes. Drain and cool under cold running water.
2. Prepare the Low-Fat White Sauce and while still hot toss with the macaroni, mustard, cayenne,

low-fat cheese, milk, Parmesan, and Romano. Spoon into a casserole and bake in a preheated 350-degree oven for 10 minutes. Top with the yellow cheddar and bake another 15 minutes.

Serves 6

Nutrition Analysis:
```
Calories . . . . . . . . . . . . . .529
Carbohydrate. . . . . . . . . .67 grams
Fiber . . . . . . . . . . . . . . . .0 grams
Fat. . . . . . . . . . . . . . . . . .15 grams
Cholesterol. . . . . . . . . . .32 milligrams
Sodium. . . . . . . . . . . . . .310 milligrams
```

CHEESY MACARONI AND VEGETABLES

2 cups medium seashell macaroni, uncooked
1 cup coarsely shredded carrot
1 cup coarsely shredded zucchini
2 tbsp finely chopped onions
2 tsp cornstarch
½ tsp paprika
¼ tsp salt
¼ tsp dry mustard
¼ tsp pepper
1 cup 2% low-fat milk
1 cup (2 oz) shredded reduced-fat Monterey Jack cheese

1. Cook macaroni in boiling water 10 minutes.
2. Add carrot, zucchini, and onions; cook 1 minute. Drain well; place pasta mixture in a bowl; set aside.

3. Combine cornstarch and next four ingredients in a small saucepan. Gradually add low-fat milk, stirring with a wire whisk. Bring to a boil over medium heat, stirring constantly, and cook 1 minute.
4. Remove from heat; stir in cheese. Pour over pasta mixture; toss gently. Serve warm.

Serves 4

Nutrition Analysis:
```
Calories . . . . . . . . . . . . . .288
Carbohydrate. . . . . . . . . .47 grams
Fiber . . . . . . . . . . . . . . . .1 gram
Fat. . . . . . . . . . . . . . . . . .5 grams
Cholesterol. . . . . . . . . . .15 milligrams
Sodium. . . . . . . . . . . . . .226 milligrams
```

MUSHROOM AND SPINACH LASAGNA

1 10-oz package whole wheat lasagna, cooked and
  drained
1 tbsp olive oil
1 large onion, chopped
4 cloves garlic, minced
8 oz mushrooms, sliced
1 10-oz package frozen, chopped spinach

1 tsp salt
½ tsp freshly ground pepper
¼ tsp ground nutmeg
1 15-oz container part-skim ricotta
1 egg
1½ cups grated low-fat mozzarella
1 cup tomato sauce

1. Preheat the oven to 400°F.
2. Warm the oil in a large, nonstick skillet over low heat. Add onion and garlic. Cook until the onion is soft, about 5 minutes, stirring occasionally.
3. Add the mushrooms and turn the heat up to medium. Cook the mushrooms until almost all the liquid has evaporated.
4. Add the spinach. Increase the heat to high, and stir until almost all the liquid has cooked away. Stir in the salt, pepper, and nutmeg. Set the mixture aside.
5. Stir the egg into the ricotta.
6. To assemble: Set aside ½ cup mozzarella. Spread half the tomato sauce onto the bottom of a 9 × 12-inch glass or ceramic lasagna dish. Lay one-third of the pasta over the tomato sauce. Spread half the ricotta over the pasta and then half the spinach mixture over ricotta. Sprinkle on ½ cup mozzarella. Cover with another layer of pasta and then repeat the ricotta, spinach, and mozzarella layers. Lay the remaining pasta on top. Spread the rest of the tomato sauce over the pasta and then sprinkle the ½ cup of mozzarella on top of the lasagna.
7. Bake 45 minutes, until brown on top and bubbling.

Serves 8

Nutrition Analysis:
Calories 305
Carbohydrate. . . . . .35 grams
Fiber . . . . .13 grams
Fat. . . . . .11 grams
Cholesterol. . . . . .63 milligrams
Sodium. . . . . .74 milligrams

COTTAGE CHEESE SPREAD

⅓ cup low-fat cottage cheese
½ small onion, chopped
⅓ small green pepper, chopped
½ carrot, finely chopped
1 stalk celery, chopped
⅛ tsp pepper

1. Press cottage cheese through strainer into bowl.
2. Chop vegetables very fine.
3. Add the vegetables and pepper to the cottage cheese. Mix well.
4. Refrigerate for 1 to 2 hours.
5. Spread on whole wheat bread, toast, or crackers.

Serves 4 (⅓ cup each)

Nutrition Analysis:
Calories 32
Carbohydrate. . . . . .4 grams
Fiber . . . . .1 gram
Fat. . . . . .1 gram
Cholesterol. . . . . .2 milligrams
Sodium. . . . . .88 milligrams

MOCK SOUR CREAM

½ cup cottage cheese, uncreamed (dry)
¼ cup buttermilk
1 tbsp oil
1 tsp lemon juice
⅛ tsp salt

1. Put all ingredients into blender container; cover. Blend until smooth.
2. Serve over baked potatoes or other vegetables.

Makes about ⅔ cup

Nutrition Analysis:
Calories 208
Carbohydrate. . . . . .5 grams
Fiber . . . . .0 grams
Fat. . . . . .14 grams
Cholesterol. . . . . .7 milligrams
Sodium. . . . . .330 milligrams

POTATO VEGETABLE SALAD WITH YOGURT

2 lb red potatoes
2 cups broccoli florets
2 cups cauliflower florets
2 medium carrots, peeled
1 medium cucumber
¾ cup sliced radishes
½ cup sliced scallions
1 cup plain low-fat yogurt
3 tbsp Dijon mustard
1 tsp salt
½ tsp freshly ground pepper

1. Steam the potatoes until they are tender. While they are cooling, steam the broccoli and cauliflower until slightly cooked, about 4 minutes. Set the broccoli and cauliflower aside to cool.
2. Cut the carrots into thin slivers. Slice the cucumber. Cut the potatoes into chunks.
3. Gently stir all the vegetables together in a large mixing bowl.
4. In another bowl, whisk together the yogurt, mustard, salt, and pepper.
5. Pour the dressing over the vegetables and stir carefully until the dressing coats everything evenly. Refrigerate for 1 hour before serving.

Serves 6

Nutrition Analysis:

Calories 190
Carbohydrate. . . . . .39 grams
Fiber . . . . .7 grams
Fat. . . . . .2 grams
Cholesterol. . . . . .3 milligrams
Sodium. . . . . .714 milligrams

APPLE-CABBAGE SLAW WITH YOGURT

¼ cup plain low-fat yogurt
¼ tsp salt
dash pepper
2 tsp vinegar
¼ tsp prepared mustard
1 cup apples, unpared, thinly sliced
2 cups cabbage, shredded

1. Mix yogurt, salt, pepper, vinegar, and mustard thoroughly.
2. Lightly mix apples and cabbage.
3. Pour yogurt mixture over apple-cabbage mixture; toss lightly.
4. Serve immediately.

Serves 4

Nutrition Analysis:

Calories 36
Carbohydrate. . . . . .8 grams
Fiber . . . . .2 grams
Fat. . . . . .0 grams
Cholesterol. . . . . .1 milligram
Sodium. . . . . .151 milligrams

HARD-COOKED EGGS

1. Place 1 egg into boiling water to cover.
2. Reduce to simmer, cover, and cook for 20 minutes.
3. Remove cover, pour off water, and run cold water over egg until cool.*
4. Refrigerate immediately.

Makes 1 hard-boiled egg

*This will prevent green discoloration of the yolk.

Nutrition Analysis:

Calories 77
Carbohydrate. . . . . .1 gram
Fiber . . . . .0 grams
Fat. . . . . .5 grams
Cholesterol. . . . . .213 milligrams
Sodium. . . . . .62 milligrams

POACHED EGG

1 egg
1 qt water
1 tbsp white vinegar

1. Break egg out of shell and into a small dish or saucer.
2. Combine water and vinegar and simmer.
3. Pour egg off saucer GENTLY into the water.
4. Remove pot from range and let stand 4–6 minutes.
5. Remove egg and serve.

Makes 1 egg

Nutrition Analysis:

Calories 77
Carbohydrate. . . . . .1 gram
Fiber . . . . .0 grams
Fat. . . . . .5 grams
Cholesterol. . . . . .213 milligrams
Sodium. . . . . .62 milligrams

PLAIN OMELET (FRENCH)

1 tsp oil (or vegetable cooking spray for less fat)
2 eggs, shelled (or use 1 egg and 2 egg whites for less cholesterol and fat)
1 tsp water
⅛ tsp salt
⅛ tsp white pepper

1. Heat oil in frying pan.
2. Combine eggs, water, salt, and pepper in bowl and mix with fork.
3. Pour into omelet pan stirring in circular motion with fork and moving the pan back and forth at the same time.
4. Let the egg set for a few seconds and then lift the pan on a 45-degree angle, fold the omelet ⅓ from one direction and ⅓ from the other direction.
5. Place on dish and serve immediately.

Serves 1

Nutrition Analysis:

Calories 190
Carbohydrate. . . . . .1 gram
Fiber . . . . .0 grams
Fat. . . . . .14 grams
Cholesterol. . . . . .426 milligrams
Sodium. . . . . .382 milligrams

FOAMY OMELET

1 tsp oil or vegetable cooking spray
2 eggs, separated
1 tsp skim milk
⅛ tsp salt

1. Beat egg whites with whip until foamy. Heat oil in nonstick pan.
2. Beat yolks and add milk, salt, and mix together.
3. Gently fold egg whites into the yolk mixture.
4. Pour into heated frying pan and cook until brown on bottom.
5. Fold in half and finish cooking in oven at 350°F.

Serves 1

Nutrition Analysis:

Calories 190
Carbohydrate. . . . . .1 gram
Fiber . . . . .0 grams
Fat. . . . . .14 grams
Cholesterol. . . . . .426 milligrams
Sodium. . . . . .382 milligrams

Banana Batter French Toast

1 ripe banana, well mashed
1 egg
1 egg white
¼ cup low-fat or skim milk
½ tsp vanilla
2 tsp vegetable oil
4 slices whole grain bread

1. In a shallow dish beat together the banana, egg, egg white, milk, and vanilla.
2. Warm the oil in a large nonstick skillet over medium-high heat. Dip each piece of bread into the batter, turning them to coat both sides. Fry the French toast until brown on both sides.
3. Serve with low-fat yogurt and fresh fruit.

Serves 2

Nutrition Analysis:

Calories 310
Carbohydrate. . . . . .42 grams
Fiber . . . . .4 grams
Fat. . . . . .10 grams
Cholesterol. . . . . .140 milligrams
Sodium . . . . .330 milligrams

❖ ❖ ❖

CHAPTER ELEVEN

GRAINS AND LEGUMES

GRAINS

Grains (the proper name is cereal grains) are the seed kernels of cultivated grasses. They include wheat, corn, rice, rye, barley, and oats, among others. All cereal grains have a large center area high in starch known as the endosperm, like that shown in the illustration. At one end of the endosperm is the germ, the area of the kernel that sprouts when allowed to germinate. The bran covers both the endosperm and the germ. The seed contains everything needed to reproduce the plant: the germ is the embryo, the endosperm contains the nutrients for growth, and the bran protects it.

Most grains undergo some type of processing or milling after harvesting to make them cook more quickly and easily, be less chewy, and lengthen their shelf life. Many grains, such as oats and rice, have an outer husk or hull that is tough and inedible and must be removed. Other processing steps might include polishing the grain to remove the bran and germ (as in making white flour), cracking the grain (as in cracked wheat), or steaming the grain (as in bulgur) to shorten the cooking time. The processes of rolling or grinding a grain, such as oatmeal, also shorten the cooking time.

Whenever the fiber-rich bran and the vitamin-rich germ are left on the endosperm of a grain, the grain is called a whole grain. Examples of whole grains include whole wheat, whole rye, bulgur (whole wheat grains that have been steamed and dried), oatmeal, whole cornmeal, whole hulled barley, and brown rice. If the bran and germ are separated (or mostly separated) from the endosperm, the grain is called refined or milled. For example, whole wheat flour is made from the entire kernel of wheat, and refined wheat, or white flour as it is more commonly called, is made only from the endosperm.

Unfortunately, refined grains lose most of the fiber, oil, B vitamins, and some protein that were in the germ and bran. Whole grains are always a more nutritious choice and are good sources of fiber, complex carbohydrates, B vitamins, and minerals. Whole grains are also a good protein choice for vegetarians (and nonvegetarians) when eaten as part of a varied diet. And you get all this good nutrition with a minimum of calories and fat. To summarize their nutritional profile, grains are:

- Low or moderate in calories
- High in complex carbohydrates
- High in fiber (if whole grain)
- Low in fat
- Moderate in protein
- Full of vitamins and minerals

Most grains are cooked by stirring into a boiling liquid (may be water or broth), then reducing the heat to a simmer, covering, and cooking until the liquid is absorbed. Table 45 summarizes the cooking information for each grain.

Start putting more grains on your table by serving them as breakfast cereals and side dishes such as pilaf, and incorporated into soups, stews, casseroles, stir-fry, breads, and salads. It should

Rice grain composition

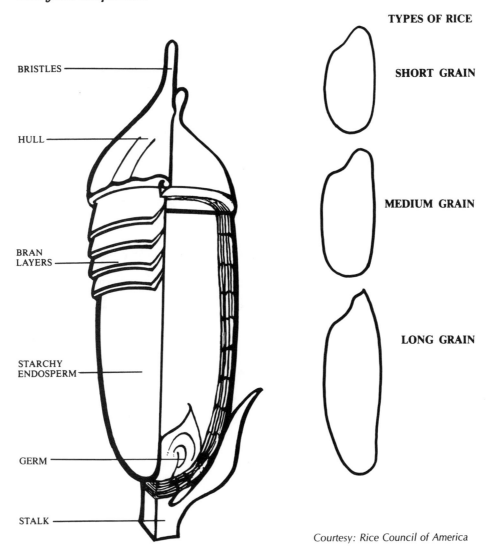

BRISTLES

HULL

BRAN LAYERS

STARCHY ENDOSPERM

GERM

STALK

TYPES OF RICE

SHORT GRAIN

MEDIUM GRAIN

LONG GRAIN

Courtesy: Rice Council of America

be easy since grains are very inexpensive, easy to store, and can be used in countless different tasty recipes. Many of them cook quite quickly as well: bulgur cooks in under 20 minutes, buckwheat kasha and quinoa in only 15 minutes.

Barley
Purchasing   When the term barley is used in a recipe, it usually refers to pearl barley. Pearl barley is white and has had the inedible husks or hulls, germ, and bran removed. Whole hulled barley is available at natural food stores and is brown-

ish gray in color due to the bran. Although whole hulled barley is more expensive than pearled barley and has to be soaked overnight prior to cooking, it is more nutritious.

Nutrition   Pearl barley is a good source of fiber, iron, potassium, niacin, and folate. Whole hulled barley contains more vitamins and minerals as well as more fiber.

Storing   Pearl barley should be stored in an airtight container and can last up to nine months on a pantry shelf. Whole hulled barley can be stored

❖ Table 45 Cooking Information for Grains ❖

Grain	Appearance	Flavor	Soaking Required	Cooking Time	Cups Liquid for Cooking	Cups Yield*	Uses	Storage
Barley, pearl	White-tan	Mild, nutty	No (but will reduce cooking time)	35–40 minutes	3	4	Soups, casseroles, stews, cooked cereals, side dishes, pilafs	Air-tight container—6–9 months at room temperature
Barley, whole hulled	Brownish-gray	Nutty, chewy	Yes	60 minutes	3	4	Same as above	Air-tight container—1 month at room temperature, 4–5 months in refrigerator
Buckwheat, whole white	Brown-white	Mild	No	20 minutes	2	2½	Side dishes	Air-tight container—1–2 months, better stored in refrigerator
Buckwheat, roasted (kasha)	Brown	Distinct, nutty, chewy	No	10–15 minutes	2	2½	Soups, side dishes, salads, pilaf, stuffing, hot cereal	Same as above
Corn, whole hominy	Yellow or white	Sweet, creamy texture	No	2½–3 hours	2½	3	Soups, stews, casseroles, hot cereal, puddings, baked goods	Air-tight container—1 month at room temperature, 5 months in refrigerator
Corn, hominy grits	Whitish-gray	Distinct	No	20–25 minutes	4	3	Hot breakfast cereal	Air-tight container, many months at room temperature
Millet	Bright gold color, small	Like corn, crunchy	No	30–35 minutes	2	3	Soups, casseroles, meat loaves, porridge, croquettes, pilaf, salads, stuffing, side dishes	Air-tight container, 6 months at room temperature
Oats, steel-cut	Off-white	Mild, pleasant	No	45–60 minutes	2	2	Hot cereal	Air-tight container—1 month at room temperature, 6 months in refrigerator
Rice, regular-milled long grain	White	Mild	No	15 minutes	2	3	Side dishes, casseroles, stews, soups, stuffing, salads	Air-tight container—many months at room temperature
Rice, regular-milled, medium or short grain	White	Mild	No	15 minutes	1½	3	Same as above	Same as above
Rice, parboiled	White	Mild	No	20–25 minutes	2–2½	3–4	Same as above	Same as above
Rice, brown	Tan-brown	Nutty	No	45–50 minutes	2–2½	3–4	Same as above	Air-tight container—1 month at room temperature, 6 months in

Grain	Appearance	Flavor	Soaking Required	Cooking Time	Cups Liquid for Cooking	Cups Yield*	Uses	Storage
Rice, wild	Dark brown	Nutty	No (but rinse it)	40–60 minutes	3	3½–4	Side dishes, stuffing, casseroles	Air-tight container— many months at room temperature
Rice, basmati	White	Nutty, spicy	Yes (rinse also)	25 minutes	1½	3	Side dishes, casseroles	Air-tight container— 1 month at room temperature, 6 months in refrigerator
Rye, whole berries	Brown, oval	Distinct rye flavor	No	1½ hours	3	3	Hot cereal, side dishes	Air-tight container— 1 month at room temperature, 5 months in refrigerator
Wheat, bulgur	Dark brown	Nutty	No	20–25 minutes	2½	2	Salads, soups, breads, desserts, with rice, meat dishes, in place of rice, pilaf, stuffing	Air-tight container in cool place, or refrigerate for 5–6 months
Wheat, whole berries	Deep brown	Nutty, crunchy	Yes (1 cup to 3½ cups cold water)	1 hour	3	2	Salads, meat loaves, croquettes, breads, side dishes	Air-tight container in cool place up to 1 month, up to 5 months in refrigerator
Amaranth	Golden	Mildly spicy, toasted sesame flavor	No	25 minutes	2	3	Hot cereal, pilaf, in baking, can be popped as a snack	Air-tight container, in cool place for many months, otherwise refrigerate for 5 months
Quinoa	Pale yellow	Nutty	No	12–15 minutes	2	2½	In place of rice	Air-tight container in cool place for 1 month, otherwise refrigerate for 5 months

*From 1 cup of uncooked grain

at room temperature for 1 month, or 4 to 5 months in the refrigerator.

Cooking Light and Healthy Either form of barley can be boiled and used in soups, casseroles, stews, cooked cereals, side dishes, or pilaf. Its taste is mild and nutty, and its texture is chewy. To cook pearl barley, put 1 cup into 3 cups of boiling water or broth, and simmer (covered) for 35 to 40 minutes. If you presoak pearl barley for 5 hours or overnight in 2 cups of water for each cup of barley, you can reduce the cooking time to 15 minutes. Whole hulled barley must be presoaked overnight—use double the amount of water as grain. Cook it like pearl barley and lengthen the cooking time to 60 minutes. Check at 30 minutes to see if it needs more water.

Buckwheat

Purchasing Although buckwheat has many grainlike characteristics, it is from an entirely different family than grains and is actually a fruit. There are two forms of buckwheat available for purchase: whole white buckwheat and roasted buckwheat, also called kasha. Kasha is packaged in four granulations: whole, coarse, medium, and fine. Roasting gives the buckwheat kernels a distinct, nutty flavor that you will probably have to acquire a taste for. Meanwhile, whole white buckwheat has a mild flavor and can replace rice or pasta at meals. Kasha can be used in soups, side dishes, and salads. Whole and coarse kasha can be used interchangeably and are good for pilafs, stuffing, and soups. Medium and fine kasha cook quicker, are less chewy, and are best for hot cereal. Buckwheat can generally be found at natural food stores.

Nutrition   A nutritional uniqueness of buckwheat is the quality of the protein it contains. The proteins in buckwheat are the best source of protein found in any plant food, even better than soybeans! Buckwheat is also a good source of fiber and magnesium.

Storing   Buckwheat should be stored in airtight containers, away from sunlight, and can only be held at room temperature for one to two months. It is better stored in the refrigerator or freezer. Cooked kasha or buckwheat can be refrigerated up to one week or frozen up to six months.

Cooking light and healthy   Most cooking instructions for kasha call for combining uncooked kasha kernels with egg (one egg to one to two cups of kasha) and then cooked for two to three minutes in a skillet over a medium heat (stir constantly to keep them from burning) until dry. The whites of the egg can be used if you are watching cholesterol. This step is usually suggested because the egg coating seals the uncooked kasha that helps the kernels remain separate and retain their individual shapes when cooked. Egg also adds to the protein value of the cooked kasha. Next, add two cups of water for each cup of kasha, cover, and cook over a low heat for 10 to 15 minutes until the water is absorbed. Remove from heat and let stand 10 minutes.

Whole white buckwheat does not require an egg wash. Simply combine the buckwheat with any seasoning until well coated, then add liquid (2 cups to each cup of buckwheat) and cook until

it boils. Reduce the heat to low and cook, covered, for about 20 minutes.

Millet

Purchasing   Millet is grown and used in the Far East and China. Although the millet raised in the United States is mostly used to feed animals and birds, millet has been eaten by people in other parts of the world since Old Testament times. Millet is a very important component of the diet for many Africans, Indians, and Chinese; it contains a high-quality protein. It can be purchased in natural food stores as a whole grain. Millet that is used for cooking has had the inedible hull (that the birds just love!) removed as well as an outer bran layer that is also inedible. Look for millet that has a bright gold color. If the millet has more than a mild odor, it is old.

Nutrition   Millet is a good source of protein, fiber, folate, magnesium, niacin, and thiamin.

Storing   Millet has excellent storage qualities and is very resistant to bugs or mold. It can be stored at room temperature in a tight-fitting container for up to six months.

Cooking light and healthy   It can be boiled and used in soups, casseroles, meat loaves, porridge, croquettes, pilaf, salads, stuffings, or as a side dish. To cook millet, add 1 to 2 cups of boiling water or broth, cover, and cook over low heat for 30 to 35 minutes until all of the liquid is absorbed. Remove from heat and let stand for 10 minutes. Millet tastes something like corn and is crunchy.

Oats

Purchasing   Oats are a very unique grain: when they are milled, only the inedible hull is removed and the bran and germ are left with the kernel. Whichever of the following forms of oats you buy, you are getting whole grain nutrition.

- Steel-cut oats are unrefined oats that have been hulled, dried, and sliced with steel blades. Because they have not been heat-treated (as the other forms are), they retain more of the B vitamins.
- Rolled oats, or "old-fashioned oats," are made by cutting up raw oats into a product that is

then steamed, shaped into flakes, and dried. Rolled oats only require 5 minutes cooking time.

- **Quick oats** start out as rolled oats, but are sliced finer and slightly precooked so they cook quicker—in about one minute.
- **Instant oats** are cut even smaller and result in a product that only needs to be mixed with boiling water.

Nutrition Whole grain oats are a source of protein, iron, and many vitamins and minerals. The popularity of **oat bran** skyrocketed when it was found that it seems to help decrease cholesterol levels and thereby lower the risk of heart attacks. Ever since, oat bran has been making a steady appearance: in muffins (see recipe on page 000), cereals, and various recipes.

Storing Oats contain a natural antioxidant that keeps them from going stale. An opened container of oats can stay on the shelf for about 1 year. After opening, seal the top.

Cooking light and healthy To cook steel-cut groats, stir 1 cup into 2 cups of boiling water, stock, or milk. Reduce heat, cover, and simmer for about 45 minutes, or simmer for 15 minutes, remove from the heat, and let stand for 45 minutes. The latter method saves energy, prevents burning, and makes the product fluffier. The other forms of oats should be prepared according to package directions. Oats can be used in soups, stews, and many baked goods.

Oat bran is somewhat easier to cook and bake with than wheat bran. Luckily oat bran does not have quite the crisp bite that wheat bran has and it is also water-soluble, meaning that you can cook unprocessed oat bran into a palatable hot cereal.

Rice

Rice, perhaps the first grain ever to be cultivated by man, is a semi-aquatic member of the grass family. Its edible seed is the staple grain for over half the world's population.

Purchasing Rice is classified by the shape of the grain: short-grain, medium-grain, or long-grain.

- **Long-grain rice** is four to five times as long as it is wide. The cooked grains are separate and fluffy and used in side dishes, entrees, salads, pilaf, and so on.
- **Medium-grain rice** is a little shorter and plumper than long-grain rice; after cooking the rice is more moist, tender, and has a greater tendency to cling together than long grains. Both medium-grain and short-grain rice are a good choice for making dishes that are creamy, such as rice pudding, risotto, molds, or croquettes.
- **Short-grain rice** is a little shorter than medium-grain rice; the shorter the grain the more tender and clinging it cooks. Short-grain rice is not as easy to find as long- or medium-grain but it usually can be found in markets specializing in Oriental or Caribbean foods. The boiled rice used in Japanese cuisine is short-grain.

As described in the accompanying explanation, rice undergoes varying degrees of processing to come in four forms: regular milled white rice, parboiled or converted rice, instant or precooked rice, and brown rice. In addition, some specialty rices are noted below.

- **Arborio rice** is one of several Italian varieties of a type of short-grain rice that is essential for making the highest-quality risotto.
- **Aromatic rice** has a flavor and aroma similar to that of roasted nuts or popcorn. Aromatic rices naturally contain aromatic substances that are found in all rice but that they contain in higher concentrations. There are two kinds of aromatic rice grown in the United States: a Della-type which cooks separate and fluffy, and a Jasmine-type which cooks more moist and tends to cling together.
- **Basmati rice** is a flavorful variety of extra long-grain rice with a unique nutty flavor that is popular with Indian food.
- **Sweet rice**, also called waxy or glutinous, is a short, plumpy rice with a chalky white, opaque kernel. When cooked, this rice is very sticky and chewy. It is used for several special dishes, including desserts, in Chinese and Japanese cuisines. It is more often used in commercial

FORMS OF RICE

1. Regular-milled white rice (also called white or polished rice)
   - The most common form of rice
   - The outer husk is removed and the layers of bran milled away until the grain is white
   - Requires about 15 minutes to cook
2. Parboiled or converted rice (such as Uncle Ben's®)
   - A specially processed long-grain rice
   - Has been partially cooked under steam pressure, dried, and then milled to remove the outer hull and bran; the parboiling process results in a grain that is harder, more compact, shiny, and more nutritious
   - The parboiling process also results in rice that is extra separate and fluffy
   - Requires about 25 minutes to cook (takes longer than regular-milled white rice)
3. Precooked, quick cooking, or instant rice (such as Minute Rice®)
   - Has been milled, completely cooked, then dried
   - Preparation involves adding boiling water that penetrates the grains and rehydrates them in a short time
   - Its texture is not as appealing as other rices
   - If overcooked or held too long, the grains become mushy
4. Brown rice
   - The least processed form of rice
   - The outer hull (it's inedible) is removed but it still retains the bran layers that give it the characteristic tan-brown color, nut-like flavor, and chewy texture
   - Has a longer cooking time than regular-milled rice (about 50 minutes) since the outer bran layers act as a barrier to heat and moisture
   - Available as short-, medium-, or long-grain
   - Has a shorter shelf life than white rice because the oil in the bran layer can become rancid; refrigerator storage is recommended for longer shelf life
   - Is more expensive than white rice because the grain must be higher in quality and a uniform, characteristic color

frozen products than in recipes. The starch and flour from waxy rice is used frozen as a binder for gravies, sauces, and fillings, because it is resistant to breakdown during freezing and thawing.

Wild rice is not a true rice; it is the grain of an aquatic grass that grows wild in the Great Lakes region of the United States. Wild rice is dark brown in color and, when cooked, has a nutty flavor. Real wild rice is quite expensive and is considered a luxury food. Wild rice comes in three different grades: giant long-grain (the highest grade), fancy medium-grain (an excellent choice), and select short-grain (stick with the fancy quality).

Rice cakes are a low-calorie rice snack most often made with puffed rice. They can be eaten plain or topped with peanut butter and jelly, cheese, bean dip, or guacamole much like regular crackers. Most rice cakes have only 35 calories per cake and some brands come in delicious flavors such as cheddar cheese, apple and cinnamon, and taco-flavored.

Nutrition Rice is an excellent source of complex carbohydrates and only contains a trace of fat and no cholesterol. Brown rice is also a source of fiber.

Table 46 is a nutritional comparison of the four different forms of rice. Brown rice, because it is a whole grain, contains more nutrients than regular-milled white rice, converted, or instant rice. Specifically, it contains more zinc, phosphorus, potassium, niacin, vitamin E, and fiber than enriched white rice. Most U.S.-grown and processed white rice is enriched with iron, niacin, and thiamin by applying a coating of nutrients (don't wash rice before cooking or you will wash

❖ **Table 46 Nutrition Information** ❖
for Cooked Long-Grain Rice
(per ½ cup serving)

	Brown	Regular-Milled White (enriched)	Parboiled (enriched)	Precooked White (enriched)
Kilocalories	111	131	100	80
Carbohydrate (g)	23	28	22	17
Protein (g)	3	3	2	2
Total fat (g)	1	0.3	0.2	0.1
Saturated fatty acids (g)	0	0	0	0
Cholesterol (mg)	0	0	0	0
Fiber (g)	1.7	0.5	0.5	0.6
Sodium (mg)	3.0	2.0	2	2

off the coating). Converted rice has a higher nutrient content than regular-milled white rice because the steaming process dissolves the vitamins and minerals in the bran layer and then carefully controlled pressure drives the freed minerals and vitamins into the kernel (before the bran is removed), resulting in a recapture of over 80 percent of the natural nutrients of the whole grain. Instant rice provides the least in amounts of nutrients (yet costs the most!).

Storage The best storage method for rice is to keep it in an airtight container so that dust, moisture, and other contaminants are kept out. White rices can be stored for many months in an airtight container without a significant loss of nutrients or quality. Brown rice, though, is a different story. Because it contains natural oils that will eventually go rancid, it can be stored for only one month at room temperature, or up to six months in the refrigerator.

Wild rice should be stored in a tightly covered container and can be held for many months at room temperature. During warm, humid months store wild rice in the refrigerator to avoid mold and bugs.

All forms of cooked rice can be refrigerated for six to seven days, or frozen for six months. Be sure to store the cooked rice in a tightly covered container or sealable plastic bag so the grains won't dry out or absorb flavors of other foods.

When reheating rice, for each cup of cooked rice, add 2 tablespoons liquid. Cover and heat on top of the range or in the oven for about five minutes until heated through. If reheating in a microwave oven, cover and cook on high power about one minute per cup of rice. Frozen rice may be cooked two minutes on high power for each cup.

Cooking See the guidelines for how much liquid and cooking time is necessary to cook various types of rice on top of the range. For liquid, you can use water, broth, consomme, and even vegetable juice.

To reduce the cooking time of brown rice or wild rice, you can soak it overnight using a water-to-rice ratio of 2½ to 1. Soak the rice in a covered pot for six hours or overnight in the refrigerator and then cook in the soaking water so nutrients are not lost. This should reduce cooking time to about 20 minutes.

You can also prepare rice in a conventional oven or microwave oven. Using your conventional oven is an efficient use of energy when other foods are baking. Combine boiling liquid, the rice, and any other ingredients in a baking dish or pan and stir. Cover tightly and bake at 350° for 25 to 30 minutes (30 to 40 for parboiled, 1 hour for brown rice). Fluff with fork. Using the microwave oven saves energy and clean-up time.

See the additional rice cooking tips, as well

Rice Dish	Seasonings
Rice pilaf	Coriander, curry powder, red pepper, saffron
Rice and vegetable casserole	Tarragon
Risotto	Nutmeg
Spinach risotto	Nutmeg, rosemary, bay leaf
Greek rice	Mint
White rice	Allspice, parsley, turmeric
Wild rice	Thyme

HOW TO PREPARE RICE

❖ ❖ ❖

For best results, always follow package directions. When not available, use this easy method.

Combine 1 cup rice, liquid, 1 teaspoon salt (optional), and 1 tablespoon butter or margarine (optional) in 2- to 3-quart saucepan. Bring to a boil; stir once or twice. Reduce heat, cover, and simmer. Cook according to time specified on chart. If rice is not quite tender or liquid is not absorbed, replace lid and cook 2 to 4 minutes longer. Fluff with fork.

1 Cup Uncooked Rice	Liquid (cups)	Cooking Time (minutes)
Regular-milled long-grain	1¾–2	15
Regular-milled medium- or short-grain	1½	15
Brown	2–2½	45–50
Parboiled	2–2½	20–25
Precooked, flavored, or seasoned mixes	Follow package directions	

MICROWAVE INSTRUCTIONS

Combine 1 cup rice, liquid, 1 teaspoon salt (optional), and 1 tablespoon margarine (optional) in 2- to 3-quart deep microproof baking dish. Cover and cook on high 5 minutes or until boiling. Reduce setting to medium (50% power) and cook 15 minutes (20 minutes for parboiled rice and 30 minutes for brown rice). Fluff with fork.

as the following list of spices that complement different rice dishes.

Wild rice should always be washed before cooking. For cooking, add 3 cups of water for each cup of wild rice. Simmer for 40 minutes (for short-grain varieties) or until the grains burst open. Long-grain varieties take longer to cook—up to 60 minutes. To get more mileage from this expensive ingredient, cook some long-grain white rice separately and mix together.

Basmati rice should be washed and picked over for small stones before cooking.

Some popular rice dishes include these four.

- Jambalaya—A traditional Louisiana rice dish, highly seasoned, and flavored with sausage, ham, seafood, pork, chicken, or other meat
- Paella—A traditional Spanish dish of saffron-flavored rice, shellfish, chicken, chorizo, vegetables, and seasonings

- Pilaf—A light and fluffy rice dish originating in the Middle East, the rice is often sauteed in oil and then cooked in a broth with onions, raisins, various spices, and sometimes meat is added
- Risotto—A rich and creamy Italian rice dish in which the rice is browned in fat or oil with onions and then cooked in broth, often flavored with Parmesan cheese

Rye
Purchasing Although rye is most well known for its flour, you can buy (at the natural food store) whole rye berries that can be cooked in liquid into a hot cereal or side dish. Rye flakes, the equivalent of rolled oats, are also available and can be cooked into a hot cereal.

Nutrition Whole rye berries are a good source of protein, phosphorus, iron, potassium, magnesium, folate, thiamin, and niacin.

RICE COOKING TIPS

❖ ❖ ❖

1. Measure the amounts of rice and liquid.
2. Time cooking accurately.
3. Keep lid on tightly during cooking to prevent steam from escaping.
4. At end of cooking time, remove lid and test for doneness. If rice is not quite tender or if liquid is not absorbed, cook 2 to 4 minutes longer.
5. When rice is cooked, fluff with fork or slotted spoon to allow steam to escape and to keep the grains separate.

Storing   Rye berries should be stored in an air-tight container and can last up to six months on a pantry shelf, a few months longer in the refrigerator.

Cooking   Rye berries are cooked by adding 1 cup to 3 cups of boiling liquid and simmering, covered, for 1½ hours. They can be used as a hot cereal or side dish and have a tangy taste.

Wheat

Wheat is the most important food grown in the world—and a very rich source of nourishment. Wheat is, of course, used to make flours, breads, cereals, and pastas, which are discussed in Chapter 13. Other forms of wheat will be discussed here.

Whole wheat grains that have been steamed, dried, and cracked into small pieces are called **bulgur.** Depending on how it was processed, some or all of the bran may be removed. Check the bulgur you want to purchase to see if the dark brown bran is still on. It has a nutty flavor that is excellent by itself or can be mixed with rice. Its uses are numerous—from salads to soups, from breads to desserts. It is also a nutritious extender and thickener for meat dishes and soups. One-third cup bulgur can be used to each pound of ground meat in recipes such as hamburgers or meat loaf. Bulgur will absorb twice its volume in water and can be used in place of rice in any recipe. It can be bought in three different sizes: coarse, medium (all-purpose), and fine grind. The largest size is good for pilafs and stuffings, the medium for salads and cooked vegetable dishes, and the smallest for Middle Eastern tabbouli and for use in other recipes such as breads and desserts.

Bulgur can be cooked by putting one cup with 2½ cups liquid in a pan and cooking over low heat about 20 to 25 minutes. Fine grind bulgur will cook more quickly than coarse or medium grind. When the liquid is completely absorbed, remove it from the heat and let stand for 10 minutes. Fluff with a fork before serving. Bulgur can also be cooked by presoaking 1 cup in 4 cups of boiling water for 1 to 2 hours.

Bulgur can be stored in an air-tight container at room temperature in a cool dry area, or better yet, put it in the refrigerator where it can last five to six months, as it is more fragile in storage than other grains. Bulgur can also be frozen.

Wheat bran is available either unprocessed or processed and is used as an ingredient in cooking or baking. It makes a high-fiber addition to baked goods such as breads and muffins and can be substituted for bread crumbs in most recipes. Wheat bran is known for its laxative effects. **Unprocessed bran** comes in flakes that look like (and taste like) sawdust. In other words, they are made edible only when used in a recipe. Unprocessed bran is available in natural food stores and also in many supermarkets (a Quaker brand is available). **Processed brans** include breakfast cereals such as All-Bran®, which is cooked under steam and baked. Although some people may complain that All-Bran® looks like twigs in their cereal bowls, and requires much chewing, it is excellent when used in cooking or baking.

Wheat germ is separated out from the wheat grain and can be purchased at the supermarket either toasted or raw. Wheat germ has a nutty, crunchy texture and can be added to cereal, pancakes, baked goods, casseroles, salads, and breading. It can replace half the bread crumbs in breading for a satisfactory product. Wheat germ can sit unopened for 8 to 12 months. Once opened, it must be stored in the refrigerator in an air-tight container because it contains oil, which can turn rancid.

Wheat berries are the actual whole wheat kernel. They are available at natural food stores and are quite inexpensive. Most wheat berries you will find are from hard wheat. When purchasing, make sure the grains are a uniform deep brown color and they feel smooth to the touch to make sure the husk has been removed. Don't purchase wheat berries that feel damp. Wheat berries are also available cracked, as **cracked wheat**, in coarse, medium, or fine qualities. They can be used as whole wheat berries and will cook a little quicker. Cracked wheat is particularly popular in breads.

It is best to soak wheat berries overnight (3½ cups cold water to 1 cup of wheat berries) before using in a recipe. To cook them, boil them in the soaking water for 50 to 60 minutes. Add more water as needed as they cook. Wheat berries can also be used as a meat extender, in casseroles, and in baking. They have a nutty flavor and chewy texture.

They are best stored in clean, air-tight containers in a cool area. Cooked wheat berries will keep up to a week in an air-tight container in the refrigerator.

Some Newer Grains: Amaranth and Quinoa
Amaranth is one of the newer grains on the market, yet it has been around for at least 5,000 years! It was a very important part of the Aztec diet many years ago. It contains a high-quality protein, and one cup (cooked) contains as much calcium as found in one cup of milk. Amaranth is also a good source of vitamin A, Vitamin C, and folate. It is a mildly spicy grain with a slightly peppery taste. Amaranth seeds can be cooked to make hot cereal, pilaf, or popped to make a snack or cold cereal. To cook amaranth, first rinse, then add 1 cup to 2 cups of cold water or broth, and heat to boiling. Reduce the heat, cover, and cook over low heat for 25 minutes. It is a good idea to use a nonstick

pan. Amaranth has a long shelf life but if your kitchen is too warm, put it in the refrigerator. If amaranth gets stale, it smells like linseed oil, so just throw it out!

Quinoa is a pale yellow seed that is technically not a cereal grain, but a dried fruit. Whereas amaranth was popular with the Aztecs, quinoa was a staple of the Incas in Peru. Like amaranth, quinoa is rich in complete protein and calcium. Quinoa also, unlike grains in general, contains an appreciable amount of oil (5 grams/1 cup cooked). There are three varieties or grades of quinoa, and the top-rated variety, known as altiplano, gives you a product that is sweet and pale ivory in color. It is your best choice as lower grades lack consistent quality.

To cook quinoa, first rinse, then add 1 cup to 2 cups of hot water or broth and heat to boiling. Reduce the heat, cover, and cook over low heat for 12–15 minutes. Quinoa has a nutty flavor and can be substituted for rice in recipes. Because of its high oil content, quinoa can be kept at a cool room temperature for only one month. If the kitchen is too warm, put it in the refrigerator.

LEGUMES

Legumes include all sorts of dried beans and peas such as kidney beans, navy beans, and split peas. Lentils, an old-world legume, will be discussed in a separate section because they cook much faster than most dried beans and peas.

Beans
Dried beans are among the oldest of foods and today are considered an important staple for millions of people. Beans were once considered to be worth their weight in gold—the jeweler's "carat" owes its origin to a pealike bean on the east coast of Africa. Beans also once figured very prominently in politics. During the age of the Romans, balloting was done with beans. White beans represented a vote of approval and the dark beans meant a negative vote.

Before reaching the consumer, beans are cleaned to remove pods, stems, and other debris. Special machines separate debris by gravity and then screen the beans by size. Discolored beans are removed by machines equipped with photo-sensitive electric eyes.

Purchasing Many varieties of beans may be found on the grocery shelf. Here are some of the more popular varieties and their uses.

- Black beans have an oval shape and a black skin. They are used in thick soups and in Oriental and Mediterranean dishes.
- Black-eye peas (also called black-eye beans or cow peas) are small, oval-shaped, and creamish white with a black spot on one side. They are used primarily as a main dish vegetable. Black-eye peas are really beans.
- Garbanzo beans (also called chick-peas) are nut-flavored and commonly pickled in vinegar and oil for salads. They are round, beige to yellow in color, and hard in texture. They can also be used as a main dish vegetable in the "unpickled" form.
- Great Northern beans are larger than but similar to pea beans, and are used in soups, salads, casserole dishes, and especially in baked beans.
- Kidney beans are large and have a red color and kidney shape. They are popular for chili con carne and add zest to salads, soups, and Mexican dishes.
- Lima beans, although not widely known as dry beans, make an excellent main dish vegetable and can be used in casseroles. They are broad and flat and come in different sizes.
- Navy beans is a broad term which includes Great Northern, pea, flat small white, and small white beans.
- Pinto beans are of the same species as the kidney and red beans. Beige-colored and speckled, they are used mainly in salads, refried beans, and chili.
- Red and pink beans have a more delicate flavor than red beans. Both are used in many Mexican dishes and chili.

Table 47 describes additional types of beans.

Soybeans are one of the best sources of vegetable protein. Forty percent of the bean's dry weight comes from protein. Because boiled soybeans have a strong taste with a metallic aftertaste, soybeans are made into a wide variety of products such as soy flour, soy milk (made from cooked soybeans), tofu (curdled soy milk), tempeh (fermented soybeans), bean sprouts, and textured vegetable protein (also called TVP). TVP is formulated as flakes and used as a meat extender in hamburgers, for instance, or fashioned into imitation meats such as imitation franks, sausage, and bacon.

When purchasing beans, check that the beans are of similar color and size. When beans get old, they lose their color. Look for beans without any obvious defects, such as cracks or pinholes that may indicate insect damage, and make sure field debris (such as stones, twigs) are not in the bag.

Nutrition Table 48 shows the nutritional profile of cooked dry beans. Dry beans are:

- High in complex carbohydrates
- High in fiber
- A good protein source (particularly when combined with grains or a small amount of animal protein such as milk, eggs, or fish)
- Low in fat
- Cholesterol free
- Rich in potassium, iron, and folate
- Good source of other vitamins and minerals
- Low in sodium (only 10 milligrams per serving)

Although beans are inexpensive, tasty, and full of nutrients, some people hesitate to eat them because of the intestinal gas and bloating they cause. This problem is more apparent for those people who eat beans infrequently. To avoid this embarrassing problem, do the following.

- Always cook beans thoroughly, as cooking breaks down the starches that cause the problem.
- Always discard the soaking water before cooking them.
- Lima beans, split peas, and lentils are the most easily digested, so start with them.
- Eat small servings initially, then slowly increase your intake.
- Chew well and slowly.
- Whenever you increase your fiber intake, you need to be sure to drink at least 8 to 10 glasses of water each day (this includes the water in

Bean, Pea, or Lentil	Size/Shape/Color	Flavor	Soaking Required	Cooking Time	Cups Liquid for Cooking	Yield*	Uses
Black beans (Turtle beans)	Small, pea-shaped, black	Full, mellow	Yes	1½ hours	4	2	Mediterranean cuisine, soups (black bean soup), chilis, salads, with rice
Black-eye peas (Cowpeas, black-eyed beans)	Small, oval, creamy white with black spot	Earthy, absorb other flavors	No	50–60 minutes	3	2	Casseroles, with rice, with pork, Southern dishes
Chick-peas (Garbanzo beans, ceci beans)	Round, tan, large	Nutty	Yes	3 hours	4	4	Salads, soups, casseroles, hors d'oeuvres, hummus and other Middle East dishes
Fava beans, whole	Large, round, flat, off white or tan	Full	Yes	3 hours	2½	4	Soups, casseroles, salads
Great Northern beans	Large, oval, white	Mild	Yes	2 hours	3½	2	Soups, casseroles, baked beans, and mixing with other varieties
Kidney beans	Large, kidney-shaped, red or white (red is much more common)	Rich, meaty, sweet	Yes	1–1½ hours	3	2	Chili, casseroles, salads, soups, a favorite in Mexican and Italian cooking
Lentils	Small, flat, disc-shaped, green, red, or brown, split or whole	Mild, earthy	No	30–45 minutes	2	2¼	Soups, stews, salads, casseroles, stuffing, sandwiches, spreads, with rice
Lima beans	Flat, oval, cream or greenish, large or baby size	Large—full; Baby—mild	Yes	1½ hours (large) 1 hour (baby)	2	1¼	Soups, casseroles, side dishes
Navy beans (Pea beans)	Small to medium, round to oval, white	Mild	Yes	1½ hours	3	2	Baked beans, soups, salads, side dishes, casseroles
Peas, split	Small, flat on one side, green or yellow	Rich, earthy	No	1 hour 30 minutes	3	2¼	Soups, casseroles
Peas, whole	Small-medium, round, yellow or green	Rich, earthy	Yes	1 hour 40 minutes	3	2¼	Soups, casseroles, Scandinavian dishes
Pinto beans	Medium, kidney-shaped, pinkish brown	Rich, meaty	Yes	1½ hours	3	2	A favorite for chili, refried beans, and in other Mexican cooking
Pink beans	Medium, oval, pinkish brown	Rich, meaty	Yes	1 hour	3	2	Popular in barbecue style dishes
Soybeans	Medium, oval-round, creamy yellow	Distinctive	Yes	3½ hours or more	3	2	Soups, stews, casseroles

*From 1 cup of uncooked bean, pea, or lentil.

❖ **Table 48 Nutritional Profile** ❖
of Cooked Dry Beans and Lentils (1 cup)

Nutrient	Cooked Dry Beans	Cooked Lentils
Calories	230 calories	231 calories
Protein	16 g	18 g
Fiber	9 g	10 g
Fat	1.5 g	Trace
Cholesterol	0	0
Sodium	10 mg	4 mg
Iron	5.4 mg	6.6 mg
Zinc	2.1 mg	2.5 mg
Folate	63 micrograms	358 micrograms
Magnesium	92 mg	71 mg
Copper	0.5 mg	0.5 mg
Manganese	1.0 mg	1.0 mg
Potassium	620 mg	731 mg

drinks like tea and juice) because fiber takes water out of the body with it.

Storing Once a package of beans has been opened, transfer them to an air-tight container and store in a cool, dry spot—but not in the refrigerator. They can be stored at room temperature for one year. Once cooked, you can cover and refrigerate for one to two days. Bean leftovers and mashed beans keep very well in your freezer. You may want to add a little moisture or seasoning after thawing to restore flavor and consistency.

Cooking light and healthy To prepare beans, wash carefully and pick over to remove any foreign particles. Beans have to be soaked in order to rehydrate them with water and cook them to a tender texture. See the instructions given for soaking and cooking on the next page.

Casseroles, stews, stuffings, sandwich spreads, salads, and soups can all be prepared with beans as the central ingredient and no one will miss the meat.

Peas
Purchasing Dry peas are an interesting and versatile food that add variety to meals. Dry peas may be green or yellow and may be bought either split or whole. Whole dry peas are available but many cooks prefer to start with the half-circles of split

peas. How do split peas get split? Specially grown whole peas are dried and their skins are then removed by a special machine. A second machine then breaks the peas in half.

- Green dry peas have a more distinct flavor than yellow dry peas.
- Split peas (green and yellow) have had their skins removed and are very popular in soups. Split peas are also great in side dishes such as salads and pilafs. Main dishes can start with split peas too, such as peas with Italian seasonings, mozzarella cheese, and tomatoes.

Green and yellow whole peas and green and yellow split peas, although they vary in taste, are used interchangeably in many recipes and in making soups. Individual preference is the deciding factor here.

When purchasing peas, check that they are of similar color and size. When peas get old, they lose their color. Look for peas without any obvious defects, such as cracks or pinholes that may indicate insect damage, and make sure field debris (such as stones, twigs) are not in the bag.

Nutrition Dry peas contain less calories ounce for ounce than meat and are a good source of protein, especially if eaten with grains, nuts and seeds, or small amounts of animal proteins such as in milk and fish. Dry peas are:

- High in complex carbohydrates
- High in fiber
- Low in fat (only a trace)
- Cholesterol free
- Rich in potassium and other minerals (and vitamins too)
- Low in sodium (only 5 milligrams per serving)

They are also a nutrition bargain as they are quite inexpensive compared to meat, poultry, or fish.

Storing Once a package of peas has been opened, transfer them to an air-tight container and store in a cool, dry spot—but not in the refrigerator. They can be stored at room temperature for one year. Once cooked, you can cover and refrigerate for up to five days. Dishes made with peas can be frozen.

SOAKING AND COOKING BEANS

❖ ❖ ❖

SOAKING

Soak beans before cooking to make them easier to digest. Use 2½ quarts of water to each pound of beans. Remember, beans will rehydrate to at least twice their dry size. Use a pot that's large enough to accommodate the soaking water and the beans in their expanded form.

Before soaking, beans should be sorted to remove any damaged beans or foreign materials.

Traditional Method: Wash beans. Add to water. Soak 6 to 8 hours or overnight. Drain and rinse before cooking.

Quick Method: Wash beans. Add to boiling water; boil 2 to 3 minutes. Cover and soak 1 to 2 hours. Drain and rinse before cooking.

COOKING

Traditional Method: Add three cups water to each cup of soaked and drained beans in a large pot. Bring to a boil and simmer until tender. Most beans will be tender in an hour. Partially cover the pot; beans generally boil over if tightly covered.

Microwave Method: Cook the soaked beans in water, covered, at full power to 8 to 10 minutes or until boiling. Reduce power to 50 percent and cook another 15 to 20 minutes or until beans are tender. Drain and store for future use.

TIPS

- One tablespoon of oil added to the cooking liquid reduces foaming.
- Salt and acidic foods (vinegar, lemon juice, and tomatoes) enhance the taste of beans but slow the cooking process. Add them when beans are almost tender.
- Simmer beans gently to avoid breaking the skins.

Cooking light and healthy Whole peas should be soaked and cooked like dry beans. Split peas do not require soaking. To cook split peas, first rinse and pick over. Put into a pot and add twice as much water (or stock) as peas and heat to boiling. Reduce heat to simmer, cover, and cook until tender, about 30 minutes. For soups and purees, cook 15 minutes longer. One cup of peas (about ½ pound) yields 2 cups of cooked peas.

Dry peas are served in many ways—with margarine, for example, or pureed and made into dips, patties, croquettes, stuffed peppers, and even souffles. They go well with vegetables, pasta, fish, meat, poultry, and more. They can go in soups, salads, side dishes, main dishes, and casseroles.

Lentils

The lentil is an old-world legume that is disc-shaped and about the size of a pea. Thousands of years old, lentils were perhaps the first of the convenience foods—they do not require soaking. After rinsing and picking over, they cook in only 15 to 20 minutes. Lentils are wonderful because they are easy to store, easy to prepare, versatile, have low food cost, and blend well with many different flavors.

Purchasing Lentils come in different colors such as greenish-brown, pink, or yellow. Lentils may come whole or split (split lentils cook faster).

When purchasing lentils, check that they are of similar color and size. When they get old, they lose their color. Look for lentils without any obvious defects, such as cracks or pinholes that may indicate insect damage, and make sure field debris (such as stones, twigs) are not in the bag.

Nutrition Table 48 lists the nutritional analysis of 1 cup plain cooked lentils. They are:

CORN

We get many interesting foods from corn.

- **Cornmeal**—the ground corn kernel used in baking (muffins and cornbread) and cooking (breading), available with or without the bran and germ. It is used to make **polenta** (an Italian dish made by cooking cornmeal and water or stock), an excellent main or side dish when topped with grated cheese; it may also be refrigerated and eaten cold in slices or grilled. Polenta is available in an instant form that can be cooked in minutes.

- **Cornstarch**—a starch used frequently for thickening
- **Whole hominy** (also called samp, posole, pozole)—whole corn that has been steeped in lime solution until the hull loosens and comes off, rinsed, and either canned or dried; comes in yellow or white; sweet flavor and creamy texture; used in soups, stews, casseroles, hot cereals, pudding, and baking; available cracked as **hominy grits** in quick-cooking and instant forms—very popular as hot breakfast cereal with butter and syrup

Whole hominy and hominy grits are most commonly eaten in the southern United States.

- High in complex carbohydrates
- High in fiber
- Low in fat (only a trace)
- Cholesterol free
- Rich in potassium and iron
- Rich in folate
- Low in sodium (only 5 milligrams per serving)

Lentils are also rich in other vitamins and minerals.

Storing Once a package of lentils has been opened, transfer them to an air-tight container and store in a cool, dry spot—but not in the refrigerator. They can be stored at room temperature for one year. Once cooked, you can cover and refrigerate for up to five days. Dishes made with lentils can be frozen.

Cooking Light and Healthy Lentils do not need to be soaked. To cook lentils, just rinse and pick over, then simmer on top of the range, or covered in the microwave on high, in water, stock, broth, or almost any other liquid using two cups liquid for each cup of lentils. If you wish, add seasonings or flavorful ingredients to the cooking water, since lentils absorb flavors well. Do not add acid ingredients, such as tomatoes or lemon juice, until later since they will slow cooking. Salt should be added at the end of the cooking time for the same reason. Drain if needed and they are ready. Cooked lentils may be stored in liquids such as broth, fruit juice, or salad dressing, to boost flavor.

Lentils are an excellent partner with many foods. They make excellent side dishes and go well in soups, stews, sauces, stuffings, and salads. Consider them as you would potatoes or rice. Lentil puree, not unlike peanut butter, can be used on bread or muffins, and in sandwiches, dips, spreads, Mexican dishes, and vegetable fillings.

RECIPES

Grains

— KASHA PILAF —

2 egg whites
½ cup kasha
2 tsp vegetable oil
1 rib celery, sliced thin
1 small onion, coarsely chopped
1 cup low-sodium chicken stock or broth
freshly ground black pepper
salt, if desired
¼ cup toasted slivered almonds

1. In a nonstick saucepan beat the egg whites slightly.
2. Mix kasha with the whites. Stir frequently over medium heat until each grain is separate and dry.
3. Push kasha to one side of the pan and add oil to the pan. When it is hot, add celery and onion and saute over medium heat a few minutes until onion begins to soften and brown.
4. Add chicken stock; combine ingredients in the pan and season with salt and pepper. Reduce heat; cover pan and simmer about 15 minutes, until kasha is tender. Stir almonds into kasha.

Serves 3

Nutrition Analysis:

Calories 214
Carbohydrate. . . . . .26 grams
Fiber . . . . .4 grams
Fat. . . . . .9 grams
Cholesterol. . . . . .1 milligram
Sodium. . . . . .315 milligrams

— OAT BRAN MUFFINS —

2 cups oat bran cereal
¼ cup firmly packed brown sugar
2 tsp baking powder
½ tsp salt
1 cup skim milk
2 egg whites, slightly beaten
¼ cup honey or molasses
1 tbsp corn oil

1. Line 12 medium muffin cups with paper baking cups or spray bottoms with vegetable oil cooking spray.
2. Combine dry ingredients. Add milk, egg whites, honey, and oil; mix just until dry ingredients are moistened. Fill prepared muffin cups almost full.
3. Bake at 425°F for 15 to 17 minutes or until golden brown.

Makes 12 muffins

Variations: Add any one of the following to the muffin batter.

Raisin Muffins: ¼ cup raisins
Banana Muffins: ½ cup mashed bananas
Blueberry Muffins: ½ cup fresh or frozen blueberries
Apple Cinnamon Muffins: ½ cup chopped apple and 1 tsp cinnamon

Nutrition Analysis:

Calories 104
Carbohydrate. . . . . .20 grams
Fiber . . . . .2 grams
Fat. . . . . .2 grams
Cholesterol. . . . . .0 milligrams
Sodium. . . . . .168 milligrams

QUICK-TO-FIX PILAF

1¾ cups water
1½ cups uncooked precooked brown rice
¼ cup seedless raisins
1 tbsp dehydrated chopped onion
1 tbsp margarine
2 tsp chicken bouillon granules
¼ tsp ground white pepper
4 tbsp slivered almonds, toasted

1. Combine water, rice, raisins, onion, butter, bouillon granules, and pepper in 2- to 3-quart saucepan. Bring to a boil; stir once or twice.
2. Reduce heat, cover, and simmer 10 minutes, or until rice is tender and liquid is absorbed. Remove from heat and stir in almonds.

Serves 6

Microwave Oven Instructions
Combine water, rice, raisins, onion, margarine, bouillon granules, and pepper in 2- to 3-quart deep microproof baking dish. Cover and cook on high 5 minutes, or until boiling. Reduce setting to medium (50% power) and cook 5 to 6 minutes. Stir in almonds.

Nutrition Analysis:
Calories 242
Carbohydrate. . . . . .43 grams
Fiber . . . . .3 grams
Fat. . . . . .6 grams
Cholesterol. . . . . .0 milligrams
Sodium . . . . .337 milligrams

APPLE BROWN RICE STUFFING

1 medium red apple, cored and diced
½ cup each chopped onions and sliced celery
⅓ cup seedless raisins
½ tsp poultry seasoning
¼ tsp each dry thyme leaves and ground black pepper
2 tsp margarine
3 cups cooked brown rice (cooked in apple juice)
4 tbsp slivered almonds, toasted
¼ cup apple juice

1. Cook apple, onions, celery, raisins, poultry seasoning, thyme, and pepper in margarine in large skillet until tender crisp.

2. Stir in remaining ingredients. Use as stuffing for poultry or pork roast. To serve as a side dish, cook until thoroughly heated.

Serves 6

Nutrition Analysis:
Calories 191
Carbohydrate. . . . . .33 grams
Fiber . . . . .2 grams
Fat. . . . . .6 grams
Cholesterol. . . . . .0 milligrams
Sodium . . . . .26 milligrams

FRUITED RICE

1 cup sliced carrots
1 tbsp vegetable oil
1 cup sliced green onions
2 cups sliced, cored unpeeled apples
3 cups cooked brown rice
½ cup seedless raisins
1 tbsp sesame seeds

1. Saute carrots in oil in a nonstick pan about 10 minutes. Add onions and apples. Cook 10 minutes longer.
2. Stir in rice and raisins. Cook, stirring constantly, until rice is heated through. Add sesame seeds and toss lightly.

Serves 6

Nutrition Analysis:
    Calories 206
    Carbohydrate . . . . .42 grams
    Fiber . . . . .2 grams
    Fat . . . . .3 grams
    Cholesterol . . . . .0 milligrams
    Sodium . . . . .23 milligrams

RICE-PASTA PILAF

⅓ cup uncooked brown rice
1½ cups chicken broth, unsalted
⅓ cup thin spaghetti, broken into ½- to 1-inch
    pieces
2 tsp margarine
2 tbsp green onions, chopped
2 tbsp green peppers, chopped
2 tbsp fresh mushrooms, chopped
½ clove garlic, minced
½ tsp savory
¼ tsp salt
⅛ tsp pepper
1 tbsp slivered almonds, toasted, if desired

1. Cook rice in 1 cup of the broth in a covered saucepan until almost tender—about 35 minutes.
2. Cook spaghetti in margarine over low heat until golden brown—about 2 minutes. Stir frequently; watch carefully.
3. Add browned spaghetti, vegetables, remaining ½ cup chicken broth, and seasonings to rice.
4. Bring to boil, reduce heat, cover, and cook over medium heat until liquid is absorbed—about 10 minutes.
5. Remove from heat; let stand 2 minutes.
6. Garnish with almonds.

Notes: Toast almonds in 350-degree oven until lightly browned—5 to 12 minutes. Or, toast in heavy pan over medium heat for 10 to 15 minutes, stirring frequently.

Serves 4

Nutrition Analysis:
    Calories 138
    Carbohydrate . . . . .20 grams
    Fiber . . . . .1 gram
    Fat . . . . .4 grams
    Cholesterol . . . . .1 milligram
    Sodium . . . . .501 milligrams

MUSHROOM RICE

1 cup sliced onions
½ lb fresh mushrooms, sliced
3 tbsp chopped fresh parsley
1 tbsp vegetable oil
3 cups cooked brown rice (cooked in beef broth)
3 tbsp nutritional yeast
¼ cup wheat germ
¼ tsp basil
½ tsp cumin seeds

1. Saute onions, mushrooms, and parsley in oil, in a nonstick pan until tender.
2. Add remaining ingredients; heat thoroughly, stirring constantly.

Serves 6

Nutrition Analysis:
    Calories 180
    Carbohydrate . . . . .31 grams
    Fiber . . . . .1 gram
    Fat . . . . .4 grams
    Cholesterol . . . . .0 milligrams
    Sodium . . . . .8 milligrams

BULGUR WITH RAISINS AND APPLE SALAD

¾ cup bulgur

2 medium-size red apples, cored and diced

¼ cup raisins

6 tbsp reduced calorie sweet and spicy French-style salad dressing

1. Pour enough boiling water over bulgur to cover by at least 1 inch. Let stand for 50 to 60 minutes or until tender and doubled in volume. Drain thoroughly, pressing out excess water. (This step can be done ahead of time and bulgur refrigerated until ready to make salad.)

2. In salad bowl, combine bulgur, apples, raisins, and salad dressing.

Serves 4

Nutrition Analysis:

Calories 158

Carbohydrate. . . . . .36 grams

Fiber . . . . .5 grams

Fat. . . . . .2 grams

Cholesterol. . . . . .1 milligram

Sodium. . . . . .197 milligrams

BULGUR WITH PARMESAN

1½ cups low-sodium beef broth

¼ tsp Tabasco sauce

⅛ tsp salt

1 cup cracked wheat bulgur

¼ cup freshly grated Parmesan cheese

1. In a large saucepan, combine beef broth, Tabasco sauce, and salt, and bring to a boil. Stir in bulgur. Remove from heat and cover.

2. Let sit until broth is absorbed and bulgur is tender. Add Parmesan and toss.

Variation: Substitute couscous for bulgur.

Serves 4

Nutrition Analysis:

Calories 155

Carbohydrate. . . . . .27 grams

Fiber . . . . .8 grams

Fat. . . . . .3 grams

Cholesterol. . . . . .5 milligrams

Sodium. . . . . .431 milligrams

ZUCCHINI, TOMATO, AND WHEAT BERRY SLAW

2 cups fully cooked wheat berries, chilled

1 large shallot, minced

2 thin medium zucchini, cut into very thin slices

16–20 cherry tomatoes, cut into ¼-inch thick rounds

2 tbsp chopped fresh basil

1 clove garlic, minced

¼ tsp salt

½ tsp Dijon mustard

1 tbsp fresh lemon juice

1 tbsp red wine vinegar

1 tbsp strong beef stock

¼ cup olive oil

1. Combine the cooked wheat berries with the shallot, zucchini, tomatoes, and basil in a serving bowl. Toss gently to mix.

2. Using the back of a spoon, mash the garlic with the salt in a small bowl until a paste is formed. Whisk in the mustard, lemon juice, vinegar, beef stock, and olive oil. Pour over the salad and toss gently to mix. Let stand 15 to 20 minutes before serving.

Serves 6

Note: If you do not have beef stock on hand, reduce ¼ cup canned beef broth to 1 tbsp by simmering for 5 minutes.

Nutrition Analysis:

Calories 206
Carbohydrate. . . . . .26 grams
Fiber . . . . .2 grams

Fat. . . . . .10 grams
Cholesterol. . . . . .0 milligrams
Sodium. . . . . .145 milligrams

Quinoa Mexican Style

½ lb onions, chopped
1 tsp minced garlic
1 tbsp vegetable oil
1 cup quinoa
1 cup chicken stock
1 cup drained canned Italian plum tomatoes
1 cup tomato juice from canned tomatoes
½ to 1 whole jalapeno or serrano chili, seeded and chopped
2 tbsp chopped fresh coriander

1. Saute onion and garlic in hot oil in heavy-bottomed pot large enough to hold remaining ingredients.
2. When onion is soft, add quinoa, chicken stock, plum tomatoes, tomato juice, and chili. Bring to boil; reduce heat; cover and cook for about 10 minutes, until quinoa is tender.
3. Sprinkle coriander over quinoa mixture and serve.

Serves 3

Nutrition Analysis:

Calories 330
Carbohydrate. . . . . .53 grams
Fiber . . . . .5 grams
Fat. . . . . .9 grams
Cholesterol. . . . . .1 milligram
Sodium. . . . . .632 milligrams

Legumes

Beans and Cashew Salad

1 bag spinach
1 cup broccoli
½ cup navy or pinto beans, cooked
¼ cup dry-toasted cashew bits
½ cup no-oil Italian dressing

1. Steam broccoli until tender (or cook covered in microwave for 2 minutes) and combine with beans in dressing. Chill.
2. Wash and dry spinach, discard stems, and tear leaves into bite-size pieces. Add spinach and cashews to vegetable and bean mixture. Toss prior to serving.

Serves 2

Nutrition Analysis:

Calories 197
Carbohydrate. . . . . .23 grams
Fiber . . . . .5 grams
Fat. . . . . .9 grams
Cholesterol. . . . . .0 milligrams
Sodium. . . . . .109 milligrams

MEXICAN BEAN SANDWICH

1 tsp vinegar
¼ to 1 tsp chili powder
⅛ tsp onion powder
2 tsp salad dressing, mayonnaise-type, reduced
    calorie
¾ cup pinto or kidney beans, cooked, drained,
    unsalted, chopped
3 tbsp celery, chopped
2 flour tortillas
4 slices tomato
2 leaves lettuce

1. Mix vinegar, chili powder, and onion powder
   with salad dressing in a bowl. Add beans and
   celery; mix well.
2. Soften tortillas in heated frying pan about 1½
   minutes or microwave at high power (100
   percent) for 15 seconds.
3. Place half of bean filling onto each tortilla near
   one edge. Top with tomato and lettuce. Roll up.

Note: Canned, drained pinto beans or red kidney
beans may be used in place of cooked beans.

Serves 2

Nutrition Analysis:

Calories 203
Carbohydrate. . . . . .35 grams
Fiber . . . . .1 gram
Fat. . . . . .4 grams
Cholesterol. . . . . .2 milligrams
Sodium. . . . . .15 milligrams

CHICK-PEA SPREAD

1¾ cups cooked chick-peas or garbanzo beans
    (save liquid)
2 tbsp lemon juice
1 tbsp mayonnaise
¼ tsp garlic powder

1. Drain chick-peas, saving liquid.
2. Mash and blend chick-peas. Add 1 tbsp chick-
   pea liquid and the lemon juice, mayonnaise,
   and garlic powder. Mix until smooth.
3. If too thick, add a little more chick-pea liquid or
   water. Variation: Beans in the recipes can be
   canned or cooked from dry beans.

Serves 6

Nutrition Analysis:

Calories 138
Carbohydrate. . . . . .21 grams
Fiber . . . . .0 grams
Fat. . . . . .3 grams
Cholesterol. . . . . .1 milligram
Sodium. . . . . .22 milligrams

VEGETARIAN CHILI

1 tbsp vegetable oil
1 medium onion, chopped
2 carrots, finely chopped
4 cloves garlic, minced
1 sweet red pepper, chopped
1 green pepper, chopped
2 jalapenos, fresh or canned, finely chopped
2 tbsp chili powder

1 tsp cumin
1 cup cooked kidney beans
1 cup cooked pinto beans
1 28-oz can tomatoes, chopped; reserve juice
1 tsp salt
½ tsp freshly ground pepper
2 tbsp fresh cilantro, finely chopped (optional)

1. In a large, nonreactive soup kettle warm the oil over low heat. Add the onion, carrot, garlic, red and green peppers, and jalapenos. Cover the kettle and cook the vegetables until they are very soft, about 10 minutes.
2. Remove the lid, add the chili powder and cumin, and cook an additional 2 to 3 minutes, stirring occasionally. Add the beans and the tomatoes and their juice.
3. Increase the heat to medium and bring the chili to a simmer. Adjust the heat to maintain a simmer and let the chili cook for 20 minutes.
4. Stir in the salt, pepper, and cilantro and serve.

Serves 4

Nutrition Analysis:

Calories	.260
Carbohydrate	.40 grams
Fiber	.13 grams
Fat	.6 grams
Cholesterol	.0 milligrams
Sodium	.708 milligrams

BROCCOLI AND WHITE BEAN SALAD

1 lb broccoli
2 carrots, cut into julienne strips
1⅔ cups cooked or canned Idaho great Northern beans
½ cup chopped red onion
Lemon Dressing

1. Break broccoli into small flowerets; peel and slice stems. Boil in water 3 to 4 minutes or until barely tender; drain.
2. Boil carrots in water 6 minutes or just until tender; drain.
3. Rinse beans; drain.
4. Combine beans, broccoli, carrots, onion, and Lemon Dressing. Marinate at least 2 hours to blend flavors.

Makes 6 servings
Lemon Dressing:
Combine ¼ cup vegetable oil, 2 tbsp lemon juice, 1 clove minced garlic, ¼ tsp each grated lemon peel, crushed oregano, salt and pepper, and ⅛ tsp paprika. Makes about ⅓ cup.

Nutrition Analysis:

Calories	.177
Carbohydrate	.19 grams
Fiber	.4 grams
Fat	.9 grams
Cholesterol	.0 milligrams
Sodium	.75 milligrams

LENTIL PILAF

1 tbsp vegetable oil
1 bunch green onions, chopped
1 to 2 cloves garlic, minced
¼ cup wild rice, washed
1 cup lentils, washed
½ cup white long-grain rice
1 oz slivered almonds
2¾ cup chicken broth (low-sodium)
½ tsp thyme
½ tsp salt
⅛ tsp pepper

1. Saute the onion, garlic, rice, and lentils in the oil until onion is tender (about 3–4 minutes). Add the rest of the ingredients, bring to a boil.
2. Reduce heat; cover, simmer 30 minutes or until all the water is absorbed.

Serves 6

Nutrition Analysis:

Calories	.220
Carbohydrate	.32 grams
Fiber	.4 grams
Fat	.6 grams
Cholesterol	.1 milligram
Sodium	.443 milligrams

Lentil Burritos

1 cup lentils
2 cups water
½ cup onion, minced
1 clove garlic, minced
½ tsp ground cumin
1 dash hot pepper sauce
1 cup mild taco sauce
1 cup zucchini, chopped
1 cup green or sweet red pepper, chopped
4 oz shredded low-fat mozzarella cheese
8 flour tortillas

1. Wash lentils.
2. Place in medium saucepan with water, onion, garlic, cumin, and hot pepper sauce. Heat to boiling, cover, reduce heat, and simmer 10–12 minutes or just until lentils are barely tender.

3. Drain, if necessary. Toss lentils with taco sauce, zucchini, pepper, and cheese. Spoon about ½ cup lentil mixture down center of each tortilla. Roll up. Serve cold or wrap each burrito in dampened paper towel and heat in microwave 1 to 2 minutes each or until cheese begins to melt.

Makes 8 burritos

Nutrition Analysis:
Calories 209
Carbohydrate. . . . . .32 grams
Fiber . . . . .4 grams
Fat. . . . . .5 grams
Cholesterol. . . . . .8 milligrams
Sodium. . . . . .196 milligrams

❖ ❖ ❖

CHAPTER TWELVE

VEGETABLES AND FRUITS

The majority of Americans not only don't eat enough vegetables and fruits to meet dietary guidelines today (at least 2 servings of fruit and 3 servings of vegetables daily), but about one-quarter of Americans rarely eat them at all! Yet eating the minimum servings is really not that difficult—consider a glass of juice with breakfast, a salad with lunch, a piece of fruit for a snack, and a potato and vegetable with dinner. It's not really all that hard!

PURCHASING

Fruits and vegetables come in many forms: fresh, frozen, canned, and dried. When purchasing fresh, look for the following.

1. Check for characteristic color, which should be bright and lively.
2. Check for characteristic shape; misshapen produce is often inferior in taste and texture and harder to prepare.
3. Check for characteristic size; it should have a good weight for size.
4. Check for freshness, which may be evident by crispness, lack of wilting, and the like, depending on the item.
5. Check for bruises, blemishes, decay, cracks, frostbite.

Tables 49 and 50 give purchasing tips for many different vegetables and fruits, and see the illustrations, which show some specialty vegetables and fruits.

Frozen vegetables and fruits have much the same flavor as fresh, but the texture often changes during freezing. Vegetables and fruits are frozen at the peak of ripeness and are very convenient to use. Choose frozen vegetables and fruits that are in clean, firm packaging. If the packages are soft, the food has already lost quality.

Canned fruits are available in heavy syrup, light syrup, juice-packed, and water-packed. Syrup-packed fruit contains much sugar. Canned vegetable are generally high in sodium; some low-sodium versions are available. Canned fruits and vegetables are mostly available as Grade A or Grade B; each offers the same nutrition, but the Grade A will have a better appearance, texture, and flavor. Look for clean cans without dents, swelling, or rust. Look for dried fruits that are bright in color and firm, but pliable.

NUTRITION

Vegetables and fruits are, in general:

- Low in calories
- Low or no fat (except avocados)
- Free of cholesterol
- Fair to good sources of fiber
- Excellent sources of vitamins and minerals, particularly vitamins A and C (see the tables)
- Low in sodium (except for canned vegetables)

Also, dried fruits, such as raisins and apricots, are good sources of iron. Whole fruits and vegetables are better sources of nutrients than juices.

❖ Table 49 Purchase and Preparation of Vegetables ❖

Name	Quality Indicators	Amount to Buy	Storage	Preparation
Artichokes, globe	Compact, tight leaves; heavy for size; brown blemishes do not affect quality.	1/person	Refrigerate unwashed in plastic bag up to 1 week.	Wash. Cut 1 inch off tops. Cut off stem and lower leaves. Scrape out choke (fuzzy center) with melon ball cutter. (Removal of choke can be done before or after cooking.) Rinse well. Dip in lemon juice immediately. Trim bottoms.
Asparagus	Tightly closed tips; firm, not withered, stalks; bright green.	⅓–½ lb/person	Refrigerate unwashed in plastic bag for up to 4 days.	Break off woody lower ends. Remove lower scales, which may harbor sand, or peel lower part of stalk. Tips may be cut to uniform lengths and/ or tied in bundles for cooking. Put in cold water to rinse, remove, and drain.
Beans, green or wax	Firm and straight, with few shriveled ends; even color, without blemishes. Should be tender and crisp enough to break when bent to 45° angle. Enclosed seeds should be small, not large and bulging.	¼ lb/person	Refrigerate unwashed in plastic bag for up to 4 days.	Wash. Cut or snap off ends. Remove any spots. Leave whole or cut into desired lengths.
Beans, lima	Shelled beans should be plump, with tender skins.	¼ lb shelled or ¾ lb unshelled beans/person	Refrigerate unwashed (in pod or shelled) in plastic bag for up to 4 days.	Shell, wash, and drain.
Beets	Firm, round, uniform size; smooth skin. Tops, if any, should be fresh or just wilted, but not yellow or deteriorated. Large, rough beets are often woody.	⅓–½ lb/person	Cut off tops, leaving 1 inch of stem attached to beets. Refrigerate unwashed in plastic bag for up to 1 week.	Leave roots on. Scrub well. Steam or boil before trimming roots and stems and slipping off skin.
Broccoli	Dark green, tightly closed buds.	⅓ lb/person	Refrigerate unwashed in plastic bag for up to 5 days.	Wash well. Soak in salted water 30 minutes if necessary to remove insects. Cut stalks 3½ inches below flowerets. Cut stalks and flowerets lengthwise into spears. Cut a 1-inch slash in bottom of stalks for even cooking.

❖ Table 49 Continued ❖

Name	Quality Indicators	Amount to Buy	Storage	Preparation
Brussels sprouts	Bright green; tight heads; uniform size, firm.	¼–⅓ lb/person	Discard old, discolored leaves. Refrigerate unwashed in plastic bag for up to 3 days.	Trim bottom ends and remove yellowed outer leaves (but don't cut off too much of the bottom or you will lose too many leaves). For more even cooking, pierce base with sharp knife point. Rinse well.
Cabbage, white, green, or red	Firm head, heavy for size. Good color. Crisp leaves. Leaves finely ribbed.	¼ lb/person	Refrigerate unwashed in plastic bag for up to 1 week.	Remove coarse or discolored outer leaves. Remove core and rinse whole, or cut into quarters and then remove core. For wedges, core is left in, but with bottom trimmed, to hold sections together.
Carrots	Bright orange color; crisp, straight, and well shaped; smooth surface. Large carrots are sometimes woody.	¼ lb/person	Refrigerate unwashed in plastic bag for up to 2 weeks. If carrots have green tops, cut off first.	Trim top and bottom ends. Pare with hand peeler if desired. Scrub well. Cut as desired.
Cauliflower	White color, not yellow or brownish; fine grained, tightly closed buds; fresh green, well-trimmed leaves.	1 medium head serves 4	Refrigerate unwashed in plastic bag for up to 1 week.	Remove leaves and cut out core. Cut away discolored parts. Wash. Separate into florets, leaving portion of center stalk attached to each one, to minimize trim loss, or cook whole.
Celery	Straight, rigid, well trimmed; fresh green color.	¼ lb/person. 1 large stalk yields 1 cup sliced or diced.	Refrigerate unwashed in plastic bag for up to 2 weeks.	Cut off root end. Separate stems and scrub well. Reserve leaves and tough outer stems for stocks, soups, mirepoix. Ribbed outer side of stems may be peeled to remove strings. Cut as desired.
Celery root (knob celery or celeriac)	Firm and heavy. Large ones are often soft and spongy in center. Clean.	¼ lb/person	Refrigerate unwashed in plastic bag up to 1 week.	Wash well, peel, and cut as desired.
Corn (on cob)	Fresh, moist husks, not dry; no worm damage; kernels well filled, tender, and milky when punctured.	1 large or 2 small ears/person	Refrigerate in a plastic bag for up to 2 days.	Strip off husks, remove silk, and cut off bottom stump. Cut into 2 or 3 sections as desired. Keep refrigerated and use as soon as possible.
Cucumbers (slicing type)	Firm, crisp, dark green, well shaped. Yellow color means overmature.	Half a cucumber/ person	Refrigerate in a plastic bag for up to 1 week.	Wash. Trim ends. Peel if skin is tough or has been waxed. Cut as desired.

❖ *Table 49 Continued* ❖

Name	Quality Indicators	Amount to Buy	Storage	Preparation
Eggplant	Shiny, dark purple color; heavy and plump; without blemishes or soft spots.	⅓ lb/person	Refrigerate unwashed in plastic bag for up to 5 days.	Wash. Trim off stem end. Peel if skin is tough. Cut just before use. Dip in lemon juice (or antioxidant solution) to prevent discoloration.
Garlic	Skin may be white or pink. No brown spots, soft spots, or spoilage; dry skin; no green shoots.	As called for in recipe.	Store, without wrapping, in a cool, dark, and dry place.	Separate cloves one by one as needed, or strike whole bulb with heel of hand to separate. To peel cloves, crush slightly with side of heavy knife. Peel and trim root end. Mince or press through a garlic press to use as a seasoning.
Kohlrabi	Uniform light green color; 2–3 inches in diameter. Crisp and firm. No woodiness.	1 small to medium bulb/person	Cut off leaves and stems and refrigerate unwashed in a plastic bag for up to 1 week.	Scrub. Peel like turnips, being sure to remove full thickness of skin. Slice or dice.
Leeks	Fresh green leaves; 2–3 inches of clean white bottoms. White part should be crisp and tender, not fibrous.	About ¾ lb serves 2.	Refrigerate unwashed in plastic bag for up to 1 week.	Cut off roots and green tops. Cut deeply through white part, separate the layers slightly, and wash very carefully to remove all embedded soil. Make one deep cut lengthwise to within an inch of the root end.
Lettuce	Springy-firm heads that give slightly to gentle pressure. Avoid brown spots on leaves.	1 head provides 2½ quarts of torn pieces, 4–6 wedges, or 2½ quarts of chunks.	Refrigerate unwashed in its original wrapper. Once washed, refrigerate in a tightly sealed container.	Hold the head core-end down and rap it against a counter. Lift or twist the core out with your fingers. Rinse the head, cored-end up under cool running water, spreading the leaves slightly to allow the moisture to penetrate to the inner leaves. Drain thoroughly cored-end down in a colander.
Mushrooms	Firm, white caps, closed at the stem. Stems should be relatively short. No dark spots, bruises, or mold.	About ¼ lb/person	Refrigerate unwashed in plastic bag for up to 4 days.	Trim bottoms of stems. Just before cooking wash quickly in cold water; drain well. If you desire to keep the mushrooms white, add a small amount of acid (lemon juice, vinegar, ascorbic acid) to the rinse water. Use whole, slice lengthwise, or chop.

❖ *Table 49 Continued* ❖

Name	Quality Indicators	Amount to Buy	Storage	Preparation
Okra	Tender, full pods, not dry or shriveled. Ridges should be soft. Seeds should be soft and white. Uniform deep green color.	¼ lb/person	Refrigerate unwashed in plastic bag up to 5 days.	Wash. Trim ends. Slice or leave whole.
Onions, dry	Clean, hard, well shaped; no mold or black fungus; no green shoots. Skins should be very dry.	¼ lb/person, as called for by recipes for seasoning.	Store unwrapped in cool, dry, dark place with good ventilation for up to 3 months.	Cut off root and stem ends. Peel. Wash. Cut or slice as needed.
Onions, green (scallions)	Fresh, crisp green tops; little or no bulb formation at white part; clean, white bottoms.	As needed for seasoning, or in recipes.	Refrigerate unwashed in a plastic bag for up to 1 week.	Cut off roots and wilted ends of green tops. Amount of green left on varies with different recipes or uses.
Parsley	Bright green, unwilted leaves with no rot.	As needed for garnish, seasoning, or in recipes.	Refrigerate unwashed in a plastic bag for up to 5 days.	Wash well and drain. Remove yellow leaves and large stems (save stems for stocks). Separate into sprigs for garnish, or chop leaves.
Parsnips	Firm, smooth, well shaped, with light, uniform color. Large ones are often woody.	¼ lb/person	Refrigerate unwashed in plastic bag for up to 2 weeks.	Refrigerating for 2 weeks develops sweetness. Trim ends and peel. Rinse. Leave whole or cut as desired.
Peas (green and black-eyed)	Firm, fresh, moderately filled-out pods. Medium-size peas.	½ lb unshelled/ person	Refrigerate unwashed in plastic bag for up to 3 days.	Shell and rinse.
Peas, edible pod	Bright green color, crisp pods, no blemishes.	¼ lb/person	Refrigerate unwashed in plastic bag for up to 3 days.	Remove stem end. Pull off strings at side veins. (Both the flat, Chinese snow peas and new full-pod variety called sugar snap peas are available. Expensive.)
Peppers, sweet (green or red)	Shiny green or red color; well shaped; no soft spots or shriveling.	1 medium/person	Refrigerate unwashed in plastic bag for up to 5 days.	Wash. Cut in half lengthwise and remove core, seeds, and white membranes. Or leave whole (as for stuffed peppers) and cut out core from the end.
Potatoes, white	Fairly clean, firm, and smooth. No wrinkled skins, soft dark areas, sprouts, cut surfaces, or greenish color.	1 medium size/ person	Store in cool, dark place that's well ventilated. Don't refrigerate.	Gently scrub with vegetable brush or cellulose sponge to clean. Peel and/or cut into desired shapes.
Potatoes, sweet (including "yams")	Clean, dry surface. Firm, not shriveled or blemished.	1 medium size/ person	Store in cool, dry, dark place with good ventilation for up to 2 weeks.	Scrub, remove sprouts, and cut out decayed, discolored, or green areas. Once potatoes are peeled, put in cold water to prevent discoloring.

❖ *Table 49 Continued* ❖

Name	Quality Indicators	Amount to Buy	Storage	Preparation
				Note: There are two basic varieties of sweet potatoes. The variety that has a moister, deeper orange flesh is sometimes referred to, inaccurately, as "yam." The two varieties are interchangeable for most purposes. True yams are an entirely different vegetable, with starchy, white flesh.
Radishes	Firm, tender, and crisp, with good shape and color.	2–3/person as relish.	Refrigerate unwashed in plastic bag for up to 1 week.	Cut off root and stem ends. Wash.
Spinach	Fresh, crisp, dark green leaves. No rot or slime or badly bruised leaves. Short stems.	½ lb/person for cooked. ¼ lb/person for salads.	Wash, dry, wrap in paper towels and put in plastic bag. Refrigerate for up to 3 days.	Remove stems and damaged or yellow leaves. Wash in several changes of water. Use large quantity of water and lift spinach up and down to float off sand and dirt. Lift from water and drain well.
Squash, summer (including zucchini)	Firm, heavy, and crisp; tender skins, no blemishes.	⅓ lb/person	Refrigerate unwashed in plastic bag.	Wash or scrub well. Trim ends.
Squash, winter	Heavy and firm. Hard rind. No blemishes.	½ medium squash or ½ lb/person	Store in a cool, dry, dark place with good ventilation up to 1 month.	Wash. Cut in half. Scrape out seeds and fibers. Cut into portion sizes. For puréed or mashed squash, either steam or bake and then remove peel; or peel, dice, and then steam.
Tomatoes	Firm but not hard, with little or no green core. Smooth, without bruises, blemishes, cracks, or discoloration. If underripe, let stand 2–3 days at room temperature.	1 medium/person	Store unwashed at room temperature until ripe.	For use with skin on: wash, remove core, cut as desired. To peel: plunge into boiling water for 10–20 seconds (riper tomatoes take less time). Cool immediately in ice water. Slip skins off and remove core.
Turnips	Firm and heavy, with good color and no blemishes. White turnips over 2½ inches in diameter may be woody or spongy.	1 medium/person	Refrigerate unwashed in plastic bag for up to 1 week.	Peel heavily to remove thick skin. Cut as desired.

❖ *Table 50 Purchase and Preparation of Fruits* ❖

Fruit	Quality Indicators	Amount to Buy	Storage	Preparation
Apples	Mature apples have fruity aroma, brown seeds, and slightly softer texture than unripe fruit. Overripe or old apples are soft and sometimes shriveled. Avoid apples with bruises, blemishes, decay, or mealy texture.	3 medium-size apples (about 1 lb) yields 3 cups diced fruit.	Refrigerate unwashed in a plastic bag.	Wash. Peel (if desired), quarter and remove core, or leave whole and core with special coring tool. Use stainless steel knife for cutting. After cutting, dip in orange juice or lemon juice (or other tart fruit juice) to prevent browning.
Apricots	Accept only tree-ripened fruits, golden yellow, firm, and plump. Avoid fruit that is too soft or with blemishes, cracks, decay, or shriveled skin.	10 apricots (about 1 lb) yields 1½ cups cut-up fruit.	If unripe, ripen at room temperature. If ripe, store in refrigerator, unwashed, in plastic bag for up to 3 days.	Wash, split in half, and remove pit. Does not need to be peeled.
Avocados	Two main types: with rough green skin turning black when ripe; with smoother skin that stays green. Fresh appearance, heavy for size, turning soft when ripe. Avoid soft spots and bruises.	1 large avocado yields 1 cup mashed.	Ripen at room temperature, 2–5 days. Once ripe or cut, refrigerate in plastic bag for up to 2 days.	Cut in half lengthwise and remove pit. Peel (skin pulls away easily from ripe fruit). Dip or rub with lemon juice immediately to prevent browning. Cut as desired.
Bananas	Plump and smooth, without bruises or spoilage. Avoid overripe fruit.	3 medium-sized bananas (about 1 lb) yields 1 cup mashed.	Ripen at room temperature until all yellow with small brown flecks. Once ripe, refrigerate (the skin will turn black).	Peel and dip in fruit juice to prevent browning.
Berries (blackberries, blueberries, cranberries, currants, raspberries, strawberries)	Full, plump and clean, with bright, fully ripe color. Watch for mold or spoiled fruits. Wet spots on carton indicate damaged fruit.	One pound yields 4 cups.	Refrigerate in original container for up to 2 days. Berries do not keep well.	Sort out spoiled berries and foreign materials. Wash with gentle spray and drain well. Remove stems from strawberries. Handle carefully to avoid bruising.
Cherries	Plump, firm, sweet, and juicy, with uniform dark red to almost black color (except Royal Anne variety, which is creamy white with red blush). No blemishes or bruises.	1 pound yields 2½ cups.	Refrigerate in original container until ready to use. Use in 3 days.	Remove stems and damaged fruit. Rinse with spray and drain well. Remove pits with special cherry pitting tool.

❖ *Table 50 Continued* ❖

Fruit	Quality Indicators	Amount to Buy	Storage	Preparation
Figs	Plump, soft fruits without spoilage or sour odor. Calimyrna figs are light green when ripe. Missions are nearly black.	8 large or 12–16 small figs per pound	Very perishable. Ripen at room temperature uncovered, out of sun. Use ripe fruit right away.	Remove stem ends.
Grapefruit and oranges	Firm, smooth skins, heavy for size. Avoid puffy, soft fruits or those with pointed ends. Cut and taste for sweetness. These fruits are already ripe.	1 grapefruit yields 1½ cups of sections. 1 pound oranges is 3 medium size.	Store in refrigerator for up to 2 weeks.	For grapefruit halves, cut in half crosswise and free flesh from membranes with grapefruit knife. For sections and slices, peel and section or slice.
Grapes	Firm, ripe, well-colored fruits in full bunches that should be firmly attached to stems, and do not fall off when shaken. Watch for shriveling or rotting at stem ends. These fruits are already ripe.	1 pound yields 3 cups.	Refrigerate unwashed in plastic bag for 2–5 days.	Wash and drain. Cut in half and remove seeds (except for seedless variety).
Kiwi fruit	Firm but slightly soft to touch when ripe. No bruises, excessively soft spots, or mold.	1 large kiwi yields ½ cup slices.	Ripen at room temperature away from sunlight. Once ripe, refrigerate in plastic bag for up to 1 week.	Peel thin outer skin with paring knife. Cut crosswise into slices. Best uncooked.
Lemons and limes	Firm, smooth skins. Color may vary: limes may be yellow, and lemons may have some green on skin.	1 lemon yields 3 tablespoons of juice, 1 lime yields 2 tablespoons of juice.	Store in refrigerator for up to 2 weeks.	Cut in wedges, slices, or other shapes for garnish, or cut in half crosswise for juicing.
Mangoes	Plump and firm, with clear color and no blemishes. Avoid rock-hard fruits, which may not ripen properly.	1 mango yields ¾ cup sliced fruit.	Let ripen at room temperature until slightly soft. Once ripe, refrigerate in plastic bag for up to 3 days.	Peel and cut flesh away from center pit, or cut in half before peeling, working a thin bladed knife around both sides of the flat pit.

❖ Table 50 Continued ❖

Fruit	Quality Indicators	Amount to Buy	Storage	Preparation
Melons	Cantaloupes: Smooth scar on stem end, with no trace of stem (called "full slip," meaning melon was picked ripe). Yellow rind, with little or no green. Heavy, with good aroma. Honeydew: Good aroma, slightly soft, heavy, creamy white to yellowish rind, not green. Large sizes have best quality. Cranshaws, Casabas, Persians: Heavy, with rich aroma and slightly soft blossom end. Watermelon: Yellow underside, not white. Firm and symmetrical. Large sizes have best yield. Velvety surface, not too shiny. When cut, look for hard dark brown seeds and no "white heart" (hard white streak running through center).	1 pound of melon yields about 1 cup cubed fruit.	Ripen at room temperature. Once cut, they won't ripen further. Refrigerate ripe and cut melon in plastic bag (tie tightly) and use within 1–2 days.	Wash, cut in half, and remove seeds and fibers. Cut into wedges or cut balls with ball cutter. Watermelon: Wash, cut into desired portions, or cut in half and cut balls with ball cutter.
Papayas	Firm and symmetrical, without bruises or rotten spots. Avoid dark green papayas, which may not ripen properly.	1 medium yields 1¼ cups sliced.	Let ripen at room temperature, until slightly soft and nearly all yellow, with only a little green. Refrigerate ripe fruit in plastic bag for up to 3 days.	Wash. Cut in half lengthwise and scrape out seeds. Peel if desired, or serve like cantaloupe.
Peaches and Nectarines	Plump and firm, without bruises or blemishes. Avoid green fruits, which are immature and will not ripen well.	3 medium/lb 1 pound yields 2 cups sliced fruit.	Let ripen at room temperature. Refrigerate unwashed for up to 3 days.	Cut in half, remove pits, and drop into fruit juice, to prevent darkening. Cut as desired.
Pears	Clean, firm, and bright; no blemishes or bruises.	3 medium/lb 1 pound yields 2 cups sliced fruit.	Let ripen at room temperature. Refrigerate when ripe in plastic bag for up to 3 days.	Wash. Peel if desired, cut in half or quarters and remove core.

❖ *Table 50   Continued* ❖

Fruit	Quality Indicators	Amount to Buy	Storage	Preparation
Pineapple	Plump and fresh looking, orange-yellow color, abundant fragrance. Avoid soft spots, bruises, and dark, watery spots. Large sizes have best yield.	1 medium pineapple yields 3 cups diced fruit.	Ripen at room temperature, away from sunlight. Once ripe, use within 2 days.	May be cut in many ways. For slices, chunks, and dice, cut off top and bottom and pare like a grapefruit, using stainless steel knife. Remove all eyes, core. Slice or cut as desired.
Plums	Plump and firm but not hard, with good color and no bruises, blemishes, or shriveled skin.	1 pound yields about 2 cups sliced fruit.	Ripen at room temperature. Once ripe, refrigerate in plastic bag for up to 3 days.	Wash, cut in half and remove pits, or serve whole.
Rhubarb	Firm, crisp, tender, with thick stalks, not thin and shriveled. Rhubarb is not actually a fruit but a stem.	1 pound yields 3 cups sliced fruit.	Refrigerate unwashed in plastic bag for up to 1 week.	Cut off all traces of leaf (which is poisonous). Trim root ends if necessary. Cut into desired lengths.

STORING

Guidelines for storing fresh vegetables and fruits appear in Tables 49 and 50. All vegetables and fruits require careful handling and storage to conserve quality. Before storing, sort vegetables and fruits, discarding any that are damaged.

The saying about the bad apples spoiling the whole bunch is true: one damaged apple (or any fruit) can accelerate the decay of fruit stored with it. The same is true for potatoes. Also never store tomatoes near lettuce because tomatoes cause the lettuce to brown.

Most produce need not be washed before storing. In particular, if you wash the following vegetables and fruits, it may cause mold or wilting: strawberries, raspberries, blueberries, mushrooms, plums, lettuce, and grapes.

Some fruits are picked when they are ripe and they therefore don't ripen further after being picked. These include grapes, citrus fruit, berries, and apples. Other fruits benefit from further ripening or softening. These include avocados, bananas, kiwi, melon, peaches/nectarines, and tomatoes.

Store frozen vegetables and fruits at 0°F or below for 10 to 12 months if your freezer can maintain that temperature. Canned vegetables and fruits can be stored in a cool, dry place for as long as a year. When stored too long or at too high a temperature, canned vegetables and fruits lose quality (but are still safe to eat). Once opened, store in another container and use within 2 to 3 days. Dried fruits should be stored in tightly closed plastic bags or containers. They can last up to 1 month at room temperature or 6 months in the refrigerator.

COOKING LIGHT AND HEALTHY

When preparing and cooking vegetables and fruits, an important consideration is doing so without the loss of valuable nutrients. Five factors are responsible for most nutrient loss: high temperature, long cooking, baking soda, exposure to the air, and dissolving in water (especially water-soluble vitamins). Because the fat-soluble vitamins are insoluble in water, they are fairly stable in cooking. The water-soluble vitamins easily leach out of foods during washing or cooking. Here are tips to retain nutrients in fruits, vegetables, and other foods as well.

1. Buy food that is fresh and of high quality. Examine fresh fruits and vegetables thoroughly for appropriate color, size, and shape.
2. Store fruits and vegetables in the refrigerator

Specialty fruits and vegetables

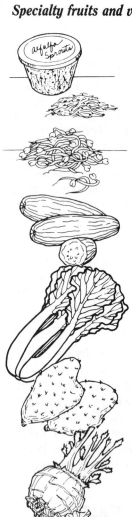

ALFALFA SPROUTS
are the tender young sprouts produced by alfalfa seeds and harvested only six days after they begin growing. They have a crunchy, nutty flavor.

BEAN SPROUTS
grow from mung beans and are harvested and sold within six days from the time they first appear. The shorter the bean sprouts, the crisper and more tender they are.

BITTER MELON
(Balsam Pear) is shaped like a cucumber, 6-8 inches long. The outer surface is clear green and wrinkled; inside it contains a layer of white or pink spongy pulp and seeds.

BOK CHOY *(Chinese Chard, White Mustard Cabbage) is a combination of chard and celery with long and broad crisp white stalks with shiny, deep green leaves. The flavor is sweet but mild.*

CACTUS LEAVES *(Nopales) grow on a cactus plant and are light green and crisp, but also tender. Served like a vegetable, they have the texture and flavor of green beans.*

CELERIAC *(Celery Root) looks like celery but only the bulb-type root is edible. The small young root knob is more tender and less woody than the larger, mature roots.*

CHARD *(Swiss Chard) is a lush green, leafy vegetable resembling spinach in appearance with flavor and texture similar to asparagus. The leaves and ribs are excellent as fresh salad greens.*

CHAYOTE *(Vegetable Pear) has a very dark green hard surface and can be either pear shaped or round. It is 3-5 inches long, looks like an acorn squash but has a more delicate flavor, and has flesh the color of honeydew melon.*

CHINESE LONG BEANS *(Dow Kwok) are pencil-thin beans, 12-25 inches long, with light green tender pods. The tiny beans inside resemble immature black-eyed peas.*

CORIANDER
(Cilantro) resembles parsley with small leafy sprigs but is more tender. The flavor is stronger than parsley and lingers on the tongue. Therefore, as a parsley substitute, less is used.

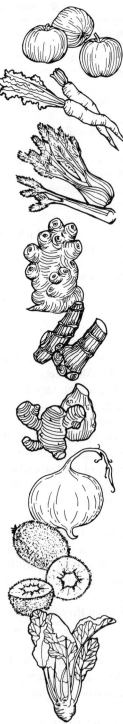

CRABAPPLES *are tiny apples with a strong, pleasing flavor for cooking and use in jellies and jams. They are too tart to eat out of hand. They can be yellow, red or green.*

DAIKON *(Japanese White Radish) is a large, tapered white radish about 8-10 inches long. It has a crisp texture and a flavor similar to an ordinary radish but sharper and hotter.*

FENNEL *(Anise) has broad leaf stalks which overlap at the base of the stem and form a firm, rounded, white bulb. The leaves are green and featherlike and the plant has a licorice aroma and flavor. The bulb as well as the inside stalks are edible.*

GINGER ROOT *is the underground stem or root of the tropical ginger plant. It is light reddish brown and knobby and is used as a tangy flavoring when shredded or mashed.*

HORSERADISH ROOT *(German Mustard) has a potent flavor and is used in small quantities. The edible part of the plant is the white root, which should be grated or shredded.*

JERUSALEM ARTICHOKES
(Sunchokes) are root vegetables of a gnarled, knotty appearance with a crisp, crunchy texture and delicious flavor. Eaten cooked or raw, they are very versatile and can be used as a substitute for potatoes.

JICAMA *is a large turnip-shaped root vegetable with a light brown peel. Inside, it is white and crisp with a delicate sweet flavor similar to water chestnuts. The peel is not usually eaten.*

KIWIFRUIT *on the outside has an unattractive brown fuzzy surface. The inside, however, is smooth, creamy, bright green flesh with a strawberry-melon flavor and tiny edible black seeds. Kiwifruit is about the size of a large egg, 3 inches long and 2 inches in diameter.*

KOHLRABI *is a green leafy vegetable with a stem which thickens above ground and looks like a bulb. The whole plant is edible. The leaves are used like spinach and the bulb (about 2-3 inches in diameter) is served cooked or raw.*

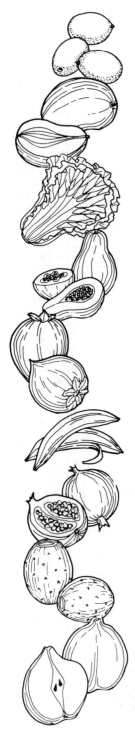

KUMQUATS *are small, orange-gold citrus fruits with sweet flavored skins and tart, tangy insides. Eaten whole, the flavors mix nicely. Remove seeds before eating.*

MANGOS *are subtropical fruits of varied size, shape and color. Their smooth skins can be green, yellow or red and their shapes vary from round to oval. Sizes can be from 2-10 inches and 2-5 pounds.*

NAPPA *(Sui Choy, Chow Choy, Won Bok, Chinese Cabbage) has broad-ribbed stalks varying in color from white to light green, resembling romaine with crinkly leaves forming a long, slender head. The flavor is mild.*

PAPAYA *is an oblong melon-like tropical fruit, green to yellow on the outside with golden yellow to orange flesh inside. A medium papaya weighs about 1 pound. The small black seeds inside are not to be eaten.*

PERSIMMONS *are a brilliant orange in color and soft to touch (like a tomato). They are about the size of an apple. Enjoy their flavorful taste by eating out of hand.*

PLANTAINS *look like large green bananas with rough, mottled peels. They are used as a vegetable and must be cooked. Never eat them raw. Black skins indicate they are sweet and fully ripe.*

POMEGRANATES *are about the size and shape of apples, golden yellow to deep red, with hundreds of kernels or seeds which are juicy and sweet. Inside, the pulp is crimson and too bitter to eat. Only the seeds are edible.*

PRICKLY PEARS *(Cactus Pear, Indian Fig, Barberry fig, Tuna) are pear-shaped with yellow to crimson skins covered with spines. Usually the spines have been removed before marketing. The flesh is yellow and sweet with a taste of watermelon; the skin is bright red when ripe. Peel back the skin to eat.*

QUINCE *looks like an apple with an odd-shaped stem end and skin which is pale yellow when the fruit is fully ripe. Quince has a distinctive biting flavor and should be served cooked in jams, jellies, sauces, puddings, etc., not eaten raw.*

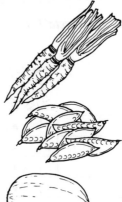

SALSIFY *(Oyster Plant) looks like parsnip with a full, grassy top, a firm gray-white root, and the juicy flavor of fresh oysters. The edible part is the carrot-shaped root which should be peeled and then cooked.*

SNOW PEAS *(Sugar Peas, China Peas) are an oriental vegetable looking like regular peas except the pods are much flatter and translucent. They have a delicate flavor and add crunch and texture to a dish. Serve hot or cold after blanching 2-3 minutes.*

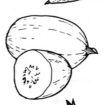

SPAGHETTI SQUASH *(Cucuzzi, Calabash, Suzza Melon) is a large edible gourd that is round to oval, about 2 feet long and 3-4 inches in diameter. The skin is pale yellow and edible; the inside forms translucent strands similar to spaghetti when cooked. Use it like pasta.*

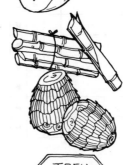

SUGAR CANE *is woody sugar stalks cut into 4-6 inch lengths. Eat by pulling away the outer covering and chewing the cane. Boil the cane for a sweet syrup topping.*

TARO ROOT *(Dasheen) is a highly digestible starchy root of mild flavor used in many different ways like a potato. It should be peeled and cooked before eating.*

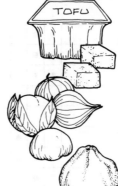

TOFU *(Soybean Curd) is similar to a very soft cheese or custard with a bland flavor and the ability to pick up the flavor of the foods with which it is cooked.*

TOMATILLOS *(Ground Tomatoes, Husk Tomatoes) are small green vegetables that grow on ground vines and look like tiny tomatoes. They turn from bright green to yellow when fully ripe but are often used unripe, raw or cooked.*

UGLI FRUIT *is an unattractive, juicy citrus hybrid, a cross between a grapefruit and a tangerine. It is the size and shape of a grapefruit with a mottled rough peel that looks loose. The rind has light-green blemishes which turn orange when ripe. The fruit has a mild, orange-like flavor.*

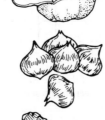

WATER CHESTNUTS *(Chinese Water Chestnuts, Waternuts) are the small edible roots of the tropical Water Chestnut plant. The deep brown skin of the roots is removed and only the white, crunchy inside is used (mainly in salads or stir-fry dishes) after blanching 2-4 minutes.*

YUCCA ROOT *(Manioc, Cassava, Casava) is the large, starchy root of the Yucca plant. Used like a potato, it must be peeled before cooking and cooked before eating. Its flavor is mild but very pleasing.*

Courtesy: United Fresh Fruit and Vegetable Association.

Selected Nutrients in Fruits and Vegetables

Fruits	Vitamin A	Vitamin C	Fiber
APPLE			■
APRICOTS (3)	●		■
BANANA			■
FIGS (2)			●
GRAPES (1 CUP)			■
GRAPEFRUIT (½)		●	■
KIWI FRUIT		●	■
NECTARINE			■
ORANGE		●	■
PEACH			■
PEAR			●
PLUMS (2)			■
PRUNES (4)			●

½ Cup Serving

	Vitamin A	Vitamin C	Fiber
CANTALOUPE	●	●	■
HONEYDEW		■	
PAPAYA	■	●	
PINEAPPLE			■
RAISINS (¼ CUP)			■
RASPBERRIES		■	■
STRAWBERRIES		●	■
WATERMELON (1 CUP)		■	

Juices ¾ Cup

	Vitamin A	Vitamin C	Fiber
ORANGE JUICE		●	
GRAPEFRUIT JUICE		●	
TOMATO JUICE		●	

Vegetables ½ Cup Cooked	Vitamin A	Vitamin C	Fiber	Cruciferous
ASPARAGUS		■	■	
BEANS, GREEN			■	
BOK CHOY	●	■	■	✔
BROCCOLI	■	●	■	✔
BRUSSELS SPROUTS		●	■	✔
CABBAGE		■	■	✔
CARROTS	●		■	
CAULIFLOWER		●	■	✔
CHILI PEPPERS (¼ CUP)	●	●		
CORN			■	
DRIED PEAS & BEANS			●	
EGGPLANT			■	
GREEN PEPPER		●		
GREENS[1]	●	■	■	
LETTUCE (1 CUP FRESH)				
SPINACH	●	■	■	
ROMAINE	■			
RED AND GREEN LEAF	■			
ICEBERG				
OKRA			■	
PEAS, GREEN			■	
POTATO (1 MEDIUM BAKED)		■	■	
SPINACH	●		■	
SQUASH, WINTER	●		■	
SWEET POTATO	●		■	
TOMATOES (1)	■	■	■	
ZUCCHINI			■	

■ These selections supply at least 25% of the U.S. RDA for vitamins A or C or at least 1–3 grams of dietary fiber per serving.

● These selections supply at least 50% of the U.S. RDA for vitamins A or C or at least 4 grams of dietary fiber per serving.

[1]Values are averages calculated using beet and mustard greens, swiss chard, dandelion, kale, and turnip greens. These foods are part of the cruciferous family.

(except green bananas, potatoes, and onions) because they contain enzymes that make fruits and vegetables age and lose nutrients. The enzymes are more active at warm temperatures.

3. Foods should not be kept in storage too long as they lose some vitamins. Keep frozen foods at or below 0°F and refrigerated foods below 45°F. Keep canned goods in a cool place.

4. When washing vegetables, do so quickly and do not soak them.

5. To retain vitamins when cooking vegetables, steaming and microwaving are the methods of choice. If boiling vegetables, the longer they are cooked, the higher will be the nutrient loss. Cook quickly. Stir-frying is also a good method for conserving nutrients.

6. Potatoes and other vegetables that are boiled or baked without being peeled retain many more nutrients than if peeled and cut. In general, the smaller the pieces into which you cut vegetables before cooking them, the higher the vitamin loss because leaching and oxidation are increased by having created more exposed surfaces. Vegetables and fruits should not be cut more than necessary.

7. Frying's high temperature can destroy vitamins in vegetables. For instance, french-fried potatoes lose much of their vitamin C.

8. Never use baking soda with vegetables as it will cause nutrient loss.

9. Use the cooking water from vegetables to prepare soup and gravy.

10. Don't make foods too far ahead of when they will be served.

Factors that destroy vitamins often spoil the color, flavor, and texture of food as well.

Vegetables can be cooked using many different cooking methods including (but not limited to) baking, broiling, stir-frying, grilling, and sauteing. Table 51 gives approximate cooking times. Following are guidelines for cooking and serving vegetables.

1. Cook vegetables for as short a time as possible. Do not overcook in order to retain an appropriate texture and the most nutrition, color, and flavor.

2. Steam or microwave vegetables where possible because they are the best cooking methods to retain nutrients, color, flavor, and texture.

3. Be very careful about timing when a vegetable is ready to come out of the steamer or microwave to avoid overcooking. Vegetables such as broccoli, cauliflower, brussels sprouts, and cabbage develop an unpleasant taste and smell when overcooked.

4. When boiling vegetables, start with boiling water to decrease the cooking time, cover, and cook in enough water to cover (to retain color and flavor) except for green and strong-flavored vegetables. Green vegetables actually need more water to keep their color, and strong-flavored vegetables need more water to help release their strong flavors. Also boil green and strong-flavored vegetables uncovered for the same reasons.

5. Do not add baking soda to vegetables because it causes a mushy texture and nutrient loss.

6. Reheat canned vegetables by bringing half of its liquid to a boil, then adding the vegetables and bringing to serving temperature. Canned vegetables are already cooked.

7. When microwaving vegetables, cover them.

Fruits are not cooked as frequently as vegetables, but they can be easily baked (baked apples), broiled (broiled bananas), sauteed (sauteed peaches), and simmered (applesauce).

Besides being cooked, many vegetables and fruits are used to make salads. The first step in making salads involves preparation of fresh fruits and vegetables, for example, cleaning and cutting up lettuce. Following are preparation guidelines.

1. Always prepare fruits and vegetables as close to serving time as possible to avoid drying out, discoloring, and nutrient loss.

2. For all vegetables, remove any yellow, heavily wilted, or discolored parts. For fruits, remove any bad parts. These dead or dying parts rob moisture and nutrients from the fruit or vegetable.

3. Wash fruits and vegetables thoroughly in cold running water to clean them and keep them moist and crisp.

4. Do not soak vegetables for very long, except

❖ Table 51 Timetable for Cooking Fresh Vegetables* ❖

Vegetable	Amount (serves four)	Boiling	Steaming	Microwaving**
Asparagus	1½ cups pieces	5–8 minutes	5–8 minutes	7–10 minutes
Green or wax beans (French style beans cook quickest)	2 cups whole or cut	15–25 minutes	20–25 minutes	13–15 minutes
Beets	3 cups diced	40–50 minutes (whole) 20 minutes (sliced or diced)	40–60 minutes	9–12 minutes
Broccoli	3 cups flowerets	8–12 minutes	8–12 minutes	4–7 minutes
Brussels sprouts	3 cups	10–15 minutes	15–18 minutes	4–6 minutes
Cabbage	4 cups	8–12 minutes (quartered) 3–8 minutes (shredded)	10–15 minutes (quartered)	9–11 minutes (quartered) 4–6 minutes (shredded)
Carrots	3 cups slices	10–12 minutes	12–15 minutes	8–10 minutes
Cauliflower	3 cups flowerets	8–12 minutes	10–15 minutes	7–10 minutes
Corn on the cob	1 ear	6–10 minutes	8–12 minutes	—
Peas, green	3 cups	10–14 minutes	12–15 minutes	6–8 minutes
Potatoes	3 cups diced	25–30 minutes	20–25 minutes	8–10 minutes
Spinach	1 pound torn	3–8 minutes	5–10 minutes	4–6 minutes
Squash, yellow or zucchini	2½ cups slices	5–8 minutes	6–10 minutes	4–5 minutes
Sweet potatoes	3 cups diced or quartered	15–25 minutes	20–30 minutes	10–13 minutes
Turnips	2½ cups diced or sliced	12–15 minutes	15–20 minutes	12–14 minutes

*Cooking times are for crisp-tender vegetables.
**When microwaving, place vegetable in microwave dish with 2 tablespoons water and cook at high power (100%). Rearrange or stir once during cooking.

for broccoli, brussels sprouts, cauliflower, and cabbage, which may be soaked for a half hour in cold water. Soaking vegetables robs them of nutrients, but may be used with these vegetables to help remove insects.

5. When cleaning leafy greens, soak briefly several times in clean water to remove sediment.
6. Wash iceberg lettuce by removing the core and running water into this area. Turn over to drain.
7. After washing leafy greens, drain well and store in a container that allows air circulation and drainage. Good air circulation is necessary to maintain crispness and drainage to prevent sogginess.
8. Peel vegetables as thinly as possible to pre-

serve nutrients which are located mostly under the skin.
9. Cut fruits and vegetables with a stainless steel knife to prevent browning of the produce, or tear with your hands. Carbon-steel bladed knives cause lettuce to brown.
10. Cut fruits and vegetables into uniform, identifiable pieces for eye appeal.
11. After cutting raw vegetables, put in ice water until used.
12. Treat vegetables which discolor with an acid such as lemon juice, or keep in water.
13. Treat fruits which discolor, such as apples, pears, peaches, and bananas, by rinsing them briefly in orange juice or lemon juice (mix 3 parts water with 1 part citrus juice).

14. Blanch vegetables by boiling or steaming briefly. Blanching is done to help vegetables keep their color and maintain freshness when, for instance, you are preparing a platter containing raw vegetables.

RECIPES

WALDORF SALAD

1 large red apple, cored and diced, but not peeled
½ cup diced celery
1 tbsp raisins
1 tsp chopped nuts
reduced calorie (or no-fat) mayonnaise

1. Combine the apple, celery, raisins, and nuts.
2. Add enough mayonnaise to hold ingredients together.
3. Serve on a bed of salad greens.

Serves 2

Nutrition Analysis:
Calories 87
Carbohydrate. . . . . .16 grams
Fiber . . . . .2 grams
Fat. . . . . .3 grams
Cholesterol. . . . . .3 milligrams
Sodium . . . . .27 milligrams

CARROT-APPLE SAUTE

3 cups diagonally sliced carrot (about 1 lb)
1 tbsp margarine or oil
⅓ cup finely chopped onion
1 large Granny Smith apple, peeled and thinly sliced
⅓ cup unsweetened apple juice
1½ tsp sugar
1 tsp lemon juice
¼ tsp salt
dash of allspice

1. Boil carrots 6 minutes or until tender; drain and set aside.
2. Melt margarine in a large skillet over medium heat. Add onion; saute 3 minutes. Add apple; saute 4 minutes. Add carrot back in along with apple juice and remaining ingredients.
3. Cover, reduce heat, and simmer 3 minutes. Serve warm.

Serves 8

Nutrition Analysis:
Calories 58
Carbohydrate. . . . . .11 grams
Fiber . . . . .3 grams
Fat. . . . . .2 grams
Cholesterol. . . . . .0 milligrams
Sodium . . . . .127 milligrams

CREAMED POTATOES

1 potato, peeled and diced
½ cup water
1 tbsp butter-flavor granules
1 tbsp onion powder
1 tsp chicken bouillon granules
½ to 1 cup skimmed evaporated milk
⅛ tsp white pepper

1. In small saucepan, combine potato and water. Bring to a boil, then cover and simmer until potato is tender, about 10 minutes.
2. Using a mixer, blend potatoes until smooth. Stir in ½ cup milk along with the remaining seasonings, blending until smooth and adding additional milk to reach a cream sauce consistency.

Makes 4½ cup servings

Suggestion: Use as a base for creamy soups, casseroles, and scalloped potato dishes.

Nutrition Analysis:
Calories 91
Carbohydrate. . . . . .15 grams

Fiber . . . . .0 grams
Fat. . . . . .1 gram
Cholesterol. . . . . .3 milligrams
Sodium. . . . . .734 milligrams

POTATO SUPREME

1½ cups fresh broccoli flowerets
½ cup sliced fresh mushrooms
¼ cup sliced green onion
¼ cup chopped sweet red pepper
1 cup diced fully cooked turkey ham
4 large potatoes, baked
½ cup nonfat plain yogurt
¼ cup skim milk
2 tsp cornstarch
1 tsp Dijon-style mustard
dash ground nutmeg
2 tbsp grated Parmesan cheese

1. In a 1-quart microwave-safe casserole, combine broccoli, mushrooms, green onion, red pepper, and 2 tablespoons water.
2. Microwave covered on 100% power (high) 3 to 5 minutes or until vegetables are tender. Drain well.

3. Add turkey ham. Cook, covered, on high 2 to 3 minutes or until heated through.
4. Stir together yogurt, milk, cornstarch, mustard, and nutmeg. Add to broccoli mixture. Cook covered on high 2 to 4 minutes or until mixture is thickened, stirring every 30 seconds. Spoon over hot baked potatoes. Sprinkle with Parmesan cheese.

Serves 4

Nutrition Analysis:
Calories 244
Carbohydrate. . . . . .41 grams
Fiber . . . . .5 grams
Fat. . . . . .3 grams
Cholesterol. . . . . .221 milligrams
Sodium. . . . . .460 milligrams

GREEN BEANS WITH MUSHROOMS

1 9-oz package frozen cut green beans
1 green onion, finely chopped, or 1 tbsp shallots, finely chopped
¼ lb mushrooms, cleaned and sliced
1 tsp lemon juice
1 tsp paprika
1 tsp flour

1. Cook green beans according to directions on package. Drain and place in a serving dish. Keep hot.
2. Meanwhile saute shallots or green onions in nonstick pan coated with vegetable spray until tender. Add sliced mushrooms and lemon juice. Cook, stirring constantly until mushrooms are tender.

3. Combine paprika and flour. Sprinkle over mushrooms and cook, stirring 1 minute. Add mushrooms to green beans in serving dish and toss lightly to mix.

Serves 4

Nutrition Analysis:
Calories 25
Carbohydrate. . . . . .6 grams
Fiber . . . . .1 gram
Fat. . . . . .0 grams
Cholesterol. . . . . .0 milligrams
Sodium. . . . . .10 milligrams

LEMON PEPPER MUSHROOMS

8 large mushrooms
1 tbsp chopped chives
2 tbsp lemon juice
1 tbsp reduced-calorie mayonnaise
1½ tsp lemon pepper

1. Select large firm mushrooms and wipe with a damp cloth. Remove stems, discard lower half, and chop upper half of the stems very fine, and in a bowl combine with the remaining ingredients.
2. Stuff mushrooms with the mixture. Bake in a shallow pan 8 to 10 minutes at 450°F. Serve immediately.

Makes 8 stuffed mushrooms

Nutrition Analysis:
Calories 17
Carbohydrate. . . . . .3 grams
Fiber . . . . .0 grams
Fat. . . . . .1 gram
Cholesterol. . . . . .1 milligram
Sodium . . . . .0 milligrams

GRAPE AND SPINACH SALAD

1 lb spinach
1 cup seedless grapes
1 apple, diced
1 tbsp dry roasted peanuts
2 tbsp chopped green onions
1 tbsp toasted sesame seeds
⅓ cup reduced-calorie Italian dressing

1. Wash and tear spinach into bite-size pieces.
2. Toss with grapes, apple, peanuts, green onion, and sesame seeds.
3. Toss with dressing to coat well.

Serves 6

Nutrition Analysis:
Calories 65
Carbohydrate. . . . . .10 grams
Fiber . . . . .1 gram
Fat. . . . . .3 grams
Cholesterol. . . . . .1 milligram
Sodium . . . . .140 milligrams

STUFFED BAKED POTATO

4 baking potatoes
½ cup lowfat cottage cheese
3 tbsp skim milk
1 tsp dried chopped chives
⅛ tsp pepper
paprika

1. Preheat oven to 425°F.
2. Wash and dry potatoes. Prick skins with a fork. Bake potatoes until tender—50 to 60 minutes. (Potatoes may be baked in a microwave oven—use the directions that came with your oven.)
3. Beat cottage cheese until smooth.
4. Slice potatoes in half; scoop out insides of potatoes and add to cottage cheese. Add milk and seasonings; beat until well blended. Fill potato halves.

Serves 4

Nutrition Analysis:
Calories 174
Carbohydrate. . . . . .35 grams
Fiber . . . . .4 grams
Fat. . . . . .1 gram
Cholesterol. . . . . .3 milligrams
Sodium . . . . .128 milligrams

Marinated Garden Vegetable Salad

⅓ cup vinegar
2 tsp oil
⅛ tsp garlic powder
pinch of pepper
½ large cucumber, cubed
2 small tomatoes, cubed
1 green pepper, sliced
⅛ small cabbage, shredded
2 small carrots, thinly sliced
12 radishes, thinly sliced
½ onion, chopped

1. Mix vinegar, oil, garlic powder, and pepper in a large bowl.
2. Add vegetables and mix well.
3. Refrigerate covered several hours or overnight to marinate. Will keep several days.

Serves 8

Variations: Chopped raw broccoli or cauliflower, diced celery, sliced zucchini, and chick-peas or other beans may be added. Fresh or dried dill weed or other herbs may also be added.

Nutrition Analysis:

Calories 38
Carbohydrate. . . . . .6 grams
Fiber . . . . .2 grams
Fat. . . . . .1 grams
Cholesterol. . . . . .0 milligram
Sodium. . . . . .13 milligrams

Sweet Potatoes with Pineapple

½ tbsp margarine
2 cups sweet potatoes, fresh, cooked, sliced (or canned)
8-oz can crushed pineapple in natural juice
¼ tsp ground cinnamon
⅛ tsp salt

1. Heat margarine in large frying pan. Add potato slices and pineapple. Sprinkle with cinnamon and salt.
2. Simmer, uncovered, until most of the juice has evaporated, about 10 to 15 minutes. Turn potato slices several times.

Serves 4

Nutrition Analysis:

Calories 141
Carbohydrate. . . . . .31 grams
Fiber . . . . .3 grams
Fat. . . . . .2 grams
Cholesterol. . . . . .0 milligrams
Sodium. . . . . .135 milligrams

Squash-Broccoli Medley

½ cup fresh mushrooms, sliced
1 tbsp margarine
1 cup fresh broccoli, cut in 1-inch pieces
1 cup yellow summer squash, sliced
¼ tsp salt
⅛ tsp pepper
½ cup water
½ tsp lemon rind, grated

1. Cook mushrooms in margarine in nonstick frying pan until lightly browned.
2. Add remaining ingredients except lemon rind.
3. Cover and boil gently until vegetables are tender, about 10 minutes. Drain.
4. Gently stir in lemon rind.

Serves 4

Nutrition Analysis:
    Calories 43
    Carbohydrate. . . . . .4 grams
    Fiber . . . . .1 gram

Fat. . . . . .3 grams
Cholesterol. . . . . .0 milligrams
Sodium. . . . . .173 milligrams

VEGETABLE-STUFFED TOMATOES

4 medium tomatoes
½ cup fresh green beans, ½-inch pieces
½ cup frozen whole kernel corn
½ cup boiling water
½ cup zucchini squash, diced
¼ cup celery, thinly sliced
2 green onions, sliced
¼ tsp salt
⅓ cup low-fat or nonfat salad dressing (such as
    French)
salad greens (as desired)

1. Cut a thin slice from top of each tomato.
   Remove cores. Scoop out as much pulp as
   possible without breaking tomato shells. Save
   firm red portion of pulp; dice and drain.
2. Drain shells. Chill until ready to fill.
3. Add beans and corn to boiling water. Cover and
   boil gently until beans are tender, about 15
   minutes. Drain.

4. Lightly mix cooked vegetables, diced tomato
   pulp, squash, celery, onions, and salt with
   dressing.
5. Chill at least 1 hour.
6. Fill chilled tomato shells with vegetable mixture.
7. Serve on crisp salad greens.

Note: For a quick and easy version, use 1½ cups
cooked unsalted frozen mixed vegetables in place
of corn, beans, and squash.

Serves 4

Nutrition Analysis:
    Calories 78
    Carbohydrate. . . . . .16 grams
    Fiber . . . . .3 grams
    Fat. . . . . .2 grams
    Cholesterol. . . . . .1 milligram
    Sodium. . . . . .315 milligrams

WINTER FRUIT CUP

½ cup grapes, halved, seeded
½ cup tangerine, sectioned
½ cup apple, unpeeled, diced
½ cup pear, unpeeled, diced
½ cup sliced banana
2 tbsp frozen orange juice concentrate, thawed

1. Mix fruit with orange juice concentrate to coat
   all pieces.
2. Serve immediately.

Serves 4

Nutrition Analysis:
    Calories 92
    Carbohydrate. . . . . .23 grams
    Fiber . . . . .2 grams
    Fat. . . . . .0 grams
    Cholesterol. . . . . .0 milligrams
    Sodium. . . . . .3 milligrams

THREE BEAN SALAD

9- or 10-oz package frozen green beans
9- or 10-oz package frozen wax beans
14 oz can kidney beans, drained
½ cup onion, diced
⅓ cup vinegar
2 tbsp vegetable oil
¼ tsp salt
⅛ tsp pepper

1. Boil, steam, or microwave green beans and wax beans until crisp and tender.
2. Combine green beans, wax beans, and kidney beans.
3. Combine onion, vinegar, oil, salt, and pepper. Pour over beans.
4. Cool and chill.

Serves 8

Nutrition Analysis:

Calories 88
Carbohydrate . . . . .12 grams
Fiber . . . . .3 grams
Fat . . . . .4 grams
Cholesterol . . . . .0 milligrams
Sodium . . . . .221 milligrams

❖ ❖ ❖

CHAPTER THIRTEEN

BREADS, CEREALS, AND PASTA

BREADS

There have been more and more types of bread appearing at the supermarket—mixed grain, oatmeal, potato, pita, and high-fiber bread, in addition to the traditional selection of white, whole wheat, rye, pumpernickel, French, Italian, and raisin bread. Bread is a staple food that is purchased and eaten frequently.

Purchasing

The most popular bread sold in the United States is **white bread**, also known as **wheat bread**. Wheat bread does not mean whole wheat, as some manufacturers might want you to think. Color is not a good indication of whole wheat bread because coloring is sometimes added to white bread to make it look more like whole wheat. Look for **whole wheat bread** and check that whole wheat flour is the first ingredient listed on the label.

Rye bread uses rye flour and wheat flour because rye flour by itself produces a very heavy, compact loaf of bread. **Pumpernickel bread** is a dark, coarse-textured, rye loaf prepared by a sour-dough process.

So-called **diet breads**, which often contain about 40 calories per slice, still contain about the same amount of fat as regular breads, but have less starch. In some cases, the manufacturer has used fiber, which has no calories, to replace the starch in the product.

Whichever style of bread best meets your needs, be sure to check the date found on the package. Breads almost always have a "sell by" date, which is the last date the bread is considered

fresh enough to be sold, and it still has several more days of storage at home before it starts to stale. In addition to checking the sell by date, it's a good idea to feel the loaf of bread. Soft-crusted breads should feel soft and spongy. Hard-crusted breads (French or Italian) should have a crisp, firm crust.

Nutrition

The nutritional content of breads appears in Table 52. Breads are about 38–45 percent starch by weight and 38 percent water. Breads are:

- An excellent source of complex carbohydrates
- A good source of fiber (if made from whole grains)
- A good source of B vitamins and iron (and even more vitamins and minerals if made from whole grains)
- Low in fat
- Cholesterol free (unless eggs are used, such as in brioche)
- Moderate in sodium content

The milling of the whole wheat kernel removes the bran and germ and produces white flour (which is mostly starch) that is used to make white bread. Because white flour, also called wheat flour, contains significantly fewer nutrients than whole wheat flour, it must (in most cases) be **enriched**, meaning that the following four nutrients are added back into the flour: thiamin, riboflavin, niacin, and iron.

Unfortunately, enrichment does not replace the fiber removed in the milling, and it only re-

❖ *Table 52* *Nutritive Value of Selected Bread Products* ❖

	Enriched White	Whole Wheat	Pumper- nickel	Pita	Reduced Calorie	Burger Bun	English Muffin	Bagel, Plain
Serving size	1 slice	1 slice	1 slice	1	1 slice	1	1	1
Calories (kcal)	67	69	82	105	40	114	133	163
Protein (g)	2	3	3	4	2	3	4	6
Carbohydrate (g)	12	13	15	21	6	20	26	31
Fat (g)	1	1	1	0.5	1	2	1	1
Total Dietary Fiber (g)	0.6	3	2	0.6	2	1	1	1
Sodium (mg)	129	178	173	215	110	241	358	198
Cholesterol (mg)	0	0	0	0	0	0	0	0

places four nutrients out of the 20 that were re-moved. Whole wheat flour (particularly if stone-ground) retains most of the original nutrients and has more fiber, vitamin B6, folacin, magnesium, and zinc than enriched white flour. Examples of whole grain breads are as follows:

- 100% whole wheat
- Stone-ground whole wheat
- Cracked wheat bread
- Multi-grain bread
- Rye bread (dark)
- Whole wheat pita bread
- Corn tortilla
- Oatmeal bread
- Whole wheat English muffins
- Whole wheat bagels

As you can see from the comparison below, most breads and bread products contain only small amounts of fat, with less than 2 grams per slice or serving, that is, if you don't spread marga-rine or mayonnaise on them! It was thought for some time that bread (at about 60 calories per slice) was fattening, when in reality, the spread (at 100 calories per tablespoon fat) was the culprit.

Some breads and bread products are made with several times the amount of fat (3–6 grams) that is found in most sliced breads. These products include biscuits, brioche, cheese bread, corn-bread, crescent rolls or croissants, and popovers. Brioche is a rich, delicate roll made with a high proportion of butter and eggs.

Storing

Soft-crusted breads actually last longer at room temperature than if put into the refrigerator (ex-cept for soft tortillas, which should be refriger-ated). Keep bread tightly sealed so it stays moist and fresh longer. If you need to keep bread for more than four or five days, wrap it air-tight (in a double thickness of foil or two plastic bags) and freeze it, where it will last up to 4 months. Frozen bread slices thaw in minutes at room temperature (leave it wrapped) and the quality is still good (unless your freezer is not doing a good job).

Hard-crusted bread is a completely different

Breads Made with Little Fat			*Higher-in-Fat Breads*
Bagel	Hot dog roll	Roman meal bread	Biscuit
Bread sticks	Italian bread	Rye bread	Brioche
Cracked wheat bread	Kaiser roll	Tortilla, corn	Cheese bread
Dinner/pan roll	Oatmeal bread	Tortilla, flour	Cornbread
English muffin	Pita pocket	Wheat bread	Crescent roll or
French bread	Pumpernickel bread	White bread	croissant
French roll	Raisin bread	Whole wheat bread	Popover
Hamburger roll	Rice cakes		

story. After one day it will become quite hard, yet if you put it into a plastic bag, the crust will become very soft and chewy. The best choice is to store it wrapped loosely in paper, preferably in a bread box, and then use it up within two days. On the second day, heat it covered in the oven for ten minutes and eat right away for best quality.

CEREALS

Cereals are made from grains, the most popular being wheat, corn, oats, and rice. Ready-to-eat cereals are made by grounding the grain into a paste, forming it into desired shapes, and toasting it to make flakes, puffs, and other familiar forms.

Purchasing

There is a huge variety of cereals on the market and sometimes choosing one is confusing. Ready-to-eat cereals come in many different forms: whole grain, refined grain, sweetened, unsweetened, plain, with fruits and nuts, flaked, or puffed. Some cereals are actually multivitamin/mineral supplements as they supply 100 percent of the RDA of various vitamins and minerals! Hot cereals come in regular, quick-cooking, and instant (just mix with boiling water) varieties. With so many choices, many consumers base their choice of cereals on nutritional considerations, such as the amount of sugar or fiber in the cereal. These are discussed in a moment.

When purchasing cereals, always look for a "use by" date on cereal boxes.

Nutrition

Table 53 takes a look at several different cereals. In general, cereals are:

- Low in calories
- High in complex carbohydrates
- Good sources of fiber (if made with whole grains or bran)
- Low in fat (except for granolas, which often contain a significant amount of fat)
- A moderate source of protein
- Full of vitamins and minerals

Most ready-to-eat cereals are fortified with at least 25 percent of the U.S. Recommended Daily Allowance for seven vitamins and iron. Other minerals may be added at lower levels.

Cereals vary in the amount of fiber, sugar, and sodium they contain, so let's look at how to choose cereals high in fiber and low in sugar and sodium.

Many grains used in making cereals have had their outer layer, referred to as the bran, removed before being made into cereals. The bran contains much fiber. Unfortunately, cereals made with refined grains contain little fiber. For example, Rice Krispies, which is made from refined rice, only contains 0.3 grams of fiber per 1-cup serving.

On the other hand, cereals made with whole grains contain the fiber-rich bran that can contribute significantly to the total fiber you eat. Examples of whole grains to look for on cereal labels include whole wheat, whole rye, and oatmeal.

❖ **Table 53 Nutritive Value of Breakfast Cereals (without milk; serving, 1 oz)** ❖

	Shredded Wheat Biscuits	Whole Wheat Flakes	Bran Flakes	Oatmeal, Uncooked	Corn Flakes	Toasted Oat O's	Sweetened Puffed Wheat
Calories (kcal)	100	99	92	109	110	111	103
Protein (g)	3	3	4	5	2	4	4
Total Carbohydrate (g)	23	23	22	19	24	20	23
Sucrose/Other Sugars	0	2	4	NA	2	1	14
Total Dietary Fiber	3	2	4	2	1	1	2
Fat (g)	Trace	Trace	Trace	2	Trace	2	Trace
Sodium (mg)	1	270	220	1	290	290	1

Oats differ from all other cereals in that the bran is not separated from the kernel during milling. Oats are flattened between heated rollers to produce rolled oats, or cut and rolled until quite thin to produce quick-cooking oats. Instant oats are precooked. Oat flour is used in some cereals such as Cheerios, originally called Cheeri-Oats.

Some examples of whole grain cereals include:

* Oatmeal and other whole grain types (see Chapter 11 for more information on whole grains; most can be cooked into a delightful hot breakfast cereal)
* Shredded wheat
* Whole grain wheat, oat, and rice flakes
* Whole grain puffed wheat, rice, and corn

Also, check on the label for the exact amount of fiber your cereal contains per serving. Remember that the recommended daily intake of dietary fiber is 20–35 grams, so try to select a cereal with at least 4 grams of fiber per serving. Table 54 compares the fiber content of different cereals.

There is also information available on most cereal boxes that tells you their **sugar** content. If you look at the label where it lists "Sucrose and Other Sugars," for every 4 grams listed, the cereal contains 1 teaspoon of sugar. Total sugar in cereal can range from less than 1 percent to more than 55 percent of the cereal by weight. Try to choose a cereal with 5 grams of sugar or less. Instead of buying presweetened cereals, make cereal naturally sweet with fresh fruit or raisins.

The amount of **sodium** varies tremendously in cereals. For instance, shredded wheat cereals contain almost no sodium, yet 1 ounce of rice crinkle-type cereal contains 340 milligrams. Read your labels well if you are watching for sodium. Among hot cereals, regular and quick-cooking types are much lower in sodium than instant cereals in individual serving packets, especially if you omit salt during cooking (it's not necessary).

A final nutritional concern is the use of the preservatives BHA and BHT in some brands of cereal. BHA and BHT may increase your risk of cancer. Luckily, they don't appear in many of the whole grain cereals. Check the label.

See the summary of cereal buying tips for more information.

❖ **Table 54   Comparison of Fiber** ❖
in Cereals

Cereal	Serving Size	Grams Fiber/ Serving
All Bran, Kelloggs	⅓ cup	8.6
All Bran with Extra Fiber, Kelloggs	½ cup	13.8
Cheerios, General Mills	1¼ cup	2.5
Cornflakes, Kelloggs	1 cup	0.5
Cream of Wheat, uncooked	2½ tablespoons	1.1
Fiber One, General Mills	½ cup	11.9
40% Bran Flakes	⅔ cup	4.3
Grapenuts, Post	¼ cup	2.8
Grits, corn, quick, uncooked	3 tablespoons	0.6
Heartwise, Kelloggs	1 cup	5.7
Nutri-Grain Wheat, Kelloggs	⅔ cup	2.7
Oat Bran, cooked, Quaker	¾ cup	4.0
Oat Bran Cereal (cold), Quaker	¾ cup	2.9
Oat Flakes, Post	⅔ cup	2.1
Oatmeal, uncooked, Quaker	⅓ cup	2.7
Product 19, Kelloggs	1 cup	1.2
Puffed Rice	1 cup	0.2
Puffed Wheat	1 cup	1.0
Quaker Oat Squares	½ cup	2.2
Raisin Bran	¾ cup	5.3
Rice Krispies, Kelloggs	1 cup	0.3
Shredded Wheat	⅔ cup	3.5
Shredded Wheat and Bran, Kelloggs	⅔ cup	2.5
Special K, Kelloggs	1 cup	0.9
Wheat Flakes	¾ cup	2.3
Wheaties, General Mills	⅔ cup	2.3

Storing

Cereals can be stored, unopened, up to one year in a cool, dry place. To keep cereal fresh once opened, fold the inner lining of the box. Opened cereal can stay fresh for two months or by "Use by" date.

Whole grain cereals, because they contain fat, turn rancid or bad more quickly than refined cereals. When the fat becomes rancid, it has an undesirable flavor and odor. To prevent this problem,

CEREAL BUYING TIPS

1. Choose whole grains such as:
   - Oatmeal
   - Shredded wheat
   - Whole grain wheat, oat, and rice flakes
   - Whole grain puffed wheat, rice, and corn
2. Select a cereal with at least 4 grams of fiber per 1 ounce serving.

3. Choose a cereal with 5 grams or less of sugar per 1 ounce serving.
4. If sodium is an important consideration, check the label. Remember that the recommended daily intake of sodium is 2400 milligrams.
5. Avoid granolas with more than 5 grams of fat per 1 ounce serving.
6. Avoid the preservatives BHA and BHT.

store whole grain cereals in air-tight containers and away from heat.

PASTAS

Pasta, from the Italian word for paste, is an edible paste or dough made from wheat flour and water that is rolled and cut into one of over 150 pasta shapes found in the United States (see accompanying illustrations for examples). Pasta has been eaten for over 5,000 years and is very closely associated with Italian cooking. Thanks to the influence of Italian cooks, Americans are eating more pasta than ever before.

Purchasing

Dried pasta includes both **macaroni and noodles**. Macaroni products are pastas made from flour and water. These include spaghetti, elbow macaroni, lasagne, ziti, and other shapes. Noodles, by law, are also made from flour and water, but must contain 5.5 percent egg solids. Noodles are usually flat, like a ribbon, and come in different widths. The three most popular pasta products are spaghetti, macaroni, and noodles.

Semolina is preferred for making dried pasta. Semolina is the roughly milled endosperm of a type of wheat called durum wheat. Durum wheat is known as a very "hard" wheat, meaning that it has a high protein content. Semolina is used almost exclusively for making pasta. Less expensive pasta products are made from a softer flour. High-

quality pasta should be yellow in color, brittle, and hold its shape well when cooked. Poor quality pasta is often a whitish-gray color and when it is cooked, it becomes soft and loses its shape.

In addition to dried pasta, **fresh pasta** is also available. Fresh pasta is made of flour and eggs, and sometimes water or oil. Fresh pasta has not been dried.

It is possible to purchase **whole wheat pasta** in a variety of shapes such as spaghetti and macaroni. Whole wheat pasta uses whole wheat flour or whole wheat durum flour as the sole wheat ingredient. Additional flours may not be used. Since whole wheat pasta is prepared from the whole grain, it contains more fiber and minerals, such as iron and zinc, than pasta made from refined flours.

It is also possible to buy **flavored pastas** (either dried or fresh) containing fresh, canned, dried, or puree of vegetables (the amount of vegetables used is quite small) such as red tomato, artichoke, beet, carrot, or spinach. They are very colorful products and the vegetables used add a subtle flavor and some additional nutrients (although they cost more!). Some pastas are flavored with herbs and seasonings such as basil or dill.

There are also **high-protein pastas** on the market that contain about double the amount of protein of regular pasta because manufacturers add protein-rich ingredients such as wheat germ or yeast.

Types of pasta

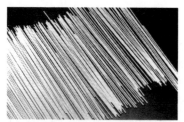

Spaghetti, Thin Spaghetti
(Spaghettini)

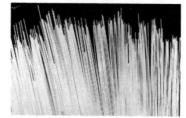

Vermicelli

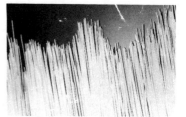

**Angel Hair, Cappellini,
Capelli Di Angelo**

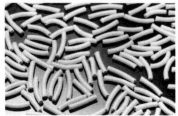

Ziti

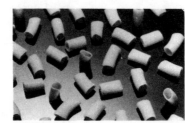

Rigatoni

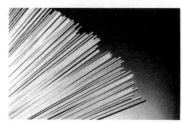

Linguine

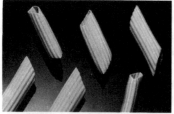

Manicotti

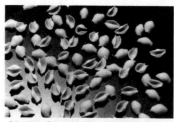

Shells, Seashells, Conchiglie
(Kon-KEEL-yeh)

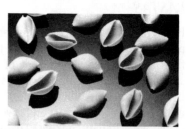

Jumbo Shells, Conchiglioni
(Kon-KEEL-yoni)

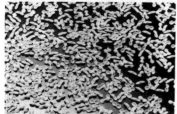

Bowties, Farfalle *(Far-FAH-leh)*
Larger size not shown

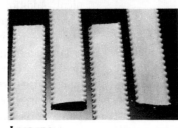

Lasagne

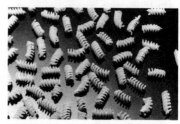

**Rotelle, Rotini, Spirals, Twirls,
Twists**

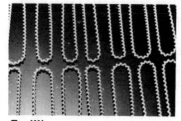

Fusilli

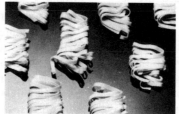

Fettuccine

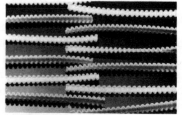

Mafalda

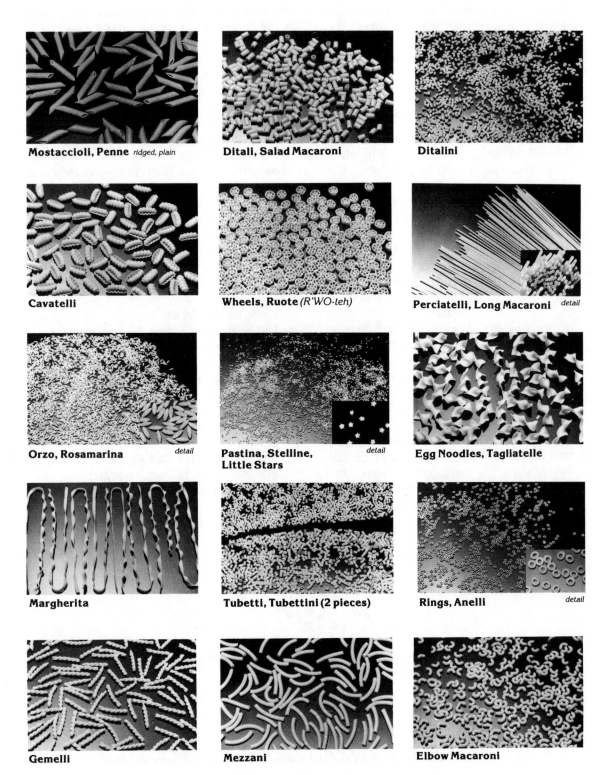

Mostaccioli, Penne *ridged, plain*

Ditali, Salad Macaroni

Ditalini

Cavatelli

Wheels, Ruote *(R'WO-teh)*

Perciatelli, Long Macaroni *detail*

Orzo, Rosamarina *detail*

Pastina, Stelline, Little Stars *detail*

Egg Noodles, Tagliatelle

Margherita

Tubetti, Tubettini (2 pieces)

Rings, Anelli *detail*

Gemelli

Mezzani

Elbow Macaroni

Asian noodles such as bean thread are also excellent in main dishes and side dishes. They can often be found in the Oriental section of the supermarket. Three basic Asian noodles are described below.

Name	Description/Uses
Bean thread (cellophane noodle, glass noodle, transparent noodle)	Clear, gelatinous noodles that work well in salads and soups. When sauteed they are a good accompaniment for poultry and seafood.
Wheat noodle	Available dried, fresh, and precooked. Can be eaten hot in soups, hot in stir-fry dishes, or cold in salads.
Rice vermicelli	Available thin and thick. Chewy noodles that add texture to soups and salads. Excellent side dish with grilled meats and seafood.

Allow 2 ounces of dried uncooked pasta per person for side dishes. This yields 1 to 1½ cups of cooked pasta. For a main course, allow 3 to 4 ounces of uncooked pasta per person. Eight ounces of spaghetti yield 4–5 cups of cooked spa-ghetti, 8 ounces of elbow macaroni yield 4½ cups, and 8 ounces of egg noodles yield 4 cups.

Nutrition

Cooked pasta is essentially starch, protein, and water (see the illustration) and is a good source of complex carbohydrates. Cooked pasta also supplies fiber, although whole wheat pasta supplies more than pasta made with wheat flour. With the exception of egg noodles, pasta is a low-fat, cholesterol-free food. Even egg noodles are low in fat (2 to 3 grams per serving). Pasta is also virtually free of sodium. The calories found in a serving of pasta are moderate—about 200 calories for one cup. Pasta made from refined wheat is often enriched with several B vitamins and iron.

Table 55 lists the nutrient content of cooked pasta. To summarize, cooked pasta is:

- moderate in calories
- low in fat (about 1 gram per cup except for egg pasta, which still has only 2 to 3 grams per cup)
- moderate in protein (about 8 grams per cup)
- cholesterol-free (except for pastas with egg, although the amount of cholesterol is probably not significant unless you are following a restricted diet)
- high in complex carbohydrates (about 42 grams of starch per cup, no sugar)
- low in sodium (less than 10 milligrams per cup)

Composition of pasta

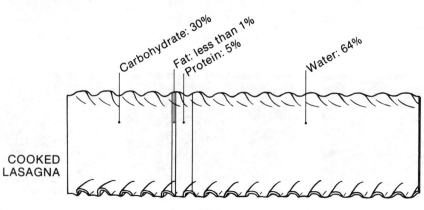

Carbohydrate: 30% Fat: less than 1% Protein: 5% Water: 64%

COOKED LASAGNA

❖ Table 55 Nutritive Value ❖
of Cooked Pasta—1 Cup Serving

	Macaroni	Spaghetti	Egg Noodles
Calories	183	190	200
Protein (g)	6	7	7
Carbohydrate (g)	37	39	37
Fiber (g)	2	2	4
Fat (g)	1	1	2
Cholesterol (mg)	0	0	50
Sodium (g)	1	1	3

Storing

Dry pasta can be stored in its own packaging at room temperature for one to two months. Better yet, store it in a tightly sealed container in a cool, dry, dark place, where it can keep for up to 12 months (except for egg noodles—they can keep up to 6 months). Fresh pasta is, in comparison, very fragile and can be stored for only two to three days in the refrigerator (or up to 1 month in the freezer). Once cooked, pasta can be held in the refrigerator for 1 to 2 days and reheated quickly in boiling water or microwaved (add water to it).

Cooking Light and Healthy

What makes pasta high calorie is when rich sauces, high-fat cheeses, too much meat, fatty sausage, or cream are used with them. Some healthier suggestions are listed here (see the recipes that follow).

- Try marinara sauce (a spicy tomato sauce) on pasta and top it with one tablespoon Parmesan cheese.
- Make your own light tomato sauce (see recipe on page 242).
- Make a sauce from a small amount of olive oil tossed with fresh vegetables such as tomatoes.
- Substitute evaporated skim milk in pasta recipes that call for cream.
- Pasta doesn't have to be served just with a sauce—dress up pasta dishes with chopped, julienned, and sliced vegetables of different textures and colors. Or add sliced mushrooms and broccoli flowerettes to your favorite tomato sauce.

- Substitute low-fat cheeses for the regular versions (see Chapter 10).

You can also cut down on calories, fat, and cholesterol in baked pasta recipes by omitting meat and using vegetables instead. Healthy revisions include zucchini lasagne, spinach-stuffed rigatoni, or broccoli and low-fat cheese stuffed shells.

For pasta salads, try low- or no-fat salad dressings or mayonnaise; or substitute plain low-fat yogurt or light sour cream in place of regular sour cream. Use plenty of vegetables.

Table 56 describes the uses of different pasta shapes. Each shape is more appropriate for certain types of dishes.

- Elbow macaroni is good in salads and soups because it retains its shape.
- Tube pastas (such as elbow macaroni) or pastas with a hollow space, such as shells, are great with meat or vegetable sauces as they trap the sauce in their hollow spaces.
- Fresh pasta, because it is softer in texture and absorbs sauce more readily than dried, is better with a smooth, light sauce that coats the pasta evenly.
- Flat noodles are also better with smooth, light sauces.
- Delicate pasta should be served with delicate sauces. Hearty pasta should be served with hearty sauces.

Dried pasta should be cooked in a generous amount of boiling water; follow the cooking directions below.

1. Bring the water to a rolling boil. Allow 3 quarts of water for 8 ounces of pasta and 4 quarts of water for 1 pound of pasta.
2. Add the pasta in batches over the course of one minute, stirring after each addition. This helps the water come to a boil again quickly. Stirring keeps the pasta from sticking together.
3. Cook the pasta until it is tender but not soft.
4. Drain immediately and serve.

The addition of salt to the cooking water for flavor is optional. Its purpose is only to add flavor,

❖ Table 56 Pasta Shapes and Uses ❖

Name	Description	Suggested Uses
Spaghetti	Long, round	With great variety of sauces, especially tomato sauces
Spaghettini	Thin, long, round	Like spaghetti, especially with olive-oil-and-seafood sauces
Vermicelli	Very thin	With light, delicate sauces and, broken, in soups
Linguine	Looks like slightly flattened spaghetti	Like spaghetti; popular with clam sauces
Fusilli	Long, shaped like a corkscrew	Thick, creamy sauces
Macaroni	Long, hollow, round tubes	Especially good with hearty meat sauces
Elbow macaroni	Short, bent macaroni	Cold, in salads; baked, in casseroles
Penne or mostaccioli	Hollow tubes, cut diagonally; may be smooth or ridged	Baked, with meat sauce or with tomato sauce and cheese; or freshly cooked, with tomato sauce
Ziti	Short, hollow tubes, cut straight	
Rigatoni	Larger tubes, with ridges	
Manicotti	Large hollow tubes, sometimes with ridges (sometimes called cannelloni, which are actually rolled from fresh egg noodle dough)	Stuff with cheese or meat filling
Fettuccine	Flat egg noodles	Rich cream sauces or meat sauces
Lasagne	Broad, flat noodles, often with rippled edges	Bake with meat, cheese, or vegetable fillings
Conchiglie	Shell shaped	With seafood or meat sauces; small sizes can be used in salads
Bow ties		With sauces containing chunks of meat, sausage, or vegetables
Pastina (little pasta)		
Ditalini	Very short, hollow tubes	In soups; cold, in salads; buttered, as a side dish
Orzo	Rice shaped	
Stelline	Tiny stars	
Acini	"Peppercorns"	

Source: *Professional Cooking* by Wayne Gisslen. Copyright © 1989, John Wiley & Sons, Inc. Reprinted by permission of John Wiley & Sons, Inc.

which can be accomplished just as easily by adding herbs and spices or a little lemon or lime juice directly to pasta's cooking water. Also, don't add oil to the boiling water to prevent sticking; simply use plenty of water—4 to 6 quarts for 1 pound of pasta.

As soon as the pasta is cooked to al dente, or firm to the bite, it should be drained. Fresh pasta cooks in 1 to 5 minutes once the water has returned to a boil, and dried pasta takes longer, at least 5 minutes or more depending on its size, shape, and ingredients. Pasta that is to be cooked further in a casserole, such as lasagne, should be

undercooked slightly so it does not become mushy during further cooking.

Cooked pasta should not be rinsed with cold water unless it is going to be used in a cold dish, such as salad, or is going to be served at a later time. If the pasta is going to be served later, toss it with a small amount of oil to prevent it from sticking together. Never store pasta in cold or hot water as it will become overcooked and mushy.

If you want to make your own pasta, use the following recipe to make enough fettuccine noodles for four, with some left over for freezing.

RECIPES

FETTUCINE NOODLES

3 cups flour (unbleached, if possible)
3 eggs, at room temperature
½ tsp salt (optional)
warm water

1. Mix the flour and salt on a clean, flat surface, or in a large mixing bowl, and make a well in the center of the flour. Break the eggs into the well. With a fork, begin beating the eggs, gradually drawing in some flour. When all the eggs are mixed in, work in the remaining flour with your hands. If the mixture is stiff, add small amounts of water, a tablespoon at a time, to get a dry dough that is not sticky. If the dough is sticky, add a little flour.
2. Gather the dough into a ball. Dust the work surface lightly with flour, and knead the ball of dough by pushing it away from you with the heels of the hand. Knead the dough until it is formed into a smooth, shiny, elastic ball—about 10 minutes should be enough.
3. Divide the dough in half with sharp knife. Form into two balls and flatten slightly. Rub each ball with a little oil to keep from drying out and put them into a plastic bag where they can rest at room temperature for at least a half hour.

4. Now comes the tricky part. On the floured surface, use a rolling pin to roll the dough as thin as possible into a long rectangle. Sift a little flour over the surface, spreading it evenly with your hands. Roll up the dough from the long side, like a jelly roll. Cut the rolled-up pasta into ¼-inch slices and quickly unroll the strips so that they do not stick together. Place the strips on floured wax paper. Repeat the process with the other half of the dough.
5. Cooking goes fast. Put the pasta in a large pot of boiling (salted) water, stir carefully, and bring the water to a second boil. At this point, taste a noodle to see if it is firm to the bite. Drain the noodles and serve immediately with your favorite sauce.

Serves 4

Nutrition Analysis:
Calories 398
Carbohydrate. . . . . .72 grams
Fiber . . . . .3 grams
Fat. . . . . .5 grams
Cholesterol. . . . . .160 milligrams
Sodium. . . . . .49 milligrams

QUICK MEAT SAUCE FOR PASTA

¾ lb very lean ground sirloin
1 26-oz jar marinara sauce
1 tsp dried oregano
2 to 3 garlic cloves
dash cayenne
freshly ground black pepper
½ tsp salt, or to taste

1. Heat a heavy, nonstick skillet over medium-high heat. Add the ground beef and saute, stirring frequently, for 4 to 5 minutes, or until meat loses its pinkness. Turn the contents of the skillet into a strainer or colander lined with paper towels and allow the fat to drain off.

2. Put the meat into a heavy 3-quart saucepan. Add the marinara sauce and stir well. Rub the oregano between the palms of your hands to powder it slightly, and add. Put the garlic through a garlic press and add, along with the cayenne, a liberal amount of black pepper, and salt to taste. Stir well, cover, and cook over gentle heat for 20 minutes, stirring occasionally. Correct the seasoning.

Serves 6

Nutrition Analysis:
Calories 154
Carbohydrate. . . . . .9 grams

Fiber . . . . .1 gram
Fat . . . . .5 grams

Cholesterol . . . . .50 milligrams
Sodium . . . . .778 milligrams

Light Tomato Sauce

1 medium onion, chopped
2 cloves garlic, minced
6 medium fresh tomatoes, peeled, seeded, and cut up
½ tsp sugar
½ tsp dried basil leaves
¼ cup red wine
⅛ tsp salt, and pepper to taste

1. Saute onion and garlic in a large nonstick skillet. Add the rest of the ingredients and simmer 15–20 minutes to cook and blend flavors. Be careful not to overcook.
2. Serve over your favorite pasta.

Makes 12 ½-cup servings

Nutrition Analysis:
Calories 26
Carbohydrate . . . . .5 grams
Fiber . . . . .1 gram
Fat . . . . .0 grams
Cholesterol . . . . .0 milligrams
Sodium . . . . .7 milligrams

Low-Fat Cheese Sauce

1 (12-oz) container low-fat cottage cheese
1 (5-oz) can evaporated skim milk
½ cup shredded American or cheddar cheese

1. Combine cottage cheese and evaporated milk in a blender; process until smooth.
2. In a small saucepan, heat mixture over medium-low heat, stirring constantly. Add cheese to hot mixture. Stir until cheese melts. Add salt and pepper.
3. Serve over your favorite pasta.

Makes 2 cups

Nutrition Analysis (per ¼ cup):
Calories 80
Carbohydrate . . . . .4 grams
Fiber . . . . .0 grams
Fat . . . . .3 grams
Cholesterol . . . . .12 milligrams
Sodium . . . . .237 milligrams

Tuna Pasta Salad

¾ cup elbow macaroni, uncooked
6½-oz can tuna, water-pack, drained
½ cup celery, thinly sliced
1 cup seedless red grapes, halved
3 tbsp salad dressing, mayonnaise-type, reduced-calorie

1. Cook macaroni according to package directions, omitting salt. Drain.

2. Toss macaroni, tuna, celery, and grapes together.
3. Mix in salad dressing.
4. Serve warm or chill until served.

Variations: Salmon Pasta Salad—Use 7½-oz can drained salmon in place of tuna. Chicken Pasta Salad—Use 1 cup diced cooked chicken in place of tuna. Beef Pasta Salad—Use 1 cup diced cooked lean beef in place of tuna.

Serves 2

Nutrition Analysis:
Calories 246
Carbohydrate. . . . . .28 grams

Fiber . . . . .2 grams
Fat. . . . . .2 grams
Cholesterol. . . . . .17 milligrams
Sodium. . . . . .522 milligrams

ITALIAN GROUND BEEF AND MACARONI

¾ lb ground beef, extra lean (you can substitute
    ground chicken or ground turkey)
½ cup chopped onion
¼ cup chopped green pepper
¼ cup chopped celery
16-oz can tomatoes
10¾-oz can tomato puree, low-sodium
1 tsp oregano leaves
1 tsp basil leaves
⅛ tsp pepper
3 cups cooked (about 1 cup uncooked) elbow
    macaroni

1. Spray frying pan with vegetable cooking spray
   and cook beef, onion, green pepper, and celery
   until beef is lightly browned and onion is clear.
   Drain.

2. Break up large pieces of tomatoes.
3. Add tomatoes, tomato puree, and seasonings to
   beef mixture. Simmer 15 minutes to blend
   flavors.
4. Stir in macaroni. Heat to serving temperature.

Serves 4

Nutrition Analysis:
Calories 358
Carbohydrate. . . . . .41 grams
Fiber . . . . .4 grams
Fat. . . . . .12 grams
Cholesterol. . . . . .52 milligrams
Sodium. . . . . .220 milligrams

❖ ❖ ❖

CHAPTER FOURTEEN

STOCKS AND SOUPS

MAKING STOCK

As with the creation of any complex project, the background and foundation must be solid in order to support the structure of the project. The same holds true when making stocks and soups. A stock is a clear, unthickened liquid flavored by substances extracted from meat, poultry, fish, vegetables, and seasonings. To make a stock, these ingredients (the exact ingredients depend on the type of stock) are basically simmered in water to extract out flavor, then the ingredients are removed, leaving a clear flavorful liquid that is the basis of most good soups and sauces.

A common practice many years ago was for a restaurant to make its own stock from leftover bones and fresh vegetables. The stock would simmer for many hours, sometimes left on a range, 24 hours per day! The chef would continually add fresh bones and vegetables. In today's food services, few operators make their own stock. Many use an alternative: convenience condensed soup bases available in chicken, fish, brown, white, and vegetable flavors. These products resemble the dried bouillon or broth mixes available at the supermarket. The main problem associated with these bases (and dried bouillon and broth mixes as well) is they contain high amounts of salt. The basic flavor of the prepared base needs the addition of a "mirepoix" (equal quantities of carrots, onions, and celery) to enhance the flavor. If you want to prepare a homemade stock, it can be done with relative ease.

Remember that the quality of the stock depends on many factors—one in particular is that the ingredients should be fresh.

The bones Bones for the stock must be purchased. The type of bones will depend on which type of stock you want to make.

Stocks are categorized according to the kind of bones used and their color.

- **White stock** is made from beef or veal bones or both.
- **Brown stock** is made from the same bones as white stock, only the bones are browned in an oven before being put into the stock.
- **Chicken stock** is made from chicken bones.
- **Fish stock** is made from fish bones and fish trimmings.
- **Vegetable stock** is a vegetarian stock that does not contain any meat products and derives its flavors from vegetables.

At one time, some caterers would specialize in prime ribs of beef as a main entree. They would purchase the rib with its bones in the size of a 16 cut. The butcher would remove some of the top layer of fat, which in turn would be bought by the "fat man," an affectionate term given to the person who resells the fat to companies that will process it into cleaners and soaps. On top of the rib is a triangular piece of meat known as the "deckle" which would be used as a london broil. The rib would be removed from the rib cage and would be used as a main entree. The meat between the bones would be removed and used in beef stroganoff, and the bones would be used for the stock.

Before the bones are placed into the stock pot, remember to "blanch" them in boiling water for a few seconds to clean any residue and remove any harmful bacteria off the bones. This will help to reduce the "scum" formation that naturally occurs during the preparation of a stock.

The vegetables The fresh vegetables should be neatly trimmed and can be cut in as large as 1-inch cubes. The combination of vegetables, known as a "mirepoix," consists of celery, carrots, and onions (usually ½ pound onions to ¼ pound celery and ¼ pound carrots). You may wish to substitute some leeks for part of the onions. Leeks add a milder onion flavor than onions.

The seasonings You then prepare a "bouquet garni" and combination of spices and herbs consisting of bay leaf, thyme, and other favorite herbs. The term "bouquet" originated because the fresh spices would be tied together in a bouquet and allowed to float in the stock, and be removed prior to use. Another method is wrapping the spices in cheesecloth and tying it with string, removing it prior to use. Of course you may also just place the spices into the stock and use a very fine strainer to filter out all ingredients prior to its use. Salt is not added to stocks because stocks are always used as ingredients in other dishes and will be appropriately flavored then.

The general procedure for making stock is as follows.

1. Cut the bones into 4-inch pieces to expose area from which flavors can be extracted.
2. Rinse the bones in cold water and blanch in boiling water.
3. Place bones in pot and cover with cold water.
4. Bring water to a boil, then reduce to simmer.
5. Add the mirepoix and bouquet garni.
6. Watch that the stock does not boil, skim off the fat as it comes to the surface, and make sure the bones stay under water.
7. Simmer for 6 hours for white and brown stock, 3 to 4 hours for chicken stock, 2 hours for vegetable stock, and ½ to 1 hour for fish stock.
8. When the stock is done, it can be drained via the pot's spigot through a fine sieve or strainer. If this type of pot is not available, you should dip several times into the pot to remove the stock while placing it into a strainer. Avoid picking up the pot and pouring it directly into the strainer—this will promote a somewhat cloudy stock.
9. Cool the stock quickly.

A stock does not have to be watched constantly during cooking—just peek at it from time to time.

The final stock should have a deep flavor and good color. While a stock is simmering, the pot should not be moved or stirred. In fact, some chefs like to add some egg whites to stocks in order to better filter out the impurities and improve the taste and color.

It is recommended that you either freeze the stock immediately in small quantities, or keep it under refrigeration for only a few days. Once a stock is refrigerated or frozen, heat to boiling and reduce to simmer for a few minutes prior to its use.

Recipes for chicken, beef, white vegetable, and red vegetable stock appear on pages 248–250.

MAKING SOUP

One of the most gratifying foods we consume is a soup because its flavor and texture can be varied as desired. A soup is a food that is primarily liquid and is composed of many substances, either vegetable and/or animal. Soup can be served either hot or cold at any time of the year. Although many recipes encourage the use of leftovers, you must remember that the preparation of a soup requires the same care and quality of ingredients as any other food prepared. Ingredients should be high quality and fresh.

A soup is an excellent appetizer. It can be served at the beginning of the meal as an appetizer to help take the "edge off the appetite." In winter, the soup provides the effect of a "warming sensation" when consumed hot after coming in from the cold. A cold soup in the summer is refreshing prior to a meal. Soups that are served as a main course generally are thick and contain protein foods. The food service industry finds the use of soups on the menu to be one of economic advantage—ease in preparation, versatility within the menu, and relatively inexpensive to prepare with good markup.

Soups are categorized according to their consistency, their use, and even their ethnic heritage. Soups range in consistency from being thin to thick with many degrees of consistency.

Thin soups, also called clear soups, include broths (also referred to as bouillons), vegetable soup, and consomme. A **broth** or bouillon is a clear soup without any solid ingredients. A **vegetable soup** is a clear, seasoned stock or broth with vegetables and possibly meats, poultry, or starches added (such as in chicken noodle soup). A **consomme** is basically the same as a broth except that it is prepared to the point of being very clear (or transparent). The key to preparing a clear consomme is the use of egg whites, not stirring the pot once residue floats to the top of the pot, and straining the soup through several layers of good quality cheesecloth.

As its name implies, the thick soup is classified according to its consistency. Thick soups differ from the thin soup not only in consistency, but also in terms of color, being nontransparent. Also, thick soups are thickened either naturally or with the use of different thickeners.

Cream soups are thickened with flour and fat (called roux) or other thickener and usually contain milk and/or cream. They are often named according to the primary food that makes up the soup, such as broccoli. Care must be taken when combining the base (cream or sauce) with the desired stock. Always use a wire whisk to add the hot stock to the base in small amounts, beating slowly, but constantly. This will help to ensure that the ingredients blend correctly and avoid curdling or breaking down of the soup. Favorite cream soups include those made from tomatoes, mushrooms, broccoli, and chicken, among others.

Pureed soups differ from cream soups in two basic ways; pureed soups are thickened naturally due to the starchy nature of the vegetable or beans used, and can be pureed via a food processor. The pureed soup does not have the smooth consistency of the cream soup and its contents are less identifiable. Split pea or potato soup are two examples.

Although the traditional **chowder** is thought to be made from shellfish (clams), chowders such as corn or potato are also popular. Chowders that have a heavy consistency are generally thickened with the use of a thin white sauce or light cream. The New England Clam Chowder (white sauce base) and the Manhattan Clam Chowder (tomato base) are time-honored favorites. Chowders made with clams generally contain a variety of vegetables.

A **bisque** differs from a chowder in that it has a smooth consistency, contains a variety of shellfish (lobster, crabs, etc.), usually does not contain pieces of distinct vegetable, and is thickened with the use of cream and eggs. Bisques are very similar to basic cream soups.

Some soups are categorized according to possible origin. The minestrone soup is an Italian favorite. It is a combination of many flavors, both meat and vegetable. It contains a combination of beef and chicken stock, pasta, tomatoes, carrots, celery, legumes, and peas. It is a very heavy soup that can be given a thicker than normal consistency if desired. The Vichyssoise is a French favorite characterized by being served cold. It is a very thick soup produced by the use of either light cream or a thin white sauce combined with pureed boiled potatoes. Other types of soups that are unusual include oxtail soup, turtle soup, and cold fruit soup, to name a few.

Soup is generally served in one cup measures or small soup bowls if served as an appetizer or large soup bowls if served as an entree or main course. If serving soup hot, you may want to heat the cups slightly. If serving soup cold, you may wish to place the cups under refrigeration prior to use.

Cold soups are potentially more hazardous in terms of spoilage than hot soups. During preparation some cold soups are subjected to heat as part of the cooking process. Upon completion of the cooking, the object is to chill down the soup as quickly as possible in order to preserve its flavor and be sure that it is safe to eat. The following are the best ways to chill down a creamed soup that will be served cold (or a creamed soup that will be served no later than 24 hours later):

- Ice/Water Bath. Place the pot of creamed soup (or divide the soup into smaller pots) in a clean kitchen sink. Place as much ice as is available around the pot of soup. If the level of ice is not at the same level as the soup, add water until the water and ice are at the level of the soup. Stir frequently and cover and refrigerate soup when it is at approximately 45°F. Add more ice during the chilling process, if necessary. DO NOT place the pot of hot soup directly into the refrigerator. If no ice is available, use cold, potable, running water.
- Shallow Pans. Pour the soup into a shallow pan(s). The depth of the soup should be no deeper than one inch thick. Place uncovered in the refrigerator on the uppermost rack until it has reached an internal temperature of 45°F. Cover the soup immediately upon being chilled.

MAKING QUICK AND HEALTHY STOCKS AND SOUPS

Making your own stocks and soups does not have to mean slaving in the kitchen on a lovely Saturday afternoon while everyone is out having fun. With good planning, you can make healthy and tasty soups without spending hours in the kitchen. Here are some ideas.

Stock

1. Plan to make 1 gallon of stock each time so you can make lots of small containers that can be put into the freezer.
2. Plan to start stock at a time when you are going to be in the kitchen for some time anyway, such as while starting to prepare dinner. This way, the stock can continue to cook while you are eating and cleaning up. If time is really short, try vegetable stock—it cooks in only 2 hours. Chicken stock takes about twice as long. See recipes for both on pages 248–250.
3. Once the stock is prepared, refrigerate it in shallow pans until cool and then remove the white-colored fat that congealed on the surface.

Soup

4. For a quick homemade vegetable soup, thaw frozen stock in the refrigerator or microwave, add vegetables—fresh, frozen, or canned—and simmer until they are tender.
5. For a quick cream-style soup, puree a lightly cooked (or sauteed—it brings out the flavor) vegetable (such as broccoli, squash, or spinach) in the blender or food processor. This pureed vegetable will act as the base and thickener. Next add 1% milk (the small amount of fat is important for some body) or evaporated skim milk (it has less than 0.5% fat) with water, and some herbs and spices for added flavor (see the list below for matching vegetables and seasonings). Simmer for about 30 minutes. You can also use stock instead of milk. These soups taste even better when refrigerated and warmed up a day later.
6. For a real quick soup, use a canned soup product and extend it with liquid and solid ingredients. This way, you can decrease the amount of fat and sodium per serving. For example, use a can of chicken rice soup, add water (or homemade stock), leftover chicken or turkey, and leftover vegetables or starches.
7. Vegetable purees can be used to thicken many kinds of soup because they are bulky. Examples include pureed beans (lentils and split peas are excellent), potato, carrot, and tomato. The amount needed to thicken a soup will vary depending on which one you use—simply add it in small amounts until the proper consistency is reached.

See the list of soup cooking tips for more ideas.

Vegetables	Seasonings
Carrots, yams, winter squash	Allspice, cinnamon, cardamon, nutmeg
Beans, cauliflower, greens (such as kale and spinach), onions, potatoes	Chili powder, coriander, cumin, garlic
Cabbage, tomatoes, onions, peppers	Basil, bay leaf, oregano, thyme

Soup Cooking Tips

1. Don't overcook soups because flavor is lost through evaporation and vegetables lose flavor and color. Also, cream soups may curdle or break.
2. Always simmer, don't boil, a soup to doneness for the best flavor, texture of ingredients, and consistency.
3. Just prior to serving, check soups for flavor, texture of ingredients, and consistency, adjusting as necessary.
4. When using vegetables and beans in a soup, make sure they all come to doneness at the same time so none of the ingredients are overcooked.
5. Cut vegetables into uniform pieces that can be readily identified for even cooking and visual appeal.
6. Canned vegetables, because they are already cooked, should be added toward the end of cooking.
7. Starchy ingredients, such as rice or pasta, should be cooked separately and added at the end because they will cloud a clear soup.
8. Do not boil soups after milk or cream has been added because the soup will curdle.
9. Do not add cold milk (or cream) to simmering soup; heat the milk or cream first to prevent curdling.

BUYING HEALTHY CANNED BROTHS AND SOUPS

Canned broths, like many canned soups, are very high in sodium. Most contain a small amount of fat, under 2 grams, but the major problem is sodium. Low-sodium products are available, but if you have ever substituted one for its regular counterpart, you probably had a pretty bland tasting dish. There are basically two solutions to this problem: make your own stock (see above) or be prepared to spice up the low-sodium product, and if possible, refrigerate it overnight to meld the flavors.

Regular canned soups are high in sodium, and most contain quite a bit of fat. Fortunately, there are a number available that have some (or all, in a few cases) of the sodium and/or fat removed. For example, Campbell's Healthy Request Soups all contain 3 grams of fat or less and under 500 milligrams of sodium per serving. Although 500 milligrams is about 20% of the recommended daily limit of 2400 milligrams, it is still better than typical canned soups that often have twice the amount of sodium. Campbell's, as well as other brands, also make other soups with even less sodium.

RECIPES

The nutritional content of stock is not given because each batch of stock is always a little different. These stocks are low in calories, fat, cholesterol, and sodium.

CHICKEN STOCK

4 lb chicken (use necks and backs or the whole chicken)
5 qt cold water
1 large onion, chopped
2 celery stalks, chopped
2 carrots, peeled and chopped
1 leek (root and green top trimmed), washed and chopped

1 garlic clove, minced
1 medium bunch parsley
5 or 6 fresh thyme sprigs or 1 tsp dried
1 bay leaf
1 tbsp black peppercorns or 1½ tsp coarsely ground pepper

1. Wash the chicken parts thoroughly and, if using a whole bird, cut it into pieces at the joints.
2. Place the chicken in a large pot, add the water, and bring to a boil over high heat. As the water nears a boil, skim off foam as it forms.
3. Add the vegetables and garlic to the stock, return to a boil, then immediately reduce the heat.
4. Simmer the stock slowly, uncovered, for 3 hours, skimming off the foam occasionally. Add more water, if needed.
5. Add the parsley, including stems, thyme, bay leaf, and peppercorns, and simmer the stock for 1 hour more.
6. Strain the stock into a bowl and separate into smaller containers for freezing. Refrigerate until cool and remove any fat that congeals on the surface.
7. Store in the freezer for up to 3 months.

Makes 1 gallon

BEEF STOCK

5–6 lb beef or veal bones (shank or knuckle bones)
5–6 qt cold water
4 large onions, coarsely chopped
5 medium carrots, quartered
4 bay leaves
3 whole cloves
1½ tsp dried thyme
5 or 6 peppercorns
2 bunches fresh parsley

1. Preheat oven to 400°F.
2. Place bones in a roasting pan and bake 25 to 30 minutes, turning bones once. Pour off fat.
3. Transfer bones and remaining ingredients to a large stockpot. Simmer 4 to 6 hours. Watch that it doesn't boil and regularly skim the fat off the top.
4. Strain through a strainer lined with cheesecloth.
5. Refrigerate until the fat hardens on the surface and can be removed.
6. Store in the freezer for up to 3 months.

Makes 1 gallon

WHITE VEGETABLE STOCK

1 lb leeks (white only), rough-cut
1 lb onions, rough-cut
2 lb celeriac (or hearts of celery only), rough-cut
1 lb white turnips, rough-cut
4 bay leaves
2 tbsp garlic, chopped
¼ cup white peppercorns, cracked
5 qt water

1. Place all ingredients in a large stockpot and simmer for 2 hours.
2. Strain.

Makes 1 gallon

Notes: The ingredient proportions in this recipe are only guidelines. Vegetable stocks can be made from any kitchen vegetables. However, some vegetables, especially in the cruciferous family (cabbage, broccoli, cauliflower, etc.), may create a bitter taste if cooked too long and should be avoided in reduced stocks. Stocks that are made quickly and used right away can utilize these vegetables. This white vegetable stock has a wider range of applications than red or darker stocks because it will add very little color to the final product.

RED VEGETABLE STOCK

1 lb leeks, rough-cut
1 lb onions, rough-cut
2 lb celery, rough-cut
2 lb tomatoes, rough-cut
2 lb carrots, rough-cut
4 bay leaves
2 tbsp garlic, chopped

2 tbsp black peppercorns, cracked
2 tbsp white peppercorns, cracked

1. Place all ingredients together into a large stockpot and simmer for 2 hours.
2. Strain.

Makes 1 gallon

BLACK BEAN SOUP

2 cups dry Idaho black beans
water
½ cup each chopped onion and celery
2 cloves garlic
1 tbsp vegetable oil
1 can (10½ oz) condensed beef broth
¼ cup dry white wine
2 tbsp lemon juice
1 bay leaf
dash each pepper and dried thyme
salt as needed

1. Soak beans overnight in 6 cups water. For quick-soak method, bring beans and water to boil and boil 2 minutes. Cover and let stand 1 hour. Drain and rinse beans.
2. Saute vegetables and garlic in oil. Combine all ingredients with 5 cups water; cover and

simmer 40–45 minutes or until beans are tender.
3. Drain beans; reserve liquid. Puree beans in blender or food processor or put through sieve. Add reserved liquid to pureed beans to reach desired consistency; salt to taste. Heat thoroughly.

Serves 6

Nutrition Analysis:

Calories	215
Carbohydrate	34 grams
Fiber	5 grams
Fat	4 grams
Cholesterol	1 milligram
Sodium	281 milligrams

PUREE OF BROCCOLI SOUP

2 tsp vegetable oil
3 cups chopped broccoli
1 large onion, chopped (1 cup)
⅔ cup chopped celery
1½ cups diced peeled potato
1 clove garlic, minced (1 tsp)
½ tsp sugar
4 whole cloves
freshly ground black pepper to taste
4 cups chicken broth

1. In a large saucepan, heat the oil, and add the broccoli, onion, celery, potato, garlic, and sugar.

Cover the pan, and cook the vegetables over low heat for about 10 minutes, stirring them occasionally.
2. Add the cloves, pepper, and broth, and bring the soup to a boil. Reduce the heat, and cook the soup, partially covering the pan, for about 20 minutes or until the vegetables are soft. Remove and discard the cloves.
3. Puree the soup in batches in a blender or food processor.

Serves 6

Nutrition Analysis:

Calories 114
Carbohydrate. . . . . .18 grams
Fiber . . . . .1 gram

Fat. . . . . .3 grams
Cholesterol. . . . . .1 milligram
Sodium. . . . . .583 milligrams

FISH CHOWDER

1 lb haddock fillets, fresh or frozen, without skin
1½ cups potatoes, ¼-inch diced
2 tbsp onion, chopped
1 cup boiling water
2 tbsp flour
2 tbsp water
2 cups skim milk
½ tsp salt
dash pepper
1 tbsp margarine

1. Thaw frozen fish in refrigerator overnight.
2. Cut fish into 1-inch pieces.
3. Add fish, potatoes, and onion to boiling water. Cover and simmer until potatoes are just tender, about 10 minutes. Drain.
4. Mix flour with 2 tbsp water until smooth. Stir into milk.
5. Add milk mixture, salt, and pepper to fish mixture. Cook, stirring gently, until thickened.
6. Stir in margarine.

Serves 4

Nutrition Analysis:

Calories 210
Carbohydrate. . . . . .19 grams
Fiber . . . . .1 gram
Fat. . . . . .2 grams
Cholesterol. . . . . .67 milligrams
Sodium. . . . . .421 milligrams

VEGETABLE SOUP

1 cup potatoes, diced
1 cup cabbage, chopped
½ cup onion, chopped
½ cup celery, diced
½ cup carrots, sliced
½ cup frozen green beans
¼ tsp oregano leaves
¼ tsp marjoram leaves
¼ tsp salt
1 bay leaf
dash pepper
2 cups water
1 cup (½ 16-oz can) tomatoes

1. Place all ingredients except tomatoes in a saucepan. Cover and boil gently for 10 minutes.
2. Break up tomatoes; add to vegetable mixture and continue cooking until vegetables are tender—about 20 minutes.
3. Remove bay leaf before serving.

Serves 4

Nutrition Analysis:

Calories 67
Carbohydrate. . . . . .15 grams
Fiber . . . . .3 grams
Fat. . . . . .0 grams
Cholesterol. . . . . .0 milligrams
Sodium. . . . . .257 milligrams

❖ ❖ ❖

CHAPTER FIFTEEN

FATS AND OILS

Because the nutritional aspects of fats and oils are so important, they will be discussed before, instead of after, tips on purchasing.

NUTRITION

Ninety percent of the fat in foods is in the form of triglycerides, a compound made of three fatty acids attached to glycerol. Fatty acids may be one of three different types:

- Saturated
- Monounsaturated
- Polyunsaturated

All fats in foods are made up of mixtures of these three types of fatty acids. If a food contains mostly saturated fatty acids, it is considered a **saturated fat**; if it contains mostly monounsaturated fatty acids, it is a **monounsaturated fat**; if it contains mostly polyunsaturated fatty acids, it is a **polyunsaturated fat** (see Table 57).

Saturated fat raises your blood cholesterol (and your chances of having heart disease) more than anything else in your diet, so let's take a look at the foods in which it is found. Animal products are a major source of saturated fat in the typical American diet, as can be seen in the following list of saturated fats.

- The fat in whole milk dairy products such as milk, cream, and cheese
- Beef fat, chicken fat, and lard (rendered pork fat)
- Butter (which is made from cream)
- The fat in egg yolks

Fats high in monounsaturated fats are liquid at room temperatures but become hard when refrigerated. Examples of monounsaturated fats include olive oil, peanut oil, and canola oil. Like other vegetable oils, these are used in salad dressings and for cooking oils.

Polyunsaturated fats, like the monounsaturated fats, tend to reduce blood cholesterol levels. Polyunsaturated fats are found in greatest amounts in vegetable oils such as safflower, corn, soybean, cottonseed, sesame, and sunflower oils. These oils are commonly used in salad dressings and for cooking oils. Nuts and seeds also contain polyunsaturated fats, enough to make nuts and seeds a rather high-calorie snack food depending on serving size. Another type of polyunsaturated fat is found in the oils of fish and shellfish. The omega-3 fatty acids found in fish oil may be beneficial in preventing heart disease.

A few vegetable oils—**coconut oil, palm kernel oil,** and **palm oil** (collectively called the **tropical oils**)—are high in saturated fat. Although recently the food industry has largely discontinued the use of these fats in many foods, they may be used for commercial deep fat frying and in foods such as cookies and crackers, whipped toppings, coffee creamers, cake mixes, and even frozen dinners.

There are two products we have not mentioned yet: **vegetable shortening** and **margarine**. Vegetable shortening is made from vegetable oils in which some or all of the oil undergoes a chemical process called **hydrogenation**. This process is used for two reasons: now that the oil is solid, it can be

❖ Table 57   Fatty Acids in Fats and Oils   ❖

Fats and Oils (1 tablespoon)	Saturated Fatty Acids (grams)	Monounsaturated Fatty Acids (grams)	Polyunsaturated Fatty Acids (grams)
Fats with large amounts of saturated fatty acids include:			
Coconut oil	11.8	0.8	0.2
Palm kernel oil	11.1	1.5	0.2
Cocoa butter	8.1	4.5	0.4
Butter	7.1	3.3	0.4
Palm oil	6.7	5.0	1.3
Lard	5.0	5.8	1.4
Fats with large amounts of monounsaturated fatty acids include:			
Olive oil	1.8	9.9	1.1
Canola oil	0.9	7.6	4.5
Peanut oil	2.3	6.2	4.3
Fats with large amounts of polyunsaturated fatty acids include:			
Safflower oil	1.2	1.6	10.1
Corn oil	1.7	3.3	8.0
Soybean oil	2.0	3.2	7.9
Cottonseed oil	3.5	2.4	7.1
Sunflower oil	1.4	6.2	5.5
Margarine, liquid	1.8	3.9	5.1
Margarine, soft tub	1.8	4.8	3.9

used successfully in commercial baking of many products. The process also extends the product's shelf life (vegetable oils go bad pretty quickly). Now this sounds fine except that hydrogenation also makes an unsaturated vegetable oil **more saturated**. The saturated fat content of vegetable shortening is higher than that found in corn oil or margarine, but is still less than that found in lard, butter, or coconut oil.

The process of hydrogenation is also used to make a spreadable product, called margarine, from vegetable oils. Although margarine and butter both contain about 100 calories and 11 grams of fat per tablespoon, only 2 or 3 grams of the fat in the stick margarine is saturated, compared to 7 grams of the fat in butter.

As Table 58 shows, all oils, whether saturated or not, contain about the same number of calories: 120 per tablespoon with 13 grams of fat. Although many Americans have switched to eating more monounsaturated and polyunsaturated fats and oils, they are not eating fewer calories. As a matter of fact, their total fat intake has not changed very much at all. Although it certainly is better to choose more healthful fats and oils, it is also important to moderate your use of all fats and oils, even the "good guys."

PURCHASING

There are several different types of margarine on the market besides stick margarine.

- **Soft tub margarine**—these are all vegetable oils with no milk solids; easier to spread than stick margarine
- **Whipped margarine**—soft margarine that has been whipped so it contains more air and therefore fewer calories per tablespoon (don't substi-

❖ Table 58   Total Calories and Fat   ❖ in Selected Fats and Oils

Fat or Oil	Calories/ Tablespoon	Grams Fat/ Tablespoon	Grams Saturated Fat/Tablespoon
Coconut oil	120	13	12
Palm kernel oil	120	13	11
Palm oil	120	13	7
Butter, stick	108	12	7
Lard	115	13	5
Cottonseed oil	120	13	3
Olive oil	119	13	1
Canola oil	120	13	1
Peanut oil	119	13	2
Safflower oil	120	13	1
Corn oil	120	13	2
Soybean oil	120	13	2
Sunflower oil	120	13	1
Shortening	106	12	3
Margarine, stick	101	11	2
Margarine, soft tub	102	11	2
Margarine, liquid	102	11	1–2
Margarine, whipped	70	8	1–2
Margarine spread	77	8	1–2
Margarine, diet	50	6	1

tute it for regular butter or margarine in recipes—it contains a lot of air and water)

- **Liquid margarine**—these are packaged in squeeze bottles in which the margarine is truly liquid, even in the refrigerator
- **Margarine spread**—these are soft margarines with water added; have about 50 to 75 percent fat (don't substitute it for regular butter or margarine in recipes—it contains a lot of water)
- **Light margarine**—more water is added to this product which contains about 40–60 percent fat (again, don't substitute it)
- **Diet or reduced-calorie margarine**—has about 40 percent fat and therefore more air and water than other margarines (don't substitute it for regular butter or margarine in recipes or use it for frying—it's not the same)

A nutritional comparison of these margarines appears in Table 58. For fewer calories, less fat and saturated fat, choose a margarine with 6 grams or less fat and 1 gram or less saturated fat per tablespoon. Check for a dating code.

When choosing vegetable oils, choose those high in polyunsaturated fats, such as corn oil, safflower oil, and sunflower oil, or monounsaturated fats, such as olive oil. Table 59 gives information on different oils. Some other purchasing tips are:

- Canola, corn, cottonseed, safflower, sunflower, and soybean oils are good all-purpose oils for the kitchen.
- Oils labeled "vegetable oils" are often soybean oil or a blend of several of the oils just mentioned.
- Be prepared to spend more money for the more exotic oils such as almond, hazelnut, sesame, and walnut oils. Because these oils tend to be cold pressed (meaning they are processed without heat), they are not as stable as the all-purpose oils and should be purchased in small quantities (you don't need to use much of them anyway because they are strong). Don't purchase these oils to cook with—they burn easily.

Vegetable oil is also available in a convenient spray form that can be used as a nonstick spray coating for cooking and baking pans with a minimal amount of fat (usually only 1 gram of fat is used). It is available flavored with butter or olive oil.

Butter is available in several forms.

- **Salted**—salt acts both to flavor and help preserve butter. The amount of salt varies by brand.
- **Unsalted or sweet**—made from fresh cream without any added salt, frequently used for baking and cooking
- **Whipped**—contains fewer calories per tablespoon because of the air whipped into it, more spreadable than stick butter

Butter is graded as USDA AA (the best—smooth texture and sweet), USDA A (has a pleasing flavor and fairly smooth texture), and USDA B (the lowest grade—made from sour rather than fresh cream). When purchasing butter, make sure it is cold and in clean, undamaged packaging. It should smell fresh and have a sweet aroma. Check for a dating code.

STORING

The enemies of fats and oils are exposure to air, heat, and light. Therefore, store them tightly sealed and in cool and dark places. Other guidelines include the following:

- The all-purpose oils (canola, corn, cottonseed, safflower, sunflower, and soybean oils) can be stored unopened for one year on a kitchen shelf. Once opened, they can generally last 6 months.
- The exotic oils (such as walnut and sesame) should be refrigerated (they are more fragile) and can last up to 3–4 months in the refrigerator.
- Olive oil should be stored in air-tight dark containers and kept in a cool, dark place. Use within 6 months. It can also be kept in the refrigerator for up to 1 year.
- Vegetable shortening, once opened, can be stored on a kitchen shelf for up to one year.

❖ *Table 59 Vegetable Oils* ❖

Oil	Characteristics/Uses	Oil	Characteristics/Uses
Canola oil	Light yellow color Bland flavor Good for frying, sauteing, and in baked goods Good for salad dressings	Peanut oil	Pale yellow color Mild nutty flavor Good for frying and sauteing Good for salad dressings
Corn oil	Golden color Mild flavor Good for frying, sauteing, and in baked goods Too heavy for salad dressings	Safflower oil	Golden color Bland flavor Has a higher concentration of polyunsaturated fatty acids than any other oil Good for frying, sauteing, and in baked goods Good for salad dressings
Cottonseed oil	Pale yellow color Bland flavor Good for frying, sauteing, and in baked goods Good for salad dressings	Sesame oil	Light golden color Distinctive, strong flavor Good for sauteing Good for flavoring dishes and in salad dressings Use in small amounts Expensive
Hazelnut oil	Dark amber color Nutty, smoky flavor Not for frying or sauteing as it burns easily Good for flavoring finished dishes and salad dressings Use in small amounts Expensive	Soybean oil	More soybean oil is produced than any other type, used in most blended vegetable oils and margarines Light color Bland flavor Good for frying, sauteing, and in baked goods Good for salad dressings
Olive oil	Varies from pale yellow with sweet flavor to greenish color and fuller flavor to full, fruity taste (color and flavor depend on olive variety, level of ripeness, and how they were processed) Extra virgin or virgin olive oil—don't cook with because it burns, good for flavoring finished dishes and in salad dressings, strong olive taste Pure olive oil—can be used for sauteing and in salad oils, not as strong an olive taste as extra virgin or virgin	Sunflower oil	Pale golden color Bland flavor Good for frying, sauteing, and in baked goods Good for salad dressings
		Walnut oil	Medium yellow to brown color Rich, nutty flavor For flavoring finished dishes and in salad dressings Use in small amounts Expensive

- For butter and margarine, check dating on packaging. Butter can stay fresh for 2 to 3 weeks past the date code but should be wrapped tightly in plastic if not used in a few weeks of purchase because it readily absorbs odors (such as onions) in the refrigerator. Butter can be frozen (double wrap it first) for 6 to 8 months. Margarine can be stored for 4 to 5 months in the refrigerator and, like butter, needs to be well wrapped. Diet margarines can only be stored for 2 to 3 months. Regular, soft, and liquid margarines can be frozen for up to 1 year (double wrap again).

Sometimes when oils are refrigerated, they may become cloudy and thick. This usually clears up

FAT SUBSTITUTES

❖ ❖ ❖

Did you know there is a frozen dessert in your local supermarket made to taste like ice cream, but has no fat? Well, there is. Simple Pleasures® is a frozen dessert made with Simplesse, the first fat substitute approved by the Food and Drug Administration (FDA). In fact, legally, Simple Pleasures can't be called ice cream because FDA's standards require that ice cream contain at least 10 percent butterfat. Both Simple Pleasures and Simplesse are products of Nutra-Sweet Co., which also makes aspartame, the popular sugar substitute.

Simplesse is made from egg white and milk protein blended and heated in a process called microparticulation, in which the protein is shaped into microscopic round particles that roll easily over one another. The aim of the process is to create the feel of a creamy liquid with the texture of fat. Because the components of Simplesse have long been used as foods, the FDA, on February 23, 1990, affirmed Simplesse as "generally recognized as safe" for use as a thickener or texturizer in frozen dessert products. Safety studies were not required.

NutraSweet plans to seek FDA approval for use of Simplesse in additional products such as mayonnaise, salad dressing, yogurt, dips, sour cream, butter, margarine, and cheese spreads. Simplesse can't be used in cooking because baking or frying causes it to lose its creaminess. NutraSweet says, however, that "products made with Simplesse can be enjoyed with many hot foods." For example, it can be used in an imitation butter spread on toast or in a sour cream-type sauce used to top a baked potato.

Other fat substitutes are under development or awaiting FDA approval. Procter and Gamble's fat substitute Olestra, however, is a different matter. Developed for use in hot foods as well as cold, it is a new substance that, according to the company, is "almost a carbon copy of regular fat, but with a molecule of sugar at its core instead of glycerol, and up to eight fatty acids attached to the core instead of the customary three."

Because it is a new molecular structure that does not break down to its component parts during digestion, Olestra must be approved as a new food additive, which means that studies must be done to ensure its safety.

It remains to be seen, however, whether consumers will, indeed, become healthier by using products with fat substitutes. Some nutritionists are concerned that people who eat products made with fat substitutes will feel freer to eat more of other high-fat foods, rationalizing that they are saving on those made with substitutes. A more basic, as yet unanswered question is whether nonfat foods will satisfy as well as the traditional foods they replace and, therefore, whether they will really help people reduce fat consumption. With more and more companies working on developing fat substitutes, only time will tell!

after they are left at room temperature again for a few minutes or they are put under warm water.

Cooking Light and Healthy

Here are some nutritious tips on using fats and oils at home.

• If you are in the habit of putting margarine on bread, you can cut out 100 calories and 11 grams fat for every tablespoon you don't use! If you can't handle plain bread, at the very least try to use less margarine and use a margarine with less fat. Other alternatives include using small amounts of jams, jellies, and fruit spreads.

• Use fruit butter, instead of butter or margarine, on pancakes, waffles, and French toast. Fruit butters do not contain any fat; they are made of fruit and sugar and they start out with much more fruit, and much less sugar, than jams, jellies, preserves, and spreads.

- Instead of using a high-fat spread on a sandwich such as mayonnaise, try loading on some fresh vegetables such as lettuce, tomato, onions, peppers, and whatever else you like.
- Instead of using a fat to flavor vegetables, use herbs, spices, flavored vinegars, or lemon juice. (See Chapter 18 on herbs and spices.)
- Make your own oil and vinegar salad dressing using a flavored vinegar such as raspberry or balsamic or fresh herbs such as basil, dill, or parsley. Use as little oil as possible.
- Instead of frying or sauteing with butter or margarine, use a nonstick pan and coat the pan with a cooking spray (only 7 calories!) or saute in lemon juice, broth, wine, or flavored vine-gars. If you have to use some fat or oil, choose olive or canola oil in very small amounts.
- See Chapter 16 for how to decrease the amount of fat (and saturated fat) in various baking recipes.

Different oils can be paired with foods as follows.

Food	Appropriate Oils
Chicken	Corn, cottonseed, peanut, sesame seed, or soybean oil
Veal	Olive oil
Fish	Peanut oil
Vegetables	Corn, olive, peanut, safflower, soybean, or walnut oil

❖ ❖ ❖

CHAPTER SIXTEEN

DESSERTS AND BASIC BAKING

DESSERTS

As we attempt to control our food intake, the thought of giving up baked goods is somewhat depressing. Although we associate desserts with lots of calories, the reality is that there are many nutritious choices available, and even if they are not nutritious, we can consume amounts that are reasonable.

Commercial cakes, pies, and cookies are often high in fat, saturated fat, and calories. In addition, some are quite high in cholesterol. These are some that are acceptable.

- Baked goods specially made without (or with little) fat is a fast-growing section in the supermarket—and one that has some good-tasting choices. Some brand names to look for are Entenmann's, Sara Lee, Pepperidge Farm, and Health Valley.
- Angel food cake or sponge cake (used to make jelly roll) uses little or no fat.
- Fig bars, gingersnaps, graham crackers, and animal crackers have less fat than many other cookies.

To keep down the amount of fat in baked goods, try to select cakes and pies with 5 grams or less of fat per serving and cookies with 4 grams or less of fat per ounce.

Fruit-based desserts vary from simply serving fresh fruit or canned fruits (use those that are packed in juice to cut down on sugar) to baking fruit into dishes such as baked apples (see recipe on page 274) or baked bananas, fruit compote, or

crumbles. Crumbles (also called crisps) are made of cut-up fruit placed in a baking dish, topped with a streusel-type topping, and baked until the fruit is soft and the top crunchy. Recipes for Peach Crisp and Apple-Pear Crisp appear on page 283. Although streusel toppings are typically high in fat, they need not be, as these recipes show. When baking fruit, it is important not to use too high a heat or to overcook them.

Puddings and custard are also popular dessert items. Puddings are soft desserts with a thick, creamy consistency or a spongy texture. Other kinds of puddings are commonly thickened with cornstarch and may include ingredients such as rice or tapioca.

Puddings made chiefly of eggs, milk, sugar, and flavorings are called custards. In making custards, use low heat and don't overcook. Cooking at too high a temperature for too long a time will curdle the milk and toughen the eggs. All custard puddings other than bread pudding should be cooked in a water bath, meaning that the custard cups or pan are placed into a pan of water for baking (the water should be almost level with the custard in the cup or pan). The water bath prevents curdling of the milk and eggs which can occur when they are exposed to heat for some time.

To keep down the amount of fat in puddings, it is possible to use skim milk. This works particularly well when you are using a pudding mix, and results in a low-fat, tasty dessert. It can also be done when making puddings from scratch (see the recipe for Raisin Whole Wheat Bread Pudding on page 274). Custards can be made with fewer eggs and skim milk.

Meringues are stiffly beaten mixtures of egg whites and sugar that are baked in an oven. They make wonderful, fat-free shells in which you can place fresh fruit or fruit sauces for a colorful dessert. See the recipe for Soft Meringue on page 275.

The category of frozen desserts includes the dairy products: ice cream, ice milk, and frozen yogurt (all are discussed in Chapter 10). Other frozen desserts include sherbet, sorbet, water ice, and fruit bars.

Sherbet is a fruit-based soft dessert that, unlike sorbet and fruit bars, contains some milk fat, generally only 1 to 2 percent. Sherbet makes a refreshingly smooth and light dessert and can be served with fresh fruit.

Sorbet, a fruity ice, is an international dessert, appetizer, and snack. It is typically made of fruit, fruit juice, water, and sugar. Some recipes call for egg white or gelatin, which are used as thickeners. It does not contain milk so it is a fat-free, relatively low calorie dessert.

Water ice, such as lemon ice, is basically water, sugar, and flavorings. It contains no fat but quite a bit of sugar (as does sorbet).

There are a variety of frozen **fruit bars** available in the freezer section of your supermarket: fruit and juice bars, fruit-flavored bars, fruit and cream bars, or real fruit bars. If there are so many varieties, then what is the difference between them? Well, most contain very little fat (1 gram, if that) and most are under 90 calories. Where they do vary is how much of the sweetness comes from real fruit and how much comes from added sugar. For the least amount of refined sugar, purchase a brand that does not list a form of refined sugar (see Table 8 in Chapter 2).

BAKING BASICS

The use of grain products is as old as the records of mankind. As a result of years of experimentation and contributions from many cultures, we have a wide variety of cakes, pies, cookies, and numerous breads that are unique to all parts of the world.

Baked goods do not have to contain excessive amounts of calories, fat, saturated fat, sugar, or cholesterol. In other words, you can make adjustments to many traditional baking recipes, including cakes, cookies, and pies, and come up with a leaner product that is still tasty. By doing your own baking, you can control the amount of sugar, fat, saturated fat, and cholesterol in your finished products. Table 60 is a list of substitutions you can make when baking to create a product lower in fat, saturated fat, and/or cholesterol.

Equipment

"A handful of this, and a handful of that!" may properly describe instructions from people you've known who had the ability to create bakery masterpieces with little equipment and a sharp eye for measurements. Although the acquired skills to be a good baker are notable, baking is a fine skill that can be acquired with persistence and a strong understanding of basic principles.

Knowledge of equipment and how to properly use the equipment is of paramount importance. Baking requires precision—from measuring exact amounts, to following a precise procedure in

❖ *Table 60 Baking Substitutions* ❖
to Reduce Fat, Saturated Fat,
and/or Cholesterol

Instead of:	Use:
1 whole egg	2 egg whites
2 whole eggs	1 whole egg plus 2 egg whites
Regular milk	Skim or 1% milk
1 cup heavy cream	1 cup evaporated skim milk
1 cup light cream	1 cup low-fat yogurt
1 cup whipped cream	Whip ⅓ cup heavy cream and add ⅔ cup nonfat yogurt
1 tablespoon butter or lard	1 tablespoon margarine
1 cup shortening	⅔ cup vegetable oil
½ cup shortening	⅓ cup vegetable oil
1 cup sour cream	1 cup reduced-fat sour cream or 1 cup low-fat yogurt
1 tablespoon cream cheese	1 tablespoon Baker's cheese or Neufchatel cheese
1 ounce baking chocolate	3 tablespoons cocoa and 1 tablespoon vegetable oil

terms of technique, to baking at a precise temperature for a certain period of time. Remember that the equipment should be spotlessly clean to ensure the best possible product in terms of taste and safety.

Organizing the equipment for baking can be divided into several categories:

Measurement utensils The measurement utensils used for the volume measurement in baking include the standard set of measurement spoons (which are used for either wet or dry ingredients) consisting of 1 tablespoon, 1 teaspoon, ½ teaspoon, and ¼ teaspoon; a set of measurement cups (for dry ingredients) consisting of a 1 cup, ½ cup, ⅓ cup, and ¼ cup measure; a 1 or 2 cup measure for liquid ingredients that probably has weight increments on the side for liquids that weigh the same as water.

Scales The use of weight for both dry and wet ingredients as the primary form of measurement is a common practice in bakeries. The reason is that weighing an ingredient is much easier and more accurate than the many variables in technique that are possible in volume measurement (commonly known as cups, pints, quarts, gallons, etc.). Nevertheless, standard measures (volume) are used in most homes, rather than the use of a scale, and with careful technique, you can still prepare a very good product.

Mixing utensils In order to properly blend baked products you should use the proper utensils. If blending cake batters, remember to use either a spoon (with a specified number of strokes) or if using an electric beater (stationary or handheld), set at the proper speed and for a specific length of time. If the recipe calls for "folding," use a rubber spatula.

Containers (bowls) for mixing Determine which bowl is best for use. Do not use a bowl that is too small, or the ingredients will not blend properly.

Baking pans Most recipes indicate the type and size of pan that should be used for a particular recipe. If in doubt about the size of a pan, simply measure it to confirm the size. If you have a simi- lar but not exact size pan, be aware that this will probably change the cooking time—either longer or shorter. Above all, be sure that the pan is properly prepared. Vegetable oil spray is fine for bakeware, and in some cases, flouring the pan will also be necessary.

The oven The oven temperature must be exact and constant in order to achieve a high level of proficiency in baking. To check your oven temperature, simply place a portable oven thermometer (available in any hardware store for under $5.00) into the oven, turn the oven on; and check that the actual oven temperature matches what you set the oven at. Electric ovens are notorious for needing longer preheating and stabilization times than gas ovens. Remember, the oven temperature is a critical part of the success of baking.

Racks for cooling Wire racks for cooling are very important. Proper cooling of a baked item will ensure even outer texture and promote a good appearance.

Ingredients

As a standard rule, all ingredients should be fresh.

Flours The most important ingredient in most baked goods is flour because it provides structure for baked products. When flour is mixed with liquid, proteins in the flour are turned into gluten, an elastic protein that is responsible for the structure of baked goods. Most people use all-purpose flour, either bleached or unbleached, available in the local supermarket. This type of flour will yield a very good product and is acceptable in many baked products. Other types of flour include bread, cake, and pastry flour, and these are described in the chart of Baking Ingredients.

Sugars Sugar does much more in baking than just make a sweet product. Sugar also makes a fine-textured and tender product, prevents staling by holding onto water, provides leavening when creamed, and helps the crust to brown. In yeast breads, sugar provides food for the yeast to eat so they produce carbon dioxide gas that makes bread rise. Sugars used in baking are generally granulated, either white or brown. Other sweetening agents may include the use of syrups, such as honey or molasses.

Liquids Liquid such as milk should be fresh and properly measured. Various types of juices and water also are used. Once again, do not discount the effect of flavors that liquids can contribute. Liquid is important for gluten development.

Eggs In addition to the use of milk as a primary ingredient for blending ingredients in many baked products, eggs are also commonly used. Eggs provide structure, moisture, flavor, and color when used in baked goods. Egg whites, when whipped, are an important leavener in products such as angel food cake. Eggs should be fresh and not too cold. Many recipes suggest that the eggs be at room temperature. This does not mean to leave the eggs out of the refrigerator overnight prior to use. It is best to remove the eggs from the refrigerator approximately 2 hours prior to usage.

Fats Fats are important for making tender baked goods that are rich-tasting. They prevent staling of baked goods and provide leavening when creamed with sugar. Common fats used in baking include butter (sweet and salted), shortening, margarine, and vegetable oil. Once again make sure that the fats are not "rancid," a condition that does not appear to be spoiled, but causes a poor taste in the end product. Use of fresh ingredients is the best assurance that the fats are fresh.

Leavening agents Freshness is most important for ingredients used for leavening. Leavening agents include:

- Yeast—a live fungi that produces carbon dioxide gas when it feeds on the sugars in a dough; may be purchased dry (it comes in little foil envelopes—always check the freshness date on them) or compressed (it comes as small moist cakes that must be refrigerated and used within two weeks)
- Baking powder—a mixture of acid and alkali (the alkali is baking soda) that reacts with liquid by foaming and creating bubbles that raise the dough; double-acting baking soda has two acids—one that foams at room temperature, another that foams at oven temperatures

- Baking soda—an acid ingredient, such as buttermilk, must be in the dough in order for baking soda to raise the dough

These leavening agents do lose some of their leavening power over a period of time. When you purchase them, mark the date of purchase with a marker on the side of the package. Allow no more than a storage time of 6 months for baking powder in a dry environment, 18 months for baking soda, and up to the date on the label of dry yeast. If you question whether your baking powder is okay to use, simply measure 1 teaspoon into 1/3 cup hot water. If it is still good, the mixture will actively fizz and bubble. If you question whether your yeast is alive, check for bubbles when the yeast is combined with lukewarm water in your recipe.

Other forms of leavening include the use of steam (as in cream puffs) and air (as in the mixing process).

Salt and flavorings Salt is a common additive for providing flavor to many baked goods. In yeast breads, salt also keeps the yeast from producing too much carbon dioxide gas and possibly ruining the final product. Flavorings may also come from other sources—extracts (such as vanilla), various fruits, liquids, nuts, seasonings, to name a few. If you are developing your own recipe (or trying to decipher Grandmother's recipe!) you will probably have to make the item several times to determine the correct flavor. Keep track of the amounts with accurate measurements to establish the flavor desired.

See the lists of common baking terms and functions and types of ingredients used in baking.

YEAST BREADS

Yeast breads are one of the most favorite forms of food that offer a great accompaniment with virtually any meal. Most breads are made primarily of flour, water, salt, and yeast, with little or no fat added. For example, French bread usually contains no fat. There are some breads, however, that use increased amounts of fat, sugar, and sometimes eggs. These include rich dinner rolls, brioche, danish pastry, croissants, and sweet rolls such as cinnamon rolls. If you follow some basic

BAKING TERMS

Cream—to work fat and sugar together with the back of a spoon to a light and fluffy texture in order to incorporate air (for leavening) in doughs and batters for cakes, cookies, and icings

Whip—to beat rapidly, usually with a whip, to incorporate air and increase volume (such as whipping cream)

Cut in—to cut fat into flour using a pastry knife or two knives when making pie crust so that small pieces of fat are coated with flour

Fold—to combine a whipped or delicate ingredient with another using an under and over motion with a flat utensil

Knead—to manipulate dough with your hands to develop gluten

Batter—a semiliquid mixture of flour (or other starch) and liquid ingredients used to make baked goods such as cakes and quick breads

Dough—a mixture of flour and liquid which is stiffer than a batter and is used to make baked goods such as bread, cookies, and pastries

Make up—to form or shape a dough or batter into a certain shape and size before baking

Gluten—the protein that provides structure in baked goods; it forms when flour is moistened

---

rules of breadmaking, you will enjoy many successes in this area and will receive many compliments.

Make sure that the ingredients are correctly measured and combined in the proper order. In all cases of using yeast, take caution NOT to kill the yeast by using water that is too hot. Yeast grows best between 100°–110°F. If at a lower temperature, it takes longer for the yeast to grow, and perhaps the bread will not rise as much as desired. If the water is too hot, much of the yeast will die—thus, the bread will not rise. If you do not have a thermometer, you can test the water if some is placed on your wrist (just like testing a baby's bottle!). The dough is properly mixed when it is no longer sticky. If it is still sticky, more flour (in small amounts) should be mixed in.

After the bread dough is mixed (whether by hand or machine), place the dough on a lightly floured table for kneading. Kneading is the process of working dough into a smooth mass by pressing and folding to develop the gluten and mix the ingredients. If you use a mixer with a "dough hook" attachment, this will do your kneading, or you can use the food processor for

kneading using the plastic dough-kneading blade. To knead by hand, do the following.

1. Place the round of dough in front of you and bring the top half of the dough over toward you.
2. Turn the dough a quarter turn, and repeat the process.
3. Continue turning the dough a quarter turn and repeating the kneading process until the dough is very soft.

If the dough feels sticky while kneading it, add a sprinkling of flour.

The purpose of kneading is to develop the gluten in the dough so that the gas produced by the yeast will be captured. When the dough is not kneaded enough, the gas is not contained, and the resulting bread tends to be heavy and small in volume. The length of kneading time varies, but 5 to 8 minutes is usually enough, or until the dough becomes smooth and shiny. The quantity of dough and the type of flour used also affect kneading time.

After the dough is kneaded, place into a lightly greased bowl, cover with a damp cloth, and place

BAKING INGREDIENTS

❖ ❖ ❖

1. Flour

Function: • Provide the structure of baked goods (needed more in breads than in more tender products such as cakes)

Forms: • All-purpose—can be used in any recipe that does not specify a particular type of flour
• Bread—a high-protein flour used to make breads and pizza dough
• Cake—a low-protein flour used to make cakes and other delicate baked goods
• Pastry—its gluten content is between cake flour and bread flour, best suited to make pie dough, quick breads, biscuits, and some cookies and pastries

2. Sugars

Functions: • Add flavor
• Make a fine-textured, tender product
• Prevent staling by holding onto water
• Provide leavening when creamed
• Help crust brown

Forms: • Fine granulated (table sugar)
• Confectioners' (powdered)—white sugar ground to a fine powder; "10X" is the finest and is used in icings, toppings, and cream fillings
• Brown sugar—table sugar that is not as highly refined, contains some molasses and caramel, used for its flavor and color

3. Milk and Cream

Functions: • Add flavor
• Develop gluten
• Provide nutritional value
• Help crust brown

Forms: • Whole, low-fat, skim milk

• Buttermilk—is mildly acid; when mixed with baking soda, it produces leavening and also imparts a special flavor
• Dry milk—usually treated as a dry ingredient which is reconstituted when water is added

4. Water

Function: • Combines with flour to make gluten

5. Eggs

Functions: • Provide structure
• Provide moisture (water)
• Provide flavor and color
• Provide leavening when whipped (egg white)
• Make batter smooth (egg yolk)

Forms: • Fresh, frozen, dried

6. Fats

Functions: • Make product tender
• Add richness
• Prevent staling of baked product
• Provide leavening when creamed

Forms: • Regular shortening—has waxy texture and no taste, creams well, and is used in pie crusts, biscuits, many pastries and cookies, and breads
• Emulsified or high-ratio shortening—softer and creams better than regular shortening, used in some cakes and icings
• Butter—makes dough hard to handle because it melts at room temperature, tastes better than shortening because it melts in the mouth (shortening leaves a film in the mouth)
• Margarine—can replace butter but lacks the flavor
• Oils—rarely used in baking,

<table>
<tr><td>

used to grease pans and deep-fry donuts

7. Leavening agents

Function:
- Makes baked goods rise by producing bubbles of gas

Forms:
- Baking powder
- Baking soda and acid ingredient such as buttermilk

</td><td>

- Yeast—a live microscopic plant that eats sugar and then produces carbon dioxide gas in bread doughs

8. Seasonings and flavorings

Function:
- Flavoring

Forms:
- Includes salt, chocolate, spices, extracts, etc.

</td></tr>
</table>

in a warm, draft-free area. Let the dough rest and rise until double in size, a procedure known as "proofing." During proofing, the yeast eat the sugars and starches in the dough, resulting in carbon dioxide gas that is the bread's leavening.

When the dough has sufficiently proofed (usually it takes about 1–1½ hours), it is tested by inserting your fingers in the dough to the knuckle in several places. If the finger marks close very slowly, the dough is ready to be punched—which does not mean to hit the dough with your fist. Punching the dough is to pull up the dough on all sides, fold over the center, and press down. Then turn the dough upside down in the bowl. The dough is punched to keep it at an even temperature, expel the carbon dioxide, further develop the gluten, and bring fresh oxygen to the yeast cells for further growth.

Once punched, divide the dough (if necessary), shape into desired shapes (rolls, loaves), and place onto nonstick or lightly oiled sheet pans or other baking dish and proof again, until double in bulk. A fully proofed loaf of dough when touched gently will slowly fill out the dents made by the fingers. Rich doughs containing fat should not be allowed to reach full proof. Fat weakens the gluten structure and the dough may collapse in baking if given as full a proof as a bread dough.

After the second proofing, place directly into a preheated oven and bake until it sounds hollow when tapped. Oven temperature is again a most important factor. If bread is placed in an oven that is not hot enough, the bread will not continue to rise in the oven and will be smaller than intended.

After baking, bread is removed from the pan immediately and cooled on cooling racks that allow good air circulation. Do not cool bread in a draft or the crust may crack. Once cooled, store bread in plastic bags, except for hard-crusted breads (the crust will soften if placed in plastic). If the bread is not completely cooled when you place it in a bag, moisture will build up inside the wrapping, making the bread soggy and encouraging mold growth.

To save much time, you can purchase frozen bread dough (usually in one-pound loaves) at the supermarket that is ready to be proofed and baked. Not only are they convenient to make your own loaf of bread, they are wonderful for making a pizza crust or being cut up to make rolls, as shown in the illustrations. For pizza, all you need to do is let the dough rise in a warm spot while you lightly saute (preferably in a nonstick pan using vegetable cooking spray) some vegetables. Then assemble the pizza by spreading tomato sauce on the crust, sprinkling mozzarella cheese (made from skim milk), and spreading the vegetables evenly on top.

Good yeast breads are characterized by an even golden brown color; the bread should be light for its size; it should have a good shape and have a tender or crispy crust as desired. The interior should be soft and free from large air pockets (evidence of letting the bread proof for too long a period of time); the texture of the bread should be smooth by having very fine air cells within the interior; the aroma should be pleasing, not strong; the interior color should be off-white.

Most yeast breads use minimal amounts of fat, amounting to no more than 1 to 2 grams per slice, and provide lots of nutrients for their calories. As explained in Chapter 2, whole wheat and other

Tying a figure eight roll.

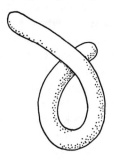

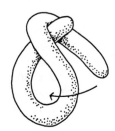

Tying a single-knot roll.

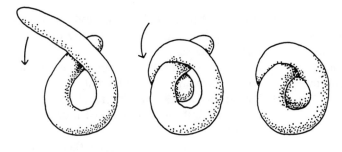

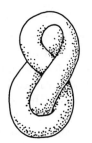

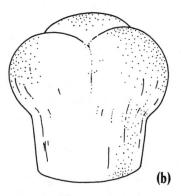

Cloverleaf rolls.

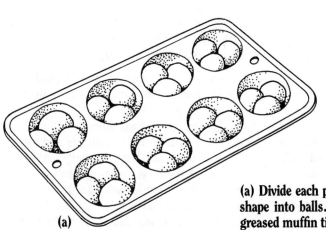

(a)

(b)

(a) Divide each piece of dough into three equal parts, and shape into balls. Place three balls in the bottom of each greased muffin tin. (b) The baked roll has this appearance.

whole grain breads contain many more vitamins, minerals, and fiber than white bread. There is a recipe for Whole Wheat Bread on page 275.

Breads such as rich dinner rolls, brioche, danish pastry, croissants, and sweet rolls such as cinnamon rolls contain more fat. Commercially made danish pastry with little or no fat is available at the supermarket, and there are sweet roll recipes that cut back dramatically on the fat but still taste great. Dinner rolls, of course, don't have to be made from a rich dough—they can be made quite easily from regular bread dough. As for brioche and croissants, they rely on fat (it's actually butter) for their flakiness, so lower-in-fat versions are simply not successful.

The amount of salt used in making bread is minimal. Don't change the amount the recipe calls for because salt is very important in controlling the growth of the yeast (and production of gases).

QUICK BREADS

Quick breads are essentially what the name implies—breads made quickly. While yeast breads require time for rising, the leavening action in a quick bread is caused by baking powder, baking soda, or steam (and sometimes combinations of all three) which cause the baked good to rise in the oven. Quick breads include muffins, certain loaf breads (such as banana bread), biscuits, pancakes, waffles, quick coffee cakes, cream puffs, and popovers. Many traditional recipes for quick breads contain more fat and sugar than necessary, but they are very adaptable to some simple modifications.

Muffins are a very popular quick bread, available in many different varieties. Following are the steps in making muffins and loaf breads.

1. Mix dry ingredients in one bowl and blend liquid ingredients in another.
2. Pour liquid ingredients, all at once, over the dry ingredients and stir together just until blended. The mixture will still be lumpy.

Following are tips for making and storing muffins and loaf breads.

- Do not overmix the batter or dough—it develops too much gluten and this results in a tough baked product with peaked tops and vertical tunnels running through it. Stir just until dry ingredients are moistened. The batter should be lumpy. The only exception to this rule is popovers—they must be beaten very well before pouring into cups for baking.
- Dried fruits, such as raisins, should be steeped in water before using them in recipes so they are plump and don't rob moisture from the batter during mixing and baking.
- Grease and flour pans, unless using nonstick pans.
- Once the batter or dough is ready, put into pans and bake right away to ensure that they rise as much as possible.
- Bake in the top third of the oven so the bottoms do not burn and they cook evenly.
- Bake until a wooden pick inserted into the center comes out clean. Overbaked muffins will be dry.
- Let muffins cool for 5 minutes then remove from pans; otherwise they will become soggy. Cool on wire racks. Loaf breads can cool in the pan.
- Store cooled baked goods in plastic at room temperature, where they can stay fresh for up to 4 days. They can also be frozen for 2 to 3 months in air-tight packaging.

Biscuits are characterized by a very rough appearance with a light golden color and cake-like interior. They use more fat, usually shortening, than most other quick breads. Biscuits generally double in size during the baking process and go well with any meal. Biscuits are made from a dough following these steps.

1. Cut shortening into the dry ingredients until the mixture becomes crumbly. Biscuits can also be made using oil.
2. Combine liquid ingredients.
3. Add liquid to dry ingredients and mix dough only until soft but not sticky and leaves the side of the bowl, forming a ball.
4. Dough is then kneaded gently.
5. Dough is rolled to about half the desired thickness of finished biscuits (usually 1 inch) and

cut into desired shapes using round cookie/biscuit cutter.

6. Dough is placed ½ inch apart on baking pan for crispy biscuits or touching each other for softer biscuits. Brush the tops with milk to enhance browning.

Cornbread is very similar to the muffin mixture, except that it is usually baked in a pan, as opposed to individual muffins.

Popovers are leavened primarily with the use of steam. When pouring them into the greased cavities of a muffin tin, place them directly into a preheated oven without delay. The popovers will rise due to the steam that they produce.

Pancakes (also known as griddle cakes) are a form of a quick bread that is characterized by a very thin, pourable batter used primarily as a breakfast food. **Crepes** (also known as French pancakes) are similar to pancakes but have a much more velvety appearance and a thinner, smoother batter. Crepes are wonderful for any meal and for desserts. They are commonly stuffed with meat, fish, fruit, and sometimes are served flambe style (flaming with the aid of brandy).

The **waffle** is very similar to the pancake batter, but is slightly thicker and somewhat richer. The use of a waffle iron is used to create the characteristic shape. Waffles should be made to order and are served with syrups, fruits, frozen yogurt, and other creation that may be your favorite.

Making Quick Breads Nutritious
Quick breads vary in how much fat they contain. Most can be made with significantly less fat or at least a less saturated fat. Muffins and loaf bread recipes are easily adaptable to using less sugar and fat; biscuits are a little harder. Here are some tips to modify recipes (also consult Table 60).

- You can decrease the fat in many of your quick bread recipes by about one-fourth to one-third of the original amount without any significant difference in quality. In recipes for muffins, quick breads, and biscuits, the minimum amount of fat is 1 to 2 tablespoons per cup of flour.
- You can substitute soft tub margarine or liquid margarine for stick margarine or butter in a recipe to get less fat and less saturated fat. You can also substitute oil for shortening (⅓ cup oil for each half cup of shortening).
- Many quick breads, especially muffins and loaf breads, are ideal candidates for fiber-rich ingredients such as fruits, raisins, wheat or oat bran, whole wheat flour, and rolled oats.
- Whole wheat pastry flour can be substituted for white flour in quick breads that use baking powder. Usually whole wheat pastry flour can replace half the white flour called for in the recipe with good results. Simply substitute an equivalent amount of whole wheat pastry flour for white flour. You may find whole wheat pastry flour at the supermarket; if not, check your natural foods store.
- You can decrease the sugar in muffin and quick bread recipes to 1 tablespoon sugar per cup of flour.
- Decrease the amount of nuts in a recipe by half. Nuts are full of fats and calories.
- When choosing muffin and loaf bread recipes, try to choose those with 5 grams or less of fat per muffin or serving. Whereas some muffins can be full of hearty, healthy ingredients such as whole wheat flour and fruits, other muffins resemble little cakes (with their high fat and sugar content).
- Biscuits do not have to be made with shortening; oil can be used (see the recipe on page 278 for Whole Wheat Biscuits).

Also, always remember to use vegetable spray to grease muffin pans (or use nonstick pans).

CAKES

Cakes are another popular form of dessert that are made from a thin batter containing flour, liquid, eggs, fat (in most cases), leavening, and flavoring. Although available in mixes (that are usually very good and are now available with less fat), the fun and pleasure of making a cake is still a favorite among those who will take the challenge. Although commercial bakeries were known to sell cakes that were exclusively made from "scratch" (a term referring to a cake made from raw ingredients), the industry has moved to the area of mixes. It may be hard to believe, but many bakeries now use mixes in the production of many of their baked goods.

Cakes are divided into three basic categories according to fat content:

Shortened or butter cake The shortened cake contains fat and requires a baking pan that has been oiled and dusted with flour prior to pouring the batter. This group generally includes the layer cakes, white cakes, yellow cakes, and pound cakes, to name a few. The shortened cake is characterized by a smooth, very lightly browned exterior. The texture is tender and moist. The steps in making a shortened cake are as follows.

1. Cream fat and sugar together until fluffy. This can be done by hand, using the back of a spoon, or at moderate speed using a mixer and paddle attachment.
2. Beat in eggs, one at a time, beating well after each addition.
3. Add one-third of sifted dry ingredients at a time into bowl and beat until smooth. Add half the liquid ingredients and beat just until well-blended. Repeat with second third of dry ingredients, second half of liquid ingredients, and end with remaining dry ingredients. Beat just until smooth and creamy. Scrape down the bowl with a rubber spatula at least once during this step for even mixing. The reason for alternately adding the flour and liquid ingredients is to make sure the flour absorbs all the liquid.

Unshortened or foam-type cake An unshortened cake contains no fat and rises due to the beaten egg whites that are part of the formula. The classic example is the angel food cake. It is a very tasty cake, low in fat and calories, and has many varieties. The baking pan for making an angel food cake is usually a tube pan. Sponge cakes are also examples of an unshortened cake. They are commonly used to make jelly roll. Unlike angel food cakes, they may have some leavening added. Unshortened cakes are characterized by being very light, free from any cracks, light brown in color, tender and moist (not dry), with an excellent shape. The steps to make an angel food cake are as follows.

1. Have the egg whites slightly warmed as they attain more volume when they are warm.
2. Sift the flour with half the sugar; this makes it easier for the flour to mix evenly with the egg whites.
3. Beat the egg whites until they form soft peaks.
4. Gradually beat in the sugar that was not mixed with the flour. Continue to beat until the egg whites form soft, glossy peaks. Do not over-beat.
5. Fold in the flour-sugar mixture just until it is completely absorbed.
6. Put into ungreased tube pan and bake immediately.

Semi-shortened cake The chiffon cake is an example of a cake that has a minimal amount of fat—usually an oil. It is relatively light and moist and has a nice spongy texture, good volume and taste. Like angel food, it is airy, but its texture is closer to a shortened cake because (unlike angel food cake) it does contain egg yolks and oil. Chiffon cake is easier to make than angel food cake and can be made in less time. It also is adaptable to adding fruit flavors, such as pineapple or raspberry.

The steps in making chiffon cake are as follows.

1. The dry ingredients are mixed in one bowl and a well is made in the center.
2. The wet ingredients (except the eggs) are mixed slowly into the dry ingredients.
3. Egg whites are beaten until foamy, then sugar is added gradually until the whites are stiff (but not dry), glossy, and just hold their shape (they should not droop). If the egg whites are underwhipped, the cake will be tough. If the egg whites are overwhipped, the cake may sink after baking.
4. Stiffly beaten egg whites are folded in gently with the batter.
5. Batter is put into an ungreased tube pan or in layer pans that have had the bottoms (not the sides) oiled and dusted with flour.

Making Cakes and Icings Nutritious

Angel food cake is a good choice as it contains no fat. Although the classic chiffon cake uses five

Tips for Making, Icing, and Storing Cakes

❖ ❖ ❖

PREPARING AND BAKING

- Preheat the oven.
- Grease and flour pans if called for, or use non-stick pans.
- The most common fault in making sponge cakes is insufficient beating of the eggs and sugar, so be sure to beat them until stiff peaks form.
- If using egg whites, they separate easier if cold but create the most volume when whipped at room temperature. Make sure the mixing bowl and utensils are free of fat as fat will create less volume. Don't use glass or plastic bowls to whip egg whites—they may also create less volume. A copper bowl and whisk are actually the best for whipping egg whites.
- If creaming fat and sugar, the fat creams better when it is about room temperature—so let it sit on the kitchen counter for about one-half hour. Cream until the mixture is the consistency of stiff whipped cream.
- Don't let cake batter sit around in the kitchen—get it in the oven or it will deflate.
- Don't fill a cake pan more than three-quarters full or else it may overflow during baking. Use a ladle or spoon for filling the pans so you are less likely to overfill.
- When loading the oven, leave space for air to circulate between pans and between each pan and the side and back of the oven.
- Bake at just the right temperature (you should have an oven thermometer to help out here). If the oven is too hot, the cake will not rise properly and the crust and bottom may brown too much, even burn. If the oven isn't hot enough, the cake will not rise properly and may fall.
- Once in the oven, leave cakes alone until the crust starts to brown. The motion involved in opening the oven door and letting cool air in could make the cake fall.
- To test for doneness, shortened cakes will pull away from the sides of the pan, the center should spring back when lightly touched, and a toothpick or cake tester will come out clean when inserted in the thickest part of the cake.
- Most cakes require 15 minutes of cooling prior to removal from the pan. Use a cooling rack so that the cooling air can circulate on the bottom of the pan and reduce the temperature quickly. In the case of unshortened cakes, you should run a metal spatula along the sides of the pan in order to help remove it from the pan. Then you can put one wire rack on top of, and one below, the cake. Invert and remove pan. For angel food cake, cool upside down on something like a soft drink bottle. Once cool, run a metal spatula along the sides of the pan and remove carefully.

ICING

- Do not attempt to ice the cake until it is completely cool; otherwise the cake will stick to your spatula and ruin the appearance of the icing.
- Dip the metal spatula into hot water for a few minutes prior to icing the cake. A warm spatula will spread the icing easier, faster, and have less of a tendency of pulling up the crumbs from the surface of the cake.
- If there is a tear in the side of the cake, mix ½ cup icing with 3 tablespoons water to make a very thin mixture. Spread over broken surface to coat evenly. Allow to dry before frosting cake.

STORING

- Shortened or butter cakes stay fresh at room temperature for up to one week or can be frozen (don't ice until later) for up to 6 months.
- Angel, sponge, and chiffon cakes only stay fresh for about four days (although chiffon can last up to two weeks) at room temperature. They can be frozen (don't ice until later) for up to 6 months.
- Cheesecake must be refrigerated and can be held up to 4 days. It can also be frozen up to 4 months.

whole eggs, these can be replaced with one whole egg and egg whites or just egg whites. On page 279, there is a recipe for Orange Chiffon Cake that uses no egg yolks. When choosing recipes or mixes for shortened cakes, try to select one with 5 grams or less per serving.

You can adjust the recipes of shortened cakes in the following ways to get a more nutritious, yet tasty, product.

1. Substitute cake flour for all-purpose flour. When you are decreasing the amount of shortening and sugar in a recipe, there is a tendency for the product to be less tender. Cake flour makes a more tender and delicate cake because it has less gluten than all other flours—gluten is what gives all baked goods their structure.

2. Decrease the fat in many of your recipes by about one-fourth to one-third of the original amount without any significant difference in quality. The minimum amount of fat in cake recipes is 2 tablespoons per cup of flour.

3. Don't substitute vegetable oil for solid fat, such as shortening or margarine, in cakes that require creaming, as the cake will be flat. Instead use unsalted margarine.

4. If you are trying to eliminate the fat from a cake recipe, substitute fruit pulps, such as applesauce, bananas, or stewed prunes, for the fat. Fruit pulps can perform the same functions as fat in cakes: add moisture and tenderness. Fruit pulps can also be substituted for part of the fat in a recipe.

5. In a cake with no fat, don't go overboard on the number of egg whites you use because they contribute to a dry product. You can probably cut back on them without ill effect.

6. When decreasing fat, you also need to decrease sugar; otherwise you will have a sticky baked good. You can decrease the sugar in many of your recipes by about one-fourth to one-third of the original amount without any significant difference in quality. You can decrease the sugar in cake recipes to ½ cup per cup of flour. Cakes with less sugar may be more like a quick bread than a cake.

Of course, grease baking pans with vegetable spray.

Most icings are high in fat and sugar. Some alternatives include:

- A sprinkling of confectioners' sugar
- No-sugar fruit spreads
- Fresh fruit or berries
- A glaze made by combining confectioners' sugar and fruit juice concentrate (try 1½ cups confectioners' sugar to 4 tablespoons juice concentrate and 1 teaspoon lemon)
- Fruit sauce (mash raw or cooked fruit with a potato masher or process in a food processor)

COOKIES

Cookies are one of the most popular baked goods available in many different varieties. Although cookies can be purchased in dry mixes and in refrigerated, ready to shape and bake forms, the fun of making cookies from scratch will yield a product that is truly unique.

The main difference between most cookie and cake batters is the lower amount of liquid in the cookie batter. Cookie doughs range from liquidy to very stiff, and these differences often call for different mixing methods, although the basic steps are much like those for shortened cakes.

For cookie sheets, use heavyweight, flat (or barely turned up edges) pans so the cookies can cook evenly. Heavyweight pans are less likely to warp, and ones made out of aluminum conduct heat nicely. Nonstick cookie sheets are fine, just be sure they are made from a heavyweight metal and are coated with a good nonstick material such as Silverstone. Insulated cookie sheets (they have air sandwiched between two sheets of aluminum) are helpful to prevent burned cookie bottoms, and cookies baked on them may sometimes require more baking time than the recipe calls for.

When baking any type of cookie, you may try to find a product known as parchment or baker's paper. This is a heat-resistant paper that is used on top of pans and requires no greasing (even if the recipe calls for it!). The main advantage of using this paper is that it reduces cleanup to a minimum. It is also useful when you need to reuse your pans during baking as you can place the

TIPS FOR MAKING AND STORING COOKIES

- Preheat the oven and make sure the temperature is accurate. Most cookies are baked quickly at a high temperature and if the temperature is too high, the cookies will burn on the edges and bottoms. If the temperature is too low, the cookie may spread too much across the pan and turn out hard, dry, and without a nice brown color.
- Your baking pans may, or may not, need to be greased. (Richer cookies often do not require greased pans.) Check the recipe. If so, lightly grease with vegetable shortening or a vegetable spray, otherwise the cookies may spread too much. Preferably, use parchment paper.
- Place cookie sheets in the upper half of the oven to prevent burned bottoms. Use the middle rack for one cookie sheet. For two cookie sheets, place side-by-side on the middle rack, if they can fit with at least one inch of space in the middle. If not, place one on one side of the middle rack, and the other sheet on the other side of a rack placed at the top of the oven. With this arrangement, you need to switch the position of both sheets halfway through baking.

- Watch cookies carefully in the oven—they will overbake much quicker than you think.
- When the edges and bottoms of the cookies are golden brown, they're done.
- When cookies are still warm, but firm enough to be handled without breaking, remove them from the pan so they won't stick. Recipes will generally tell you the cooling time needed.
- Do not cool cookies too quickly, as they might crack.
- Cookies will generally keep well in an air-tight container for up to one week, and in some cases, even longer. Only store cookies that have completely cooled and store different types of cookies separately to avoid sogginess. (Crisp cookies are noted for stealing moisture from cake-type cookies, ruining both of them!)
- Cookies can be frozen in air-tight packages for up to 3 or 4 months. If cookies need to be frosted or glazed, wait to do so until they are thawed. Brownies also freeze well.

cookie dough directly onto the parchment paper and then place the paper onto a cookie sheet. When you put cookie dough onto a hot baking sheet, the dough will spread and start to bake before being put into the oven. Baker's paper is used throughout the commercial baking industry. It is often available at a kitchen supply/cooking store.

There are many different types of cookies. Here are a few of the more popular ones.

- **Dropped cookies** are made from a soft dough or batter and are dropped onto a cookie sheet from a spoon. Two spoons are usually used: one to scoop out the batter and the other to push the batter out onto the cooking sheet. The cookies should be similar in size and shape

so they cook evenly and for the same period of time.
- **Rolled cookies** are cut out from a stiff chilled dough with cookie cutters. They tend to be rich cookies.
- **Molded and pressed** cookies are molded into the desired shapes by hand or using a cookie mold or cookie press. They also tend to be rich cookies.
- **Refrigerator or icebox cookies** are made ahead of time and stored in the refrigerator in rolls until they are needed. Then they are cut and baked.
- **Bar cookies**, like brownies, are baked in pans rather than on cookie sheets. They are generally cooled completely in the pan before removing.

Making Cookies Nutritious

Many cookies can be categorized as being crisp or soft. Crisp cookies are crisp because of their high sugar and fat content and their low proportion of liquid in the recipe. On the other hand, soft cookies have a high proportion of liquid in the recipe and lower sugar and fat content, so softer texture cookies are generally more nutritious. Select recipes that use whole grains such as whole wheat flour or oatmeal, and fruits, including dried fruits such as raisins. When choosing recipes for cookies, try to select one with 3 grams of fat or less per cookie.

The following adjustments can be made to recipes to make cookies more nutritious.

1. The fat level can usually be adjusted to 2 tablespoons per cup of flour. Decreasing the fat too much in rolled cookies can make a dough that is difficult to roll out.
2. For soft cookies, you can substitute soft tub margarine or liquid margarine for stick margarine or butter in a recipe. You can also substitute oil for shortening (⅓ cup oil for each half cup of shortening). These changes result in less saturated fat.
3. Whole wheat pastry flour can be substituted for white flour in cookies such as oat, molasses, carrot, date, and pumpkin. Usually whole wheat pastry flour can replace half the white flour called for in the recipe with good results. Simply substitute an equivalent amount of whole wheat pastry flour for white flour. Using whole wheat pastry flour in rich cookies such as shortbread doesn't work nearly as well. If the whole wheat flour causes the cookie to be too heavy, increase the proportion of white flour to whole wheat.
4. You can decrease the sugar in many of your recipes by about one-fourth to one-third of the original amount without any significant difference in quality.
5. Substitute raisins and chopped dry fruit in baking for chocolate chips.
6. Cut back by half the amount of nuts called for in a recipe. Nuts are full of fat and calories.

Also, try to use parchment paper on cookie sheets so they don't have to be greased.

PIES

Pies and pastry are among the most popular desserts. Pies are truly an American treat, with apple pie being among the most favorite. A most important aspect of good pies and pastry hinges primarily on the quality of the crust. In all instances the crust should be flaky, tender, and flavorful.

Pies are comprised of two basic parts—the crust and the filling. Many varieties can be created which may include either a one- or two-crust pie, and a variety of fruit, creams, puddings, or other fillings.

The pie dough, also known as the crust, is generally only made up of four ingredients—flour, fat, salt, and water. Unfortunately, these four ingredients can create a real challenge to the novice—ranging from perfect to a total disaster! In order to achieve a level of perfection, it is important not to let the flour develop too much gluten. This happens when the dough is handled too much. Here are the basic procedures.

1. The flour. The flour can either be all-purpose (readily available in the supermarket) or a pastry flour. The flour gives the basic structure to the dough. It should be fresh, without any lumps or bugs—look carefully. The flour is placed into a large bowl.
2. The salt. The salt lends flavor of its own to the dough and helps to color the baked crust. The salt can be added either to the flour (thoroughly mixed) or can be combined with the water (thoroughly stirred prior to addition).
3. The fat. Recipes often call for shortening, although a mixture of half shortening and half margarine (see recipe on page 282) is quite acceptable. Oil can even be used, but the crust will not be as flaky as those using solid fats. Commercial bakeries that make their own dough for pies use a form of shortening known as "high ratio shortening." This is designed specifically for baking. The fat, chilled prior to use so it does not melt during handling (resulting in a pie crust that isn't flaky), is added to the flour and salt mixture and is incorporated by a method known as "cutting in." This can be accomplished in three different ways.

1. Pastry Blender. A pastry blender is a device specifically designed for cutting the fat into the flour mixture. Its purpose is to cut the fat in such a way that the fat is broken into the shape of "garden peas" and each pea is coated with flour.

2. Two Butter Knives. The use of two butter knives used at a 90-degree angle from one another will perform the same basic task as a pastry blender. Be careful not to over-mix the dough.

3. A Metal Dinner Fork. The use of a metal dinner fork works least best of the three methods, but with practice will help to make a pie dough.

4. The water. The water should be very cold so as not to melt the fat. If you elect to add the salt to the water (instead of to the flour), stir the water just before adding it slowly to the pie dough as you are gently mixing it with a spoon or fork. As the water is being added, mix just enough to blend the ingredients together into the shape of a ball. If you overmix the dough, it will appear greasy and will yield a tough crust. Wrap the dough with clear wrap and refrigerate it for 20 minutes so it will be easier to roll out.

The metal blade of the food processor can be used to make pie dough in seconds. Simply add small chunks of fat into the flour and salt in the work bowl and pulse 3 or 4 times. Add the water through the feed tube while pulsing very rapidly (about 20–30 times) until it is just about gathered into a ball. Remove and press together.

While the dough is chilling in the refrigerator, start making your filling. After making the filling, you are ready to roll the pie dough.

1. If making a double-crust pie (top and bottom crusts), cut the dough in half, and place one half back into the refrigerator.

2. Place the dough on top of a piece of wax paper that is very lightly dusted with flour.

3. Push down on the dough, keeping it rounded, and place another piece of wax paper on top.

4. Roll out the dough in a rounded shape so that it is about 1–2 inches larger than the pie pan

(note: place the pie pan on top of the dough to approximate this distance).

5. Place the dough into the pie tin (glass is best, metal, aluminum disposable, etc.) and pour in the filling.

6. To finish the edge of the pie crust, trim the edge within ½ inch of the rim. Now, you can press the tines of a fork around the entire rim of the pie plate for a decorative finish.

When using a pie filling that is soggy, such as custard, or when the filling does not need to be cooked, the pie crust is partially or fully baked before it is filled. Follow your recipe carefully.

When making a two-crust pie, roll out the second piece of dough a little thinner than the first. Place the top crust on the filled pie, press the edges to seal with your fingers, and trim the edge to within ½ inch of the rim. You can now flute the edges using your thumb and forefinger.

To bake the pie, brush the top of the pie with milk (to help brown the crust) just prior to baking. Place the pie into a preheated oven (usually 400–425°F) and bake for the prescribed time (usually until golden brown).

Leftover pie dough pieces can be reused to make miniature tarts (along with leftover fillings). Once again, be careful not to overmix the dough or it will become very tough.

Besides the traditional pie shells, there are crumb crusts, such as graham cracker crust. They are easy and quick to make and are used only for unbaked pies, such as cream pies. Crumb crusts may also use vanilla or chocolate wafer crumbs, or gingersnap crumbs. See the recipes for lower-in-fat graham cracker and vanilla wafer crusts on page 282.

Making Pies Nutritious

The traditional pastry dough recipes use a significant amount of fat, and those that use shortening are higher in saturated fat than they need be. As the Healthier Pie Crust recipe indicates, it is possible to have a flaky crust using less total fat, and substituting half the shortening with margarine. You can also use 1 cup of flour to 3–4 tablespoons of stick margarine and 3 tablespoons of cold water. Oil can also be used to make a pie crust, as seen in the Apple Pie recipe, although oily crusts tend not to be quite as flaky as regular crusts. When making pies, avoid two-crust pies.

Now that we figured out how to make a better crust, let's take a look at fillings. Fruits, of course, make excellent fillings, and to cut down on sugar in fruit pies, use sweet fruit and six tablespoons sugar or less per pie. If you love custard or cream-filled pies, there are lower-in-fat recipes available. For a tasty cream-style pie, fill the graham cracker or vanilla wafer crusts on page 282 with pudding made with low-fat or skim milk. Top with ⅓ cup heavy cream whipped with ⅔ cup plain low-fat yogurt. Or make a pie by blending yogurt, fresh or frozen fruit, and 1 cup whipped cream. Pour into pie shell and freeze.

Instead of making pie crust, a good alternative is a fruit crumble or cobbler, as discussed in the first section of this chapter.

RECIPES

Fruit-Based Desserts

BAKED APPLES

¼ cup or less brown sugar
1 tsp cinnamon
1 tbsp vegetable oil
⅓ cup raisins
6 medium baking apples, cored

1. In a bowl, mix sugar, cinnamon, oil, and raisins. Fill center of apples and place upright in a baking dish. Pour 1 cup water around apples.
2. Bake at 375°F 45–60 minutes, basting frequently.

Serves 6

Nutrition Analysis:

Calories	159
Carbohydrate	36 grams
Fiber	3 grams
Fat	3 grams
Cholesterol	0 milligrams
Sodium	5 milligrams

Puddings

RAISIN WHOLE WHEAT BREAD PUDDING

1½ cups whole wheat bread, cut into 1-inch cubes
⅓ cup raisins
2 tbsp sugar
¾ tsp ground cinnamon
1 egg
¼ tsp vanilla
1¼ cups skim milk

1. Preheat oven to 325°F (slow).
2. Place bread cubes in 1-quart casserole. Sprinkle with raisins.
3. Mix sugar and cinnamon. Stir in egg. Add vanilla.
4. Heat milk; slowly stir into egg mixture. Pour over bread.

5. Bake until tip of knife inserted in center comes out clean—about 40 minutes.

Serves 4

Nutrition Analysis:

Calories	156
Carbohydrate	29 grams
Fiber	3 grams
Fat	2 grams
Cholesterol	55 milligrams
Sodium	190 milligrams

Meringue

SOFT MERINGUE

2 egg whites
½ tsp cream of tartar
5 tbsp granulated sugar

1. Place egg whites and cream of tartar into a small stainless steel bowl and beat with whisk until a coarse foam is formed.
2. Add ½ tbsp of sugar at a time and continue beating.
3. After addition of all sugar, continue beating until stiff peaks form and sugar dissolves.
4. Spoon meringue, using the back of a spoon, into 4-inch circles.

5. Bake at 350°F for 50 to 60 minutes until dry and firm.
6. Let cool and fill with fresh fruit or fruit sauce.

Serves 2

Nutrition Analysis:

Calories 130
Carbohydrate. . . . . .30 grams
Fiber . . . . .0 grams
Fat. . . . . .0 grams
Cholesterol. . . . . .0 milligrams
Sodium . . . . .55 milligrams

Yeast Breads

WHOLE WHEAT BREAD

6 cups whole wheat flour
1 package active dry yeast
1 tsp salt
2 cups water
¼ cup oil
2 tbsp honey

1. Mix 2 cups of the flour with yeast and salt.
2. Heat water and oil together until warm (105–115°F). Add honey. Stir into flour mixture. Beat well.
3. Mix in enough of the remaining flour to make a soft dough that leaves the side of the bowl.
4. Knead on a lightly floured surface until dough is smooth and elastic, about 15 minutes.
5. Place dough in greased bowl and turn over once to grease upper side of dough.
6. Cover and let rise in a warm place (80–85°F) until double in size, about 1 hour.
7. Grease two 9 × 5 × 3-inch loaf pans.

8. Press dough down to remove air bubbles.
9. Divide dough in half. Shape each half into a loaf. Place in pans.
10. Cover and let rise in a warm place until double in size, about 50 minutes.
11. Preheat oven to 375°F (moderate).
12. Bake until bread sounds hollow when tapped, about 30 minutes.
13. Remove bread from pans and cool on rack.

Makes 2 loaves (20 slices/loaf)

Nutrition Analysis per slice:

Calories 76
Carbohydrate. . . . . .14 grams
Fiber . . . . .2 grams
Fat. . . . . .2 grams
Cholesterol. . . . . .0 milligrams
Sodium . . . . .54 milligrams

DEEP DISH PIZZA

1 package active dry yeast
1 cup warm water (105–115°F)
1 tsp sugar
1 tsp salt
2 tbsp oil
2½ cups all-purpose or whole wheat flour
1 cup sliced vegetables
1 jar (15½ oz) pizza sauce
6 oz shredded, low-fat cheese such as part-skim
   mozzarella

1. Dissolve yeast in water.
2. Stir in sugar, salt, vegetable oil, and flour. Beat vigorously 20 strokes. Let rest about 5 minutes.
3. Saute vegetables for a few minutes in pan sprayed with vegetable cooking spray.

4. Press dough evenly on bottom and halfway up sides of greased 13 × 9 × 2-inch pan.
5. Put on sauce, vegetables, then shredded cheese.
6. Bake at 425°F for 20–25 minutes.

Makes 8 slices

Nutrition Analysis:

Calories 264
Carbohydrate . . . . .37 grams
Fiber . . . . .3 grams
Fat . . . . .8 grams
Cholesterol . . . . .12 milligrams
Sodium . . . . .645 milligrams

Quick Breads

PEANUT BUTTER APPLE MUFFINS

2 cups all-purpose flour
4 tsp baking powder
¾ tsp salt
1 tsp cinnamon
¾ tsp nutmeg
3 tbsp oil
¼ cup peanut butter
½ cup sugar
1 egg
1 cup skim milk
1 cup chopped unpeeled apple

1. Combine flour, baking powder, salt, cinnamon, and nutmeg.
2. In a separate bowl, blend oil and peanut butter together. Gradually add sugar and beat until

fluffy. Add egg and beat well. Stir in milk and apple.
3. Add flour mixture to peanut butter mixture all at once. Stir just enough to moisten ingredients.
4. Fill paper-lined muffin cups ⅔ full.
5. Bake at 400°F for 20 minutes.

Makes 16 muffins

Nutrition Analysis:

Calories 142
Carbohydrate . . . . .21 grams
Fiber . . . . .1 gram
Fat . . . . .5 grams
Cholesterol . . . . .13 milligrams
Sodium . . . . .214 milligrams

WHOLE WHEAT CORNMEAL MUFFINS

⅔ cup yellow cornmeal, degerminated
⅔ cup whole wheat flour
1 tbsp sugar
2 tsp baking powder
⅛ tsp salt
⅔ cup skim milk

1 egg, beaten
2 tbsp oil

1. Preheat oven to 400°F (hot).
2. Grease 8 muffin tins or use paper liners.
3. Mix dry ingredients thoroughly.

4. Mix milk, egg, and oil. Add to dry ingredients. Stir until dry ingredients are barely moistened. Batter will be lumpy.

5. Fill muffin tins two-thirds full. Bake until lightly browned—about 20 minutes.

Makes 8 muffins

Nutrition Analysis:
Calories 128
Carbohydrate. . . . . .19 grams
Fiber . . . . .2 grams
Fat. . . . . .4 grams
Cholesterol. . . . . .27 milligrams
Sodium. . . . . .133 milligrams

READY BAKE BRAN MUFFINS

3 cups unprocessed bran
1 cup boiling water
2 eggs, slightly beaten
2 cups buttermilk, nonfat yogurt or soured skim milk
½ cup vegetable oil
1 cup raisins, currants, or chopped pitted prunes, dried dates, or apricots
2½ tsp baking soda
½ tsp salt
⅓ cup sugar
1 cup unsifted enriched all-purpose flour
1½ cups whole wheat flour

1. Preheat oven to 425°F.

2. Mix bran and boiling water together in a large bowl, stir to moisten evenly, and set aside to cool.

3. In another bowl, mix together the eggs, buttermilk, oil, and raisins; stir into the bran mixture.

4. In third bowl, stir together the baking soda, salt, sugar, all-purpose flour, and whole wheat flour; stir into bran mixture.

5. Put in greased muffin pans and bake about 20 minutes.

Makes 24 muffins

Nutrition Analysis:
Calories 147
Carbohydrate. . . . . .23 grams
Fiber . . . . .2 grams
Fat. . . . . .5 grams
Cholesterol. . . . . .19 milligrams
Sodium. . . . . .150 milligrams

WHOLE WHEAT CORN BREAD

½ cup whole wheat flour
2½ tsp baking powder
½ tsp salt
1 tbsp sugar
1 cup yellow cornmeal
1 egg
2 tbsp vegetable oil
¾ cup buttermilk

1. Preheat the oven to 350°F.

2. Spray an 8 × 8-inch baking pan with baking spray or lightly coat it with vegetable oil.

3. Sift the flour, baking powder, salt, and sugar into a large bowl. Stir in the cornmeal.

4. In a separate bowl, beat together the egg, vegetable oil, and milk.

5. Stir the liquids into the dry ingredients quickly. Pour the batter into the prepared pan and bake until firm and nicely browned on top, about 20 minutes.

Serves 8

Nutrition Analysis:
Calories 130
Carbohydrate. . . . . .20 grams
Fiber . . . . .2 grams
Fat. . . . . .4 grams
Cholesterol. . . . . .32 milligrams
Sodium. . . . . .294 milligrams

Biscuits

WHOLE WHEAT BISCUITS

1 cup whole wheat flour
1 cup all-purpose flour
2½ tsp baking powder
½ tsp salt
⅔ cup skim milk
⅓ cup oil

1. Preheat oven to 450°F.
2. Mix dry ingredients thoroughly.
3. Mix milk and oil.
4. Make a depression in center of dry ingredients. Pour in liquid mixture all at once.
5. Stir with a fork until dough leaves the side of the bowl.
6. Knead dough gently on a lightly floured surface 18 times.
7. Roll to ½-inch thickness.
8. Cut with a 2-inch biscuit cutter.
9. Place on ungreased baking sheet.
10. Bake until lightly browned, about 12 minutes.

Makes 12 biscuits

Nutrition Analysis:

Calories	130
Carbohydrate	16 grams
Fiber	2 grams
Fat	6 grams
Cholesterol	0 milligrams
Sodium	165 milligrams

Cakes

CARROT CAKE

Oil for greasing pan
3 cups cake flour
2 tsp baking powder
1 tsp baking soda
1 tsp ground cinnamon
½ tsp salt
1 cup applesauce
1 cup light brown sugar
1 cup granulated sugar
3 egg whites
grated rind and juice of one orange
3 cups peeled, shredded carrots
1 cup raisins
Orange glaze: 1½ cups confectioners' sugar
4 tbsp orange juice concentrate
1 tsp lemon juice

1. Preheat oven to 350°F. Lightly grease bundt-style pan or 10-inch springform pan with center hole.
2. Combine flour, baking powder, baking soda, cinnamon, and salt. Set aside.
3. Beat together applesauce, sugars, egg whites, and orange rind and juice.
4. Blend in flour mixture with mixer at medium speed, beating only until smooth. Do not overheat.
5. Stir in carrots and raisins.
6. Pour batter into prepared pan and bake 50–60 minutes or until a knife inserted near center comes out clean. Remove cake from pan, or, if using springform, remove sides of pan and put cake on wire rack to cool completely. Spoon orange glaze over cake and serve.

Serves 20

Nutrition Analysis:

Calories	213
Carbohydrate	52 grams
Fiber	2 grams
Fat	0 grams
Cholesterol	0 milligrams
Sodium	146 milligrams

ANGEL FOOD CAKE

1 cup sifted cake flour
1½ cups confectioners' sugar
1 tsp cream of tartar
½ tsp salt
1½ cups egg whites (about 12) at room temperature
1 tsp vanilla extract
½ tsp almond extract
1 tsp lemon juice

1. Preheat the oven to 325°F.
2. Sift together flour and ½ cup of the sugar. Set aside.
3. Sprinkle the cream of tartar and salt over the egg whites and beat in a very large, clean bowl, using a hand-held or electric beater until stiff peaks form.
4. Sift a little of the remaining cup of sugar over the whites and gently fold in with a whisk. Repeat until all the sugar is incorporated. Then sift a little of the reserved sugar-flour mixture over and fold in. Repeat until it is all incorporated.

5. Fold in the vanilla and almond extracts and the lemon juice.
6. Turn the batter into an ungreased tube pan (10-inch).
7. Bake for one hour. Test by pressing lightly in the center—it should spring back if it is done. If not, test at 5-minute intervals.
8. Remove from oven, invert pan, and let the cake cool for 1½ hours. When thoroughly cooled, remove the cake from the pan by loosening the sides with a metal spatula.

Serves 12

Nutrition Analysis:

Calories 142
Carbohydrate. . . . . .32 grams
Fiber . . . . .0 grams
Fat. . . . . .0 grams
Cholesterol. . . . . .0 milligrams
Sodium . . . . .138 milligrams

ORANGE CHIFFON CAKE

½ cup vegetable oil plus extra for preparing pan
1½ cups sifted cake flour plus extra for preparing pan
¾ cup sugar
2 tsp baking powder
¼ tsp salt
½ cup fresh orange juice
1 tsp orange extract
3½ tbsp grated orange zest (about 2 oranges)
6 large egg whites, at room temperature
2 tbsp sifted confectioners' sugar
Orange Glaze and Garnish
1½ cups sifted confectioners' sugar
1½ tbsp fresh orange juice
1 tbsp fresh lemon juice
1 tsp grated orange zest

1. Position rack in center of oven and preheat oven to 350°F. Brush oil over the inside of a 9-inch

bundt or springform tube pan. Dust with flour and tap out the excess.
2. Sift together flour, sugar, baking powder, and salt into a large mixing bowl. Make a well in the center and add oil, ½ cup orange juice, orange extract, and 3½ tablespoons grated orange zest. Do not mix.
3. In another large mixing bowl, beat egg whites until they are white and foamy. Add 2 tablespoons confectioners' sugar and continue beating until stiff but not dry. Scrape off the beaters and, without washing them, place them in the flour-and-oil mixture and beat at low speed just until well blended. In four additions, gently fold this batter into the whites with a rubber spatula.
4. Turn the batter into the prepared pan and smooth the top with a rubber spatula. Bake for

25–35 minutes, or until the top of the cake feels springy and a cake tester comes out clean.

5. Cool the cake upright on a wire rack for 10 minutes. With a knife, loosen sides and center of cake from the pan. Invert onto the rack, lift off pan, and cool.

6. Make the orange glaze by combining the remaining ingredients and beating until smooth. Spoon glaze on top of still-warm cake, letting it drip down the sides.

Serves 16

Nutrition Analysis:

Calories 146
Carbohydrate. . . . . .19 grams
Fiber . . . . .0 grams
Fat. . . . . .7 grams
Cholesterol. . . . . .0 milligrams
Sodium. . . . . .97 milligrams

PUMPKIN CUPCAKES

1½ cups whole wheat flour
1 cup all-purpose flour
¾ cup sugar
2 tbsp baking powder
2 tsp ground cinnamon
½ tsp ground nutmeg
¼ tsp salt
3 eggs, slightly beaten
1 cup skim milk
½ cup oil
1 cup canned pumpkin
¾ cup raisins, chopped
1 tbsp vanilla

1. Preheat oven to 350°F (moderate).
2. Place 24 paper baking cups in muffin tins.
3. Mix dry ingredients thoroughly.
4. Mix remaining ingredients; add to dry ingredients. Stir until dry ingredients are barely moistened.
5. Fill paper cups two-thirds full.
6. Bake about 20 minutes or until toothpick inserted in center comes out clean.
7. Remove from muffin tins and cool on rack.
8. Freeze cupcakes that will not be eaten in the next few days.

Makes 24 cupcakes

Nutrition Analysis:

Calories 139
Carbohydrate. . . . . .21 grams
Fiber . . . . .2 grams
Fat. . . . . .5 grams
Cholesterol. . . . . .27 milligrams
Sodium. . . . . .64 milligrams

STRAWBERRY SAUCE

2½ cups strawberries (or raspberries)
2 tbsp sugar
1 tsp fresh lemon juice

1. In a blender or food processor, combine strawberries, sugar, and lemon juice. Puree until very smooth.

Makes 1 cup

Nutrition Analysis per ¼ cup:

Calories 51
Carbohydrate. . . . . .13 grams
Fiber . . . . .2 grams
Fat. . . . . .0 grams
Cholesterol. . . . . .0 milligrams
Sodium. . . . . .1 milligram

Cookies/Bars

ORANGE-APRICOT COOKIES

1 cup all purpose flour
¾ cup whole wheat flour
¼ cup sugar
2 tsp baking powder
½ tsp ground cinnamon
¼ tsp salt
¾ cup dried apricots, chopped
½ cup orange juice, fresh
¼ cup oil
1 tsp orange rind, grated
1 egg, beaten

1. Preheat oven to 375°F (moderate).
2. Mix dry ingredients thoroughly.
3. Add remaining ingredients. Mix well.

4. Drop dough by teaspoonfuls onto ungreased baking sheet, about 1 inch apart.
5. Bake about 11 minutes or until lightly browned.
6. Remove from baking sheet while still warm.
7. Cool on rack.

Makes about 4 dozen cookies

Nutrition Analysis:

Calories 37
Carbohydrate. . . . . .6 grams
Fiber . . . . .1 gram
Fat. . . . . .1 gram
Cholesterol. . . . . .4 milligrams
Sodium. . . . . .26 milligrams

OATMEAL APPLESAUCE COOKIES

1 cup all-purpose flour
1 tsp baking power
1 tsp ground allspice
¼ tsp salt
½ cup margarine
½ cup sugar
2 egg whites
2 cups rolled oats, quick-cooking
1 cup unsweetened applesauce
½ cup raisins, chopped

1. Preheat oven to 375°F (moderate).
2. Grease baking sheet.
3. Mix flour, baking powder, allspice, and salt.
4. Beat margarine and sugar until creamy. Add egg whites; beat well.

5. Add dry ingredients.
6. Stir in oats, applesauce, and raisins. Mix well.
7. Drop by level tablespoonfuls onto baking sheet.
8. Bake 11 minutes or until edges are lightly browned.
9. Cool on rack.

Makes about 5 dozen cookies

Nutrition Analysis:

Calories 38
Carbohydrate. . . . . .5 grams
Fiber . . . . .0 grams
Fat. . . . . .2 grams
Cholesterol. . . . . .0 milligrams
Sodium. . . . . .34 milligrams

Pies

HEALTHIER PIE CRUST

1 cup all-purpose flour
1½ tbsp margarine
1½ tbsp vegetable shortening
3 to 4 tbsp ice water

1. Cut cool margarine and vegetable shortening into flour in large bowl using a pastry blender or

two knives until the mixture is crumbly and the particles of shortening resemble coarse cornmeal.
2. Stir in ice cold water, 1 tablespoon at a time, with fork, adding just enough to moisten mixture.

3. Keep mixing dough with fork until pastry leaves the sides of the bowl, forming a ball.
4. Wrap in wax paper and chill 15 minutes.
5. Place dough on lightly floured surface and, using a rolling pin, start from center and roll out dough evenly with a circular motion, so pastry will retain its circular shape, to the desired diameter.

Makes 1 9-inch crust

Nutrition Analysis for ⅛ pie:
Calories 97
Carbohydrate. . . . . .12 grams
Fiber . . . . .0 grams
Fat. . . . . .5 grams
Cholesterol. . . . . .0 milligrams
Sodium. . . . . .25 milligrams

GRAHAM CRACKER CRUST

1¼ cups graham cracker crumbs
⅓ cup margarine, melted

1. Combine crumbs and margarine in 9-inch pie pan. Press firmly on sides and bottom of pan.
2. Bake at 375°F for 6–8 minutes, or until lightly browned.

Makes 1 pie crust

Nutrition Analysis for ⅛ pie:
Calories 79
Carbohydrate. . . . . .10 grams
Fiber . . . . .1 gram
Fat. . . . . .4 grams
Cholesterol. . . . . .0 milligrams
Sodium. . . . . .91 milligrams

VANILLA WAFER CRUST

1 cup vanilla wafer crumbs (about 28 vanilla wafers)
2 tbsp margarine, melted

1. Combine crumbs and margarine in a bowl. Stir well and press into a 9-inch pie plate coated with vegetable cooking spray.
2. Bake at 350°F for 10 minutes. Let cool.

Makes 1 pie crust

Nutrition Analysis for ⅛ pie:
Calories 73
Carbohydrate. . . . . .11 grams
Fiber . . . . .0 grams
Fat. . . . . .3 grams
Cholesterol. . . . . .9 milligrams
Sodium. . . . . .46 milligrams

APPLE PIE

1 cup all-purpose flour
½ tsp sugar
½ tsp salt
⅓ cup canola oil (or use safflower oil)
1½ tbsp skim milk
6 cups apples, pared and sliced
1¼ tbsp lemon juice

¼ cup sugar
⅛ tsp salt
½ tsp cinnamon
2 tbsp all-purpose flour

1. Stir flour, sugar, and salt together in a 9-inch pie pan. Drizzle oil and milk over the mixture and

lightly mix with fingertips. Using the back of a spoon, pat dough evenly around the pie pan. Crimp edges with floured fork. Cover and refrigerate 30 minutes.

2. In a bowl, toss apples with lemon juice. Combine sugar, salt, cinnamon, and flour, and mix with apples. Spoon into pastry-lined pie plate.

3. Bake at 450°F for 10 minutes. Reduce heat to 375°F and continue baking 40–50 minutes.

Makes 1 pie

Nutrition Analysis for ⅛ pie:
```
Calories . . . . . . . . . . . . . .236
Carbohydrate. . . . . . . . .37 grams
Fiber . . . . . . . . . . . . . . . .4 grams
Fat. . . . . . . . . . . . . . . . . .9 grams
Cholesterol. . . . . . . . . . .0 milligrams
Sodium. . . . . . . . . . . . . .168 milligrams
```

PEACH CRISP

vegetable oil spray
7 large peaches
2–3 tbsp lemon juice
1 tsp grated lemon zest
several gratings nutmeg
2 tbsp vegetable oil
¼ cup whole wheat flour
¼ cup uncooked rolled oats
¼ cup tightly packed light brown sugar
1 tsp ground cinnamon

1. Preheat the oven to 325°F. Spray a 9 × 9-inch ovenproof dish with vegetable oil spray.

2. Slice the peaches thinly and put the slices in the prepared dish. Sprinkle with the lemon juice, grated lemon zest, and nutmeg and toss gently.

3. Combine the remaining ingredients in a small bowl and stir well. Sprinkle over peach slices.

4. Bake for 30 minutes, or until the peaches are tender. If you would like the top to be a little browner, run the dish under the broiler for 40 seconds or so, and watch constantly. Serve at room temperature.

Serves 6

Nutrition Analysis:
```
Calories . . . . . . . . . . . . . .149
Carbohydrate. . . . . . . . .27 grams
Fiber . . . . . . . . . . . . . . . .2 grams
Fat. . . . . . . . . . . . . . . . . .5 grams
Cholesterol. . . . . . . . . . .0 milligrams
Sodium. . . . . . . . . . . . . .3 milligrams
```

❖   ❖   ❖

CHAPTER SEVENTEEN

COFFEE AND TEA

A question that invariably comes up when the topic of coffee and tea is discussed is their caffeine content. Table 61 compares the caffeine content of various beverages. As you can see, tea does contain significantly less caffeine than coffee, and brewed coffee contains much more caffeine than instant coffee. Regardless of caffeine content, coffee and tea are top-rated beverages.

COFFEE

One of the most popular drinks, second only to water, is coffee. Coffee has become a national drink since the Boston Tea Party when coffee was preferred to tea and was a measure of patriotism. Americans are great coffee drinkers and are affectionately known as "coffee lovers." Coffee any time and any place is commonplace. Americans have a special love for rich, well-brewed coffee.

Coffee beans are the berries of a tropical tree. Beans come from a variety of coffee trees found in tropical areas such as Colombia, Brazil, and Venezuela. Coffee beans are often identified by where they came from, such as Java, which is an island in Indonesia. Coffee producers use several varieties of coffee beans to produce their own distinctive blends.

Coffee beans are also often identified by the type of roast. Coffee beans, after being cleaned, skinned, and dried, are roasted to different degrees—dark, medium, light—to develop their flavor. The amount of roasting affects the color and flavor of the coffee brewed from the beans—the more the bean is roasted, the darker it is and

more strongly flavored. Most of the commercial blends of coffee are made from a light medium roast, also called American or full city roast. A very dark roast is used to make beans for espresso, a strong dark coffee.

Purchasing
When buying coffee, you may purchase **whole beans** (in bulk or in bags), **ground coffee** (in vacuum-packed cans, bags, or bulk), or **instant coffee** (in vacuum-packed jars or cans). Whole beans can be ground in the home using an electric coffee grinder (it uses stainless steel blades to pulverize the beans) or electric coffee mill (more sophisticated—uses grinding disks to ensure a more precise, uniform grind). Most coffee grinders are quite small and easy to clean. Fresh ground coffee yields a very fresh and excellent tasting product. Instant coffee is actually brewed coffee that has been dried using a method such as freeze-drying. The flavor of instant coffee depends on the blends it contains.

The **grind** of a coffee, such as coarse, medium, or fine, refers to the size of the grounds produced from the coffee beans. Coffee beans must be ground so the water can extract the flavor essences. The names of some grinds refer to the type of coffee maker suitable (see Table 62 for types of coffee makers and appropriate grinds to use for each) because it is actually the type of coffee maker that determines the best grind. The finer the grind, the more flavorings will be extracted by the water during the coffee-making process. Therefore, the size of the grind is related

❖ Table 61 Caffeine in Beverages ❖

Item	Milligrams Caffeine		Item	Milligrams Caffeine	
	Average	Range		Average	Range
Coffee (5-ounce cup)			Root beer		0
Brewed, drip method	115	60–180	Ginger ale		0
Brewed, percolator	80	40–170	Tonic water		0
Instant	65	30–120	Other regular soda		0–44
Decaffeinated, brewed	3	2–5	Juice added		0
Decaffeinated, instant	2	1–5	Diet cola		36–50
Tea (5-ounce cup)			Decaffeinated diet cola		0–0.2
Brewed, major U.S. brands	40	20–90	Diet cherry cola		0–46
Brewed, imported brands	60	25–110	Diet lemon-lime, diet root beer		0
Instant	30	25–50	Other diets		0–70
Iced (12-ounce glass)	70	67–76	Club soda, seltzer, sparkling		0
Soft Drinks (12-ounce can)			water		
Cola		30–46	Chocolate		
Decaffeinated cola		0–2	Cocoa beverage (5-ounce cup)		4
Cherry cola		36–46	Chocolate milk beverage		5
Lemon-lime		0	(8 ounces)		
Other citrus		0–64			

Source: *The Food and Drug Administration*

to the method of making the coffee. For example, if grounds are subject to hot water for a short time, a fine grind is recommended.

Decaffeinated coffee is coffee from which the caffeine has been removed. Caffeine can be removed by one of two methods: using water or using a solvent, such as methylene chloride. There has been much consumer concern about the use of questionable chemicals, such as methylene chloride, in making decaffeinated coffee. More coffee producers are switching over to the water method in response and this is often stated

❖ Table 62 Types of Coffee Makers ❖

Coffee Maker	Description	Coffee Maker	Description
Percolator	Heated water is forced up a tube in the middle of the percolator and sprayed over the coffee grounds held in a basket at the top of the pot. Make sure water level is below the bottom of the basket. **Uses regular (coarse) grind**.	Automatic Drip-Filter Coffee Makers	Enough cold water is poured into the reservoir to make the desired amount of coffee. Water in the reservoir is heated instantly as it flows past the heating element and is sprayed over the finely ground coffee in a basket lined with filter paper. **Uses drip grind or grind made for automatic drip coffee makers**.
Drip	Almost boiling water poured into a filter cone above the coffee pot drips slowly through the grounds held in a basket in the center and drips into the coffee pot. **Uses drip (medium) grind**.		

on the label. Decaffeinated coffee may be purchased as whole beans, ground coffee, or instant coffee.

The latest trend is the consumption of many **specialty coffees**, as listed below, and **flavored coffees**, which are available in specialty shops. Natural flavorings are blended with the finest beans to make coffees such as Pina Colada, Irish Cream, Cafe Amaretto, Viennese with Cinnamon, Swiss

Name	Description
Cafe au lait	Half strong coffee, half hot milk
Espresso or expresso	Strong dark coffee made from coffee beans that have been roasted until almost black, brewed in special expresso machines that force water through the ground coffee while under pressure, served in small cups after dinner
Cappuccino	Equal parts espresso coffee and steaming hot milk, often topped with whipped cream and cinnamon, served in tall cups
Demitasse	Strong coffee made from a dark roast served in small cups (demitasse means half cup) after dinner
Mocha java	A mix of regular strength coffee and hot cocoa
Irish coffee	A mix of hot coffee and Irish whiskey, topped with whipped cream
Viennese coffee	Strong, hot coffee, steeped with cloves, cinnamon sticks, and allspice, strained into cups and served with whipped cream

Chocolate Almond, Chocolate Mint, French Vanilla, and Chocolate Walnut. You can buy flavored beans, ground, or instant coffees.

As a general guide to purchasing coffee, do the following.

1. When buying coffee beans, check that they are of uniform size and color with good coffee aroma and no trace of mustiness. Buy from a reputable retailer who has fresh coffee beans. Purchase in small amounts as they don't stay fresh too long.
2. To buy ground coffee, select the proper grind for your coffee maker (see Table 62). Too fine a grind may cause bitter coffee. Too coarse a grind can produce weak, flavorless coffee.
3. When buying ground coffee, buy only enough to last one week as it keeps in the refrigerator just about that time. One pound of coffee makes about 40 cups. Unopened cans of coffee can stay on the shelf for one year.

Nutrition
Coffee does not contain any calories, or significant amounts of any nutrients. If you like cream or coffee whitener in your coffee, try skim milk instead as it contains no fat.

Storing
Coffee beans have a fairly high oil content, and when the fat becomes stale or rancid, it produces undesirable flavors (and odors too). Both air and moisture hasten rancidity, so an air-tight container is vital. The oil also has a tendency, like any oil, to pick up flavors of other foods, so that's just another reason to keep it air-tight. Store coffee beans at room temperature for 1 to 3 weeks or in the freezer for 3 to 4 months.

When storing ground coffee, store in air-tight containers in your refrigerator or freezer. Once the coffee bean is ground, the quality of the coffee goes downhill quickly for two reasons: more of the oil in the bean is now exposed to the air so it becomes rancid much more quickly and, because the flavor of coffee is so volatile, ground coffee loses flavor within days at room temperature. Ground coffee can keep in the refrigerator for 7 to

❖ *Storage Times for Coffee* ❖

Type of Coffee	Time on Shelf	Time in Refrigerator	Time in Freezer
Instant coffee			
Unopened	12 months	—	—
	(6 months if freeze-dried)		
Opened	2–3 months	—	—
Ground coffee			
Unopened	12 months	—	—
Opened	Not Recommended	7–10 days	7–10 days
Whole beans	1–3 weeks	—	3–4 months

10 days, longer in the freezer (see the guidelines above).

Making Coffee

To make good coffee, follow these guidelines.

1. Use spotlessly clean equipment because the fat found in coffee readily adheres to coffee-making equipment. This coffee residue, if not cleaned, will lead to horrible-tasting coffee as the fat becomes rancid.
2. Use fresh coffee.
3. Start with cold water. Never use hot tap water as it contains a build-up of minerals due to storage of the water in hot water tanks. This will have an adverse effect on the flavor of your coffee.
4. Measure accurately so the coffee is not too weak or too strong. For drip coffee, use 2 tablespoons or 1 coffee measure of ground coffee to each 6 ounces of water for a medium strong cup of coffee. Use less grounds for weaker coffee and more grounds for stronger coffee.
5. If using filters (paper or cloth), make sure they are clean.
6. For the best flavor, make at least three-quarters of the capacity of your coffee maker.
7. Coffee is best when served immediately. Do not hold for more than 60 minutes.
8. Remove the coffee grounds as soon as brewing is completed, for the grounds absorb aroma from the coffee.
9. Keep coffee warm but never boil it as it will turn bitter.
10. There's only one way to reheat coffee and get a decent cup—microwave it.

TEA

Tea is one of the most inexpensive and popular beverages in the world. It is easy to prepare and comes in many different varieties. Tea is the dried leaf of an evergreen shrub, named Camellia sinensis, that grows wild in places like China, Japan, and Indonesia. Tea plants flourish where it is warm and where a great deal of rain falls.

Purchasing

The types of tea fall into three main categories according to how long the tea leaves have been processed: black, green, and oolong.

- **Black tea** is the most popular form of tea in the United States. It is made by fermenting the freshly harvested tea leaves so they turn black. The tea produced has a very deep flavor and dark color.
- **Green tea** leaves are dried without fermenting so they retain their original green color. Green tea has a very light color and a weaker flavor than the black tea.
- **Oolong tea** is produced from tea leaves that are partially fermented to a brownish-green color, somewhat of a combination of black and green tea.

There are over 3,000 varieties of tea, each with its own flavor, body, color, and aroma. Like wines, they take their names from the districts where they are grown. Here are some popular regional teas:

- Assam—bright, full-bodied; rich, malty taste; grown in Northeastern India
- Ceylon—rich, pungent tea from Sri Lanka
- Keemun—elegant, smooth, flowery, the finest of China's black teas

The terms "orange pekoe" and "pekoe" do not refer to a particular variety or flavor but to the size of the leaf. Because small tea leaves brew faster than large tea leaves, teas are usually sorted by size for more efficient brewing. Souchong refers to large leaves, pekoe refers to medium leaves, and orange pekoe are the smallest leaves.

When people choose their favorite tea, they usually base their preferences on its aroma, color, and flavor. Much of the tea bought in the United States is produced by blending a number of varieties of teas, sometimes as many as 20 or more.

Tea is a variable product and by blending, a company can protect the flavor of its brand from any great changes in the quality of one variety and maintain a constant quality throughout the year. Tea packers also sometimes add flowers, herbs, spices, and flavors to their blends. Some, such as Earl Grey, Orange Spice, and Jasmine, are described in Table 63. Teas that go with certain foods are listed in Table 64.

Tea can be purchased as **loose tea** or in **tea bags** and it is brewed in boiling water. Instant tea and iced tea mixes are also available. Instant tea is made from a highly concentrated brew of tea from which the water is removed by a drying process. Iced tea mixes are a combination of instant tea and possibly sugar or sugar substitute and flavorings.

In addition to regular tea, there are also **decaffeinated teas** and **herbal teas**. Decaffeinated tea contains a maximum of 5 milligrams of caffeine

❖ *Table 63   Descriptions of Specialty Teas* ❖

Name of Tea	Description	Name of Tea	Description
Black Dragon	From the Amoy, Foochow, and Canton provinces of China and Taiwan, it has a delicate, fruity taste with a light color. It makes an excellent choice with fruit or fruity dishes.	Earl Grey	An unusual blend of India and China teas flavored with Oil of Bergamot.
		English Breakfast	A blend of India and Ceylon teas that is full-bodied and rich.
Ceylon Breakfast	A blend of teas grown on the hillsides of Sri Lanka producing a rich golden tea with superb flavor.	Irish Breakfast	A blend of teas from Kenya and India traditionally favored by the Irish for its pungent, amber brew.
China Black	The traditional blend of Keemun and other fine teas from the Chinese mainland with a mellow character and unusually distinctive smoky taste.	Jasmine	A blend of green and black teas scented with jasmine flowers.
		Lapsang Souchong	A large leaf, black tea with a distinctive smoky flavor.
China Oolong	A select blend of large leaf teas from the Orient with excellent flavor and the aroma of fresh peaches.	Lemon	Lemon scented tea produced from a Ceylon blend that is particularly enjoyable when made iced.
		Orange Pekoe	A blend of carefully selected Ceylon teas giving a smooth flavor that is particularly refreshing when served iced.
Darjeeling	A fine blend of teas, from the foothills of the Himalayas, with a subtle flowery bouquet and the delicate muscatel flavor for which the Darjeeling teas are known.	Prince of Wales	A blend of carefully selected finest Keemun black teas considered by connoisseurs to be one of the finest Chinese teas.

❖ Table 64   Matching Foods to Different Types of Tea   ❖

Food	Type of Tea	Character of Tea	Food	Type of Tea	Character of Tea
Breakfast	Breakfast teas	Brisk, rich, full-bodied		Spiced blends	Aromatic, pronounced flavor
	Traditional black tea blends	Bright, balanced		Green tea	Pungent
	Earl Grey	Fragrant, smooth	Dessert	Traditional black tea blends	Bright, balanced
Sandwiches, hamburgers	Traditional black tea blends	Bright, balanced		Flavored teas such as:	
	Darjeeling	Nutty flavor		Orange	Light
	Yunnan	Brisk		Lemon	Sweet
	Assam	Malty		Blackberry	Fragrant
	Ceylon	Bright, full of flavor		Peppermint	Refreshing
				Herbal teas such as:	
Beef, pork, spicy ethnic entrees	Traditional black tea blends	Bright, balanced		Chamomile	Delicate
				Hibiscus	Flowery
				Almond	Fragrant

per cup. Herbal tea is a misnomer because it does not contain any leaves from the tea plant. Herbal teas are made from dried buds, leaves, and flowers steeped in boiling water. They are caffeine free. Because some herbs have medicinal effects, they act like drugs in your body. Herbal teas that are safe, and not safe, to use are listed below.

Nutrition
Tea does not contain any calories, or significant amounts of any nutrients.

Storing
Air and moisture hasten the deterioration of tea. Loose tea, tea bags, and herbal tea should be

Safe Herbal Teas

Alfalfa	Linden flower
Catnip	Nettle
Chamomile	Peppermint
Chicory root	Rosehip
Elder flowers	Red and black
Fennel	raspberry
Fenugreek	Red clover
Ginger	Spearmint
Goldenrod	Slippery elm bark
Hibiscus	Yarrow
Lemon grass	

*Note: The following teas are known
to have some medicinal effect on the body.
Use them with caution.*

Barberry leaves	Burdock
Buchu leaves	Cascara Sagrada
Buckthorn bark	Dandelion

Dong Quai	Lovage
Echinacea	Mate
Eyebright	Passion flowers
Feverlew	Scullcap herb
Ginseng	Senna
Gotu Koa	Uva Ursi (bearberry)
Horsetail (shave grass)	Valerian root
	Vervain
Hydrangea	Yellow dock
Licorice	

STOP: These teas are unsafe to use.

Calamus root	Mandrake root
Comfrey	Mistletoe
Goldenseal	Oak bark
Hawthorne berries	Pennyroyal
Juniper berries	Pokeroot
Life root (ragwort)	St. John's wort
Lobelia	Wormwood

stored in air-tight containers at room temperature, where they can be stored for 6 to 9 months. Keep tea away from sunlight.

Making Tea

Use the guidelines provided for ways to make tea.

HOW TO MAKE TEA

HOT TEA

1. Use a teapot, preheating it by rinsing it out with hot water. This keeps the tea hot during the brewing.
2. Bring fresh cold tap water to a full rolling boil. Water that has been reheated gives tea a flat taste, and only boiling water can extract the full flavor and benefit from the leaves.
3. Use 1 teaspoonful of tea or 1 tea bag per cup (about 6 ounces of water) and pour the boiling water over the tea in the teapot.
4. Brew for 3 to 5 minutes. Don't judge the strength of tea by its color. It takes time for the leaves to unfold and release their flavor.

ICED TEA

Follow the rules for making hot tea but use 50 percent more tea to allow for melting ice. For example, you would use 4 tea bags to make 4 cups of hot tea, but to make 4 glasses of iced tea, you need 6 tea bags.

To make 2 quarts, use this easy method.

1. Bring 1 quart of freshly drawn cold water to a full rolling boil in a saucepan.
2. Remove from the heat and immediately add 12 tea bags or ¼ cup loose tea.
3. Stir. Cover and let stand 5 minutes.

4. Stir again and pour into a pitcher (strain if you are using loose tea) holding an additional quart of freshly drawn cold water.

Or try this cold water method for clear, cloudless iced tea.

1. Fill a quart pitcher or container with cold tap water.
2. Add 8–10 tea bags (remove tags). Cover. Let stand at room temperature or in the refrigerator.
3. After at least 6 hours, or overnight, remove tea bags, squeezing against side of container.
4. When ready to serve, pour into ice-filled glasses.

This recipe makes about 6 glasses and it may be doubled.

INSTANT TEA

Hot Tea: For 1 cup, use a level teaspoon instant tea to a teacup (about 6 ounces) of boiling water. For a potful, use 2 level tablespoons instant tea for each quart of boiling water.

Iced Tea: For 1 glass, use a rounded teaspoon instant tea for each 6–8 ounces of cold water. For a pitcherful, use 2 rounded tablespoons instant tea for each quart of freshly drawn cold water.

❖ ❖ ❖

CHAPTER EIGHTEEN

FLAVORING FOOD: A GUIDE TO HEALTHY SAUCES, HERBS, AND SPICES

HEALTHY SAUCES

A sauce is a flavorful liquid, usually thickened, that adds flavor, moistness, and appearance to a dish. Most sauces are made of three ingredients: a liquid (such as stock), a thickening agent, and seasonings. A major reason why sauces are usually fattening is that the thickener used quite often is made of butter and flour (it is called roux). There are many ways to thicken sauces (or defatted pan juices, in the case of gravy) without the use of roux.

- Evaporated skimmed milk has virtually no fat, but is thick and can thicken stock-based sauces.
- Various starches, such as arrowroot, cornstarch, and flour can be mixed with water and then added to a sauce for thickening, as described in the accompanying tips. Arrowroot is used like cornstarch and it is a high-quality (but very expensive) thickener.
- Reduction is a process of simmering a liquid, such as stock or a sauce, and as its liquid evaporates, the stock or sauce gets thicker.
- Vegetable purees, such as tomato puree used to make spaghetti sauce, are great thickeners.
- Buttermilk and yogurt are natural thickeners and can be used in some recipes instead of cream and eggs.

It isn't even necessary to stop using roux altogether: it is possible to make a reduced-calorie roux. Simply use 1 tablespoon reduced-calorie margarine to 1 tablespoon plus 2 teaspoons all-purpose flour. See the healthy sauce recipes at the end of the chapter.

Salsa is a wonderful, low-fat sauce that is very versatile. Salsa is a general term for a variety of highly seasoned sauces that are popular in Mexican cooking. They are chunky and full of tomatoes, chili peppers, onion, garlic, cilantro, and possibly other ingredients. Salsa cruda is a basic uncooked salsa found on the table of most restaurants in Mexico. Picante sauce is similar to salsa but is usually smoother and milder in flavor. Salsa is an excellent sauce to use on fish; on hamburgers, steak, and chicken; on taco salads or any salad; on baked potatoes; or on eggs. See the recipe for salsa on page 298.

Many other sauces are normally low in fat: tomato sauce, spaghetti sauce, barbecue, ketchup, mustard, cocktail sauce, and soy sauce (buy lower in sodium versions). Most jarred spaghetti sauce has about 3 to 4 grams of fat per ½ cup serving (and 500 milligrams of sodium). New varieties of spaghetti sauce are coming out, such as Healthy Choice®, that reduce the fat to almost nothing and bring the sodium down somewhat, to under 400 milligrams per ½ cup.

GUIDE TO HERBS AND SPICES

Herbs can provide creative, tasteful alternatives to salt for flavoring foods. Through the skillful use of herbs and spices, imaginative flavors can be created and simple foods made into gourmet delights.

Herbs and spices differ only in that herbs are

❖ Table 65 Matching Foods with Appropriate Herbs and Spices ❖

Food	Herbs and Spices	Food	Herbs and Spices
Soups	Bay, chervil, French tarragon, marjoram, parsley, savory, rosemary		Cranberries—allspice and coriander; cinnamon and dry mustard
Poultry	Rosemary and thyme		Strawberries or kiwi fruit—cinnamon and ginger; black pepper and nutmeg
	Tarragon, marjoram, and onion and garlic powders	Bread	Caraway, marjoram, oregano, poppy seed, rosemary, thyme
	Cumin, bay leaf, and saffron (or turmeric)	Vegetables	Beans (green)—marjoram and rosemary; caraway and dry mustard
	Ginger, cinnamon, and allspice		Broccoli—ginger and garlic powder; sesame and nutmeg
	Curry powder, thyme, and onion powder		Cabbage—celery seeds and dill; curry powder and nutmeg
Beef	Thyme, bay leaf, and instant minced onion		Carrots—cinnamon and nutmeg; ginger and onion powder
	Ginger, dry mustard, and garlic powder		Corn—chili powder and cumin; dill and onion powder
	Dill, nutmeg, and allspice		Peas—anise and onion powder; rosemary and marjoram
	Black pepper, bay leaf, and cloves		Spinach—curry powder and ginger; nutmeg and garlic powder
	Chili powder, cinnamon, and oregano		
Lamb	Garlic, marjoram, oregano, rosemary, thyme (make little slits in lamb to be roasted and insert herbs)		Squash (summer)—mint and parsley flakes; tarragon and garlic powder
Pork	Caraway, red pepper, and paprika		Squash (winter)—cinnamon and nutmeg; allspice and red pepper
	Thyme, dry mustard, and sage		Tomatoes—basil and rosemary; cinnamon and ginger
	Oregano and bay leaf	Potatoes, Rice, and Pasta	Potatoes—dill, onion powder, and parsley flakes; caraway and onion powder; nutmeg and freeze-dried chives
	Anise, ginger, and sesame		
	Tarragon, bay leaf, and instant minced garlic		Rice—chili powder and cumin; curry powder, ginger, and coriander; cinnamon, cardamom, and cloves
Cheese	Basil, chervil, chives, curry, dill, fennel, garlic chives, marjoram, oregano, parsley, sage, thyme		Pasta—basil, rosemary, and parsley flakes; cumin, turmeric, and red pepper; oregano and thyme
Fish	Cumin and oregano		
	Tarragon, thyme, parsley flakes, and garlic powder	Salads	Basil, borage, burnet, chives, French tarragon, garlic chives, parsley, rocket-salad, sorrel (These are best used fresh or added to salad dressing. Otherwise, use herb vinegars for extra flavor.)
	Thyme, fennel, saffron, and red pepper		
	Ginger, sesame, and white pepper		
	Cilantro, parsley flakes, cumin, and garlic powder		
Fruit	Apples—cinnamon, allspice, and nutmeg; ginger and curry powder		
	Bananas—allspice and cinnamon; nutmeg and ginger		
	Peaches—coriander and mint flakes; cinnamon and ginger		
	Oranges—cinnamon and cloves; poppy and onion powder		
	Pears—ginger and cardamom; black (or red) pepper and cinnamon		

HOW TO USE FLOUR, CORNSTARCH, AND ROUX TO THICKEN

❖ ❖ ❖

Following are steps to use flour to thicken.

1. Vigorously mix 1 tablespoon flour with 2 tablespoons cold water until smooth.
2. Stir into hot liquid and simmer for a few minutes until it no longer tastes starchy and liquid is thickened.

Following are steps to use cornstarch to thicken.

1. Vigorously mix 1 tablespoon cornstarch with 2 tablespoons cold water until smooth.
2. Stir into 1 cup of hot liquid, bring to a boil, and then simmer until there is no starchy taste and the liquid is clear.
3. Do not hold a product thickened with cornstarch for a long period of time because the cornstarch may break down and the product then thins out.

Following are steps used to make roux.

1. In a saucepan, melt fat, then add flour (for example, 2 tablespoons fat and 3 tablespoons flour).
2. Whip thoroughly, cooking and stirring over a low heat for just a few minutes (3 to 5 minutes) until it appears foamy and somewhat gritty.
3. Now the roux is ready to be used to thicken a liquid, such as soup.

leaves and stems of plants, and spices come from other parts of the plant such as the bark, roots, or seeds. Spices are almost always dried, whereas many people prefer to grow their own herbs to have a fresh supply throughout the growing season, thereby assuring top quality. Professional cooks prefer fresh herbs, if available. But fresh herbs are less concentrated, and two to three times as much should be used if a recipe calls for dried herbs.

If growing herbs for drying, the harvesting should be done in the morning after the dew has evaporated but before the sun is very bright. The essential oils in herbs will evaporate into the atmosphere during the day, so it is important to collect them when flavor is at its peak. Cut only the amount to be used in one day.

The herbs should be dried in bunches or laid on screens in a warm, dark, well-ventilated spot. An attic is ideal, although closets or dry basements will suffice. Ideally, the temperature should not be over 90 degrees. If it's too hot, the herbs will

cook. The length of time required for drying will vary according to the thickness of the plant parts. Herbs should be stored away from direct sunlight to prevent bleaching. Be sure they're well labeled. Most dried herbs will keep for at least one year in glass or plastic containers, but eventually they lose most of their potency and should then be thrown out. Certain herbs, such as chives, parsley, French tarragon, mint, basil, and sorrel, keep well in the freezer. Put them into individual plastic bags or small plastic jars and freeze them.

There are no strict limits to the use of herbs. A good general rule is not to mix two very strong herbs together, but rather one strong and one or more milder flavors to complement both the stronger herb and the food. The following is a breakdown of herbs by strength.

- Strong or Dominant Flavors: These should be used with care since their flavors stand out—approximately 1 teaspoon for 6 servings. They include bay, cardamom, curry, ginger, hot pep-

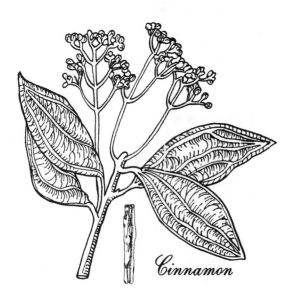

Cinnamon

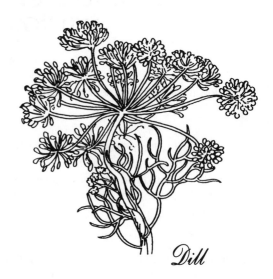

Dill

pers, mustard, pepper (black), rosemary, and sage.

- Medium Flavors: A moderate amount of these is recommended—1 to 2 teaspoons for 6 servings. They are basil, celery seed and leaves, cumin, dill, fennel, French tarragon, garlic, marjoram, mint, oregano, savory (winter and summer), thyme, and turmeric.
- Delicate Flavors: These may be used in large quantities and combine well with most other herbs and spices. This group includes burnet, chervil, chives, and parsley.

Herbs can be combined with certain foods (see Table 65) to enhance flavor. They can be added loosely or wrapped in cheesecloth and removed before serving. A number of herb blends are listed in Table 66.

Here are some tips for cooking with herbs and spices:

1. Use only good quality seasonings and flavorings.
2. Store all herbs and spices in cool, dry areas away from light and moisture, which deteriorate them at a faster rate. Store in air-tight containers. Fresh herbs can be washed, dried, and kept in the refrigerator for one week in an air-tight container. Whole dried herbs and spices can last up to 12 months on the shelf, ground herbs and spices can last only up to 6 months.
3. Whole herbs and spices need heat to release their flavors. Ground herbs and spices release their flavors quickly and should be added toward the end of the cooking process. Whole spices are excellent to use in long-cooking dishes such as stews because they take longer to release their flavor. Wrap whole spices in a cheesecloth or muslin bag for easy removal and add at the beginning of the cooking process. Too much cooking results in loss of flavors because they evaporate during cooking. The kitchen may smell wonderful, but the food is losing its taste.
4. If adding herbs and spices to cold foods such as salads and dressings, allow at least several hours or overnight for the flavors to develop.
5. Dried herbs and spices are much stronger than fresh. A useful formula is: 2–3 teaspoons fresh herbs = 1 teaspoon dried.
6. When adding herbs or spices to a dish, add ¼

❖ *Table 66 Herb Blends* ❖

Blend	Components	Blend	Components
Egg herbs	Basil, dill weed (leaves), garlic, parsley	Herb vinegars	Heat vinegar in a pan (do not let it boil), pour it into a vinegar bottle, and add one or several culinary herbs (to taste). Let the mixture set for two weeks before using. Any type of vinegar may be used, depending on personal preference.
Fish herbs	Basil, bay leaf (crumbled), French tarragon, lemon thyme, parsley (options: fennel, sage, savory)		
Poultry herbs	Lovage, marjoram (two parts), sage (three parts)		
Salad herbs	Basil, lovage, parsley, French tarragon		
Tomato sauce herbs	Basil (two parts), bay leaf, marjoram, oregano, parsley (options: celery leaves, cloves)	**Herb Blends to Replace Salt** **(These can be placed in shakers and used instead of salt.)**	
Vegetable herbs	Basil, parsley, savory	Saltless surprise	2 teaspoons garlic powder and 1 teaspoon each of basil, oregano, and powdered lemon rind (or dehydrated lemon juice). Mix well. Store in glass container, label well, and add rice to prevent caking.
Italian blend	Basil, marjoram, oregano, rosemary, sage, savory, thyme		
Barbecue blend	Cumin, garlic, hot pepper, oregano		
French herbal combinations			
Fine herbs	Parsley, chervil, chives, French tarragon (sometimes adding a small amount of basil, fennel, oregano, sage, or saffron)	Pungent salt substitute	3 teaspoons basil, 2 teaspoons each of savory (summer savory is best), celery seed, ground cumin seed, sage, and marjoram, and 1 teaspoon lemon thyme. Mix well, then powder with a mortar and pestle.
Bouquet garni mixtures	Bay, parsley (two parts), thyme. The herbs may be wrapped in cheesecloth or the parsley wrapped around the thyme and bay leaf.		
		Spicy saltless seasoning	1 teaspoon each of cloves, pepper, and coriander seed (crushed), 2 teaspoons paprika, and 1 tablespoon rosemary. Mix ingredients in a blender. Store in air-tight container.
Basic herb margarine	One stick unsalted margarine, one to three tablespoons dried herbs, ½ teaspoon lemon juice, and white pepper. Combine ingredients and mix until fluffy. Pack in covered container and let set at least one hour. Any of the culinary herbs and spices may be used.		

teaspoon at a time per pound of meat or pint of sauce or soup until the desired taste is achieved. Add only ⅛ teaspoon at a time of cayenne or red pepper.

7. Constantly test the foods being seasoned and adjust as needed.

8. To become familiar with the specific flavor of an herb, try mixing it with butter and/or cream cheese, let it set for at least an hour, and spread on a plain cracker.

Table 67 is an herb and spice equivalents chart.

❖ Table 67 Herb and Spice Equivalents ❖

Spice	Teaspoons Per Ounce	Spice	Teaspoons Per Ounce
Allspice	14	Mixed pickling spice	17
Anise	14½	Mustard	14½
Basil	35	Nutmeg	12¾
Bay leaves	136 leaves	Oregano	26
Caraway seed	9½	Paprika	13½
Cardamom seed	14½	Parsley	50
Cayenne pepper	14½	Pepper, Black	15¼
Celery seed	14	Pepper, White	13¼
Chili powder	11½	Red pepper	14
Cinnamon	17½	Crushed red pepper	16
Cloves	14½	Poppy seed	11¼
Coriander	14	Poultry seasoning	14
Cumin	14	Rosemary	35
Curry powder	12½	Saffron	35
Dill	14	Sage	22
Fennel	14	Savory	18¾
Fenugreek	14	Sesame seed	14
Ginger	14	Tarragon	50
Mace	14	Thyme	20¼
Marjoram	19½	Turmeric	12
Mint	50		

RECIPES

BROWN SAUCE

½ small onion
1 medium carrot
½ tsp dried thyme
½ bay leaf
1½ tbsp cornstarch
¼ cup white wine
5 cups brown or beef stock
¼ cup tomato puree, low-sodium

1. Finely chop carrot, onion, dried thyme, and bay leaf, and place in pan. Toss with cornstarch until evenly coated.
2. Stir in white wine and put on moderate heat. Cook for about 2 minutes to warm the mixture.
3. Stir in stock and bring to a boil over moderate heat, stirring frequently and scraping the bottom of the pot often.

4. Reduce heat to low and simmer for about 2 hours, or until the mixture is reduced to about 2 cups. Stir frequently and scrape sides and bottom of pot. Can be frozen.

Makes 2 cups

Nutrition Analysis per tablespoon:
Calories 18
Carbohydrate. . . . . .3 grams
Fiber . . . . .0 grams
Fat. . . . . .0 grams
Cholesterol. . . . . .0 milligrams
Sodium . . . . .128 milligrams

MUSHROOM SAUCE

1 tbsp oil
1½ tbsp flour
¼ tsp salt
¾ cup skim milk
2-oz can mushrooms, sliced, drained

1. Heat oil; stir in flour and salt.
2. Add milk slowly, stirring constantly; cook until thickened.
3. Add mushrooms. Heat to serving temperature.

Serves 4

Nutrition Analysis:

    Calories 58
    Carbohydrate . . . . .5 grams
    Fiber . . . . .0 grams
    Fat . . . . .4 grams
    Cholesterol . . . . .1 milligram
    Sodium . . . . .157 milligrams

LIGHT TOMATO SAUCE

1 medium onion, chopped
2 cloves garlic, minced
6 medium fresh tomatoes, peeled, seeded and cut up
½ tsp sugar
½ tsp dried basil leaves
¼ cup red wine or beef broth
salt and pepper to taste

1. Saute onion and garlic in a large skillet. Add the rest of the ingredients to vegetables and simmer 15–20 minutes to heat and blend flavors. Be careful not to overcook.
2. Serve over your favorite pasta, cooked, or other dish.

Makes 12 ½-cup servings

Nutrition Analysis:

    Calories 26
    Carbohydrate . . . . .5 grams
    Fiber . . . . .1 gram
    Fat . . . . .0 grams
    Cholesterol . . . . .0 milligrams
    Sodium . . . . .7 milligrams

LOW-FAT CHEESE SAUCE

1 (12-oz) container low-fat cottage cheese
1 (5-oz) can evaporated skim milk
½ cup shredded American cheese
salt and pepper to taste

1. Combine cottage cheese and evaporated milk in a blender; process until smooth.
2. In a small saucepan, heat mixture over medium-low heat, stirring constantly. Add cheese to hot mixture. Stir until cheese melts. Stir in salt and pepper.
3. Serve over your favorite pasta, cooked, or other dish.

Makes 2 cups

Nutrition Analysis per ¼ cup:

    Calories 80
    Carbohydrate . . . . .4 grams
    Fiber . . . . .0 grams
    Fat . . . . .3 grams
    Cholesterol . . . . .12 milligrams
    Sodium . . . . .237 milligrams

SALSA

8-oz can no-salt-added tomato sauce
1 tbsp chili peppers, canned, drained, finely
   chopped
¼ cup green pepper, finely chopped
2 tbsp onion, finely chopped
1 clove garlic, minced
¼ tsp oregano leaves, crushed
⅛ tsp ground cumin

1. Mix all ingredients thoroughly.
2. Chill before serving to blend flavors.
3. Serve with toasted pita bread, breadsticks, or
   raw vegetables.

Makes 1½ cups

Nutrition Analysis per ½ cup:
     Calories 37
     Carbohydrate. . . . . .8 grams
     Fiber . . . . .1 gram
     Fat. . . . . .0 grams
     Cholesterol. . . . . .0 milligrams
     Sodium. . . . . .55 milligrams

MUSTARD-TARRAGON SAUCE

⅓ cup beef broth, low-sodium
1 tsp Dijon mustard
1 tsp red wine vinegar
½ tsp cornstarch
½ tsp chopped fresh tarragon or ¼ tsp dry tarragon

1. Mix ingredients and warm up in saucepan.

Makes 4 tbsp

Nutrition Analysis per tbsp:
     Calories 4
     Carbohydrate. . . . . .0 grams
     Fiber . . . . .0 grams
     Fat. . . . . .0 grams
     Cholesterol. . . . . .0 milligrams
     Sodium. . . . . .25 milligrams

LOW-FAT WHITE SAUCE

2 tbsp margarine
3 tbsp flour
2 cups skim milk
1 tsp fresh lemon juice
¼ tsp freshly ground black pepper

1. In a 1-quart saucepan heat margarine over
   medium heat. Add flour and cook 1 to 2
   minutes, stirring frequently.
2. Gradually add milk, stirring constantly. Add
   seasonings and stir until mixture thickens.

Makes 1¼ cups

Nutrition Analysis per tbsp:
     Calories 23
     Carbohydrate. . . . . .2 grams
     Fiber . . . . .0 grams
     Fat. . . . . .1 gram
     Cholesterol. . . . . .0 milligrams
     Sodium. . . . . .26 milligrams

❖ ❖ ❖

RECOMMENDED DIETARY ALLOWANCES (RDA), 1989[*]

Age (years)	Weight (kg)	Weight (lb)	Height (cm)	Height (inches)	Protein (g)	(RE) Vitamin A	(µg) Vitamin D	(mg) Vitamin E	(µg) Vitamin K	(mg) Vitamin C	(mg) Thiamin	(mg) Riboflavin	(mg equiv.) Niacin	(mg) Vitamin B$_6$	(µg) Folate	(µg) Vitamin B$_{12}$	(mg) Calcium	(mg) Phosphorus	(mg) Magnesium	(mg) Iron	(mg) Zinc	(µg) Iodine	(µg) Selenium
Infants																							
0.0–0.5	6	13	60	24	13	375	7.5	3	5	30	0.3	0.4	5	0.3	25	0.3	400	300	40	6	5	40	10
0.5–1.0	9	20	71	28	14	375	10	4	10	35	0.4	0.5	6	0.6	35	0.5	600	500	60	10	5	50	15
Children																							
1–3	13	29	90	35	16	400	10	6	15	40	0.7	0.8	9	1.0	50	0.7	800	800	80	10	10	70	20
4–6	20	44	112	44	24	500	10	7	20	45	0.9	1.1	12	1.1	75	1.0	800	800	120	10	10	90	20
7–10	28	62	132	52	28	700	10	7	30	45	1.0	1.2	13	1.4	100	1.4	800	800	170	10	10	120	30
Males																							
11–14	45	99	157	62	45	1000	10	10	45	50	1.3	1.5	17	1.7	150	2.0	1200	1200	270	12	15	150	40
15–18	66	145	176	69	59	1000	10	10	65	60	1.5	1.8	20	2.0	200	2.0	1200	1200	400	12	15	150	50
19–24	72	160	177	70	58	1000	10	10	70	60	1.5	1.7	19	2.0	200	2.0	1200	1200	350	10	15	150	70
25–50	79	174	176	70	63	1000	5	10	80	60	1.5	1.7	19	2.0	200	2.0	800	800	350	10	15	150	70
51+	77	170	173	68	63	1000	5	10	80	60	1.2	1.4	15	2.0	200	2.0	800	800	350	10	15	150	70
Females																							
11–14	46	101	157	62	46	800	10	8	45	50	1.1	1.3	15	1.4	150	2.0	1200	1200	280	15	12	150	45
15–18	55	120	163	64	44	800	10	8	55	60	1.1	1.3	15	1.5	180	2.0	1200	1200	300	15	12	150	50
19–24	58	128	164	65	46	800	10	8	60	60	1.1	1.3	15	1.6	180	2.0	1200	1200	280	15	12	150	55
25–50	63	138	163	64	50	800	5	8	65	60	1.1	1.3	15	1.6	180	2.0	800	800	280	15	12	150	55
51+	65	143	160	63	50	800	5	8	65	60	1.0	1.2	13	1.6	180	2.0	800	800	280	10	12	150	55
Pregnant					60	800	10	10	65	70	1.5	1.6	17	2.2	400	2.2	1200	1200	320	30	15	175	65
Lactating																							
1st 6 months					65	1300	10	12	65	95	1.6	1.8	20	2.1	280	2.6	1200	1200	355	15	19	200	75
2nd 6 months					62	1200	10	11	65	90	1.6	1.7	20	2.1	260	2.6	1200	1200	340	15	16	200	75

[*]The allowances are intended to provide for individual variations among most normal, healthy people in the United States under usual environmental stresses. Diets should be based on a variety of common foods in order to provide other nutrients for which human requirements have been less well defined.

Source: Recommended Dietary Allowances. © 1989 by the National Academy of Sciences, National Academy Press, Washington, D.C.

❖ Estimated Safe and Adequate Daily Dietary Intakes ❖ of Additional Selected Vitamins and Minerals (United States)[a]

Age (years)	Vitamins	
	Biotin (μg)	Pantothenic Acid (mg)
Infants		
0–0.5	10	2
0.5–1	15	3
Children		
1–3	20	3
4–6	25	3–4
7–10	30	4–5
11 +	30–100	4–7
Adults	30–100	4–7

Age (years)	Trace Elements[b]				
	Chromium (μg)	Molybdenum (μg)	Copper (mg)	Manganese (mg)	Fluoride (mg)
Infants					
0–0.5	10–40	15–30	0.4–0.6	0.3–0.6	0.1–0.5
0.5–1	20–60	20–40	0.6–0.7	0.6–1.0	0.2–1.0
Children					
1–3	20–80	25–50	0.7–1.0	1.0–1.5	0.5–1.5
4–6	30–120	30–75	1.0–1.5	1.5–2.0	1.0–2.5
7–10	50–200	50–150	1.0–2.0	2.0–3.0	1.5–2.5
11 +	50–200	75–250	1.5–2.5	2.0–5.0	1.5–2.5
Adults	50–200	75–250	1.5–3.0	2.0–5.0	1.5–4.0

[a]Because there is less information on which to base allowances, these figures are not given in the main table of the RDA and are provided here in the form of ranges of recommended intakes.

[b]Because the toxic levels for many trace elements may be only several times usual intakes, the upper levels for the trace elements given in this table should not be habitually exceeded.

Source: Recommended Dietary Allowances, © 1989 by the National Academy of Sciences, National Academy Press, Washington, D.C.

❖ *Estimated Minimum Requirements of Sodium, Chloride, and Potassium* ❖

Age (years)	Sodium[a] (mg)	Chloride (mg)	Potassium[b] (mg)
Infants			
0.0–0.5	120	180	500
0.5–1.0	200	300	700
Children			
1	225	350	1000
2–5	300	500	1400
6–9	400	600	1600
Adolescents	500	750	2000
Adults	500	750	2000

[a]*Sodium requirements are based on estimates of needs for growth and for replacement of obligatory losses. They cover a wide variation of physical activity patterns and climatic exposure but do not provide for large, prolonged losses from the skin through sweat.*

[b]*Dietary potassium may benefit the prevention and treatment of hypertension and recommendations to include many servings of fruits and vegetables would raise potassium intakes to about 3500 mg/day.*

Source: *Recommended Dietary Allowances,* © *1989 by the National Academy of Sciences, National Academy Press, Washington, D.C.*

❖ *Median Heights and Weights and Recommended Energy Intakes (United States)* ❖

Age	Weight		Height		Average Energy Allowance			
(years)	(kg)	(lb)	(cm)	(inches)	REE[a] (cal/day)	Multiples of REE[b]	cal per kg	cal per day[c]
Infants								
0.0–0.5	6	13	60	24	320		108	650
0.5–1.0	9	20	71	28	500		98	850
Children								
1–3	13	29	90	35	740		102	1300
4–6	20	44	112	44	950		90	1800
7–10	28	62	132	52	1130		70	2000
Males								
11–14	45	99	157	62	1440	1.70	55	2500
15–18	66	145	176	69	1760	1.67	45	3000
19–24	72	160	177	70	1780	1.67	40	2900
25–50	79	174	176	70	1800	1.60	37	2900
51 +	77	170	173	68	1530	1.50	30	2300
Females								
11–14	46	101	157	62	1310	1.67	47	2200
15–18	55	120	163	64	1370	1.60	40	2200
19–24	58	128	164	65	1350	1.60	38	2200
25–50	63	138	163	64	1380	1.55	36	2200
51 +	65	143	160	63	1280	1.50	30	1900
Pregnant (2nd and 3rd trimesters)								+300
Lactating								+500

[a]*REE (resting energy expenditure) represents the energy expended by a person at rest under normal conditions.*
[b]*Recommended energy allowances assume light to moderate activity and were calculated by multiplying the REE by an activity factor.*
[c]*Average energy allowances have been rounded.*
Source: Recommended Dietary Allowances, © 1989 by the National Academy of Sciences, National Academy Press, Washington, D.C.

INDEX*

Please note recipe page numbers appear in italic.